The Teaching Process

Theory and Practice in Nursing

The Teaching Process

Theory and Practice in Nursing

Helen L. Van Hoozer
Barry D. Bratton
Patricia M. Ostmoe
Donn Weinholtz
Martha J. Craft
Craig L. Gjerde
Mark A. Albanese

ACC APPLETON-CENTURY-CROFTS/Norwalk, Connecticut

0-8385-8835-2

87 88 89 90 / 10 9 8 7 6 5 4 3 2 1

Prentice-Hall of Australia, Pty. Ltd., Sydney
Prentice-Hall Canada, Inc.
Prentice-Hall Hispanoamericana, S.A., Mexico
Prentice-Hall of India Private Limited, New Delhi
Prentice-Hall International (UK) Limited, London
Prentice-Hall of Japan, Inc., Tokyo
Prentice-Hall of Southeast Asia (Pte.) Ltd., Singapore
Whitehall Books Ltd., Wellington, New Zealand
Editora Prentice-Hall do Brasil Ltda., Rio de Janeiro

Library of Congress Cataloging-in-Publication Data

The Teaching process.

Includes bibliographies and index.
1. Nursing—Study and teaching. I. Van Hoozer, Helen L. [DNLM: 1. Education, Nursing. 2. Teaching—nurses' instruction. WY 18 T2528]
RT71.T345 1986 610.73'07 86-14185
ISBN 0-8385-8835-2

Design: M. Chandler Martylewski

PRINTED IN THE UNITED STATES OF AMERICA

Co-Authors

Mark A. Albanese, Ph.D.
Adjunct Assistant Professor of Biostatistics, Department of Preventive Medicine and Environmental Health; Associate Research Scientist and Interim Director, Office of Consultation and Research in Medical Education, The University of Iowa, Iowa City, Iowa

Barry D. Bratton, Ph.D.
Associate Professor, The University of Iowa, College of Education, Iowa City, Iowa

Martha J. Craft, R.N., Ph.D.
Associate Professor, The University of Iowa, College of Nursing, Iowa City, Iowa

Craig L. Gjerde, Ph.D.
Associate Professor, The University of Iowa, Colleges of Medicine and Education, Iowa City, Iowa

Patricia M. Ostmoe, B.S.N., M.S.N., Ph.D.
Dean, School of Nursing, University of Wisconsin-Eau Claire, Eau Claire, Wisconsin

Helen L. Van Hoozer, B.A., M.A.
Instructional Designer, The University of Iowa, College of Nursing, Iowa City, Iowa

Donn Weinholtz, Ph.D.
Assistant Professor, The University of Iowa, Colleges of Education and Medicine, Iowa City, Iowa

In memory of Libby Anderson, who first envisioned a work such as this.

Contents

Preface

This book is written primarily for graduate nursing students, nurse educators, and practicing nurses working in hospitals, community agencies, and home-care settings. The text links teaching and learning theory with practical application to show how theory and practice must be interrelated to promote learning. Each chapter contains learning objectives, summary sections, a posttest, suggested application activities, selected research, and bibliography. The authors have drawn information from a variety of fields, including nursing, educational and general psychology, instructional design, and educational media. This book is intended to guide the actions of the nurse as teacher; its goal is to improve teaching effectiveness to facilitate learning.

The authors are indebted to many individuals. Among the most valued contributions were the constructive criticisms and compliments received from Prentice-Hall reviewers, faculty and students at The University of Iowa College of Nursing and College of Education, and The University of Wisconsin–Eau Claire School of Nursing. Sincere gratitude is extended to Professor Geraldene Felton, Dean, and Professor Pamela J. Brink, The University of Iowa College of Nursing; Professor Bernice Wagner, Instructor Michaelene Mirr, and graduate students enrolled in nurse-educator role preparation courses at The University of Wisconsin–Eau Claire. Special thanks is extended to Denise M. Baretich and Dianne M. Haase, The University of Iowa College of Nursing, for allowing portions of their microteaching lectures to be used as examples in Chapter 3. Special acknowledgment is given to our first-draft typists, Steven Warner, Donna Sabin, and Gwen McIntosh, and to Diane Hartley for helping to prepare the final manuscript. We are indebted to our editors at Prentice-Hall, David Gordon and Dudley Kay, for their patience, interest, help, and encouragement during the preparation of this work. Last but not least, thanks is extended to Jennifer Rod for preparing some of the preliminary illustrations.

All names and situations in the text are fictitious and are included only to personalize or illustrate information. Any similarity to living persons is purely coincidental.

Introduction

Every field of human endeavor has its recurring issues, trends, and problems. Teaching is no exception. In spite of a substantial body of validated research, the criteria for excellence in teaching remain controversial. Because we are individuals, each of us has intuitive feelings and biases about what teaching is and what it should be. Probably most potential teachers have already developed a philosophy of teaching through exposure to various role models over time. Such acquired attitudes are ingrained and difficult to change.

The authors of this work attempt to provide a holistic view of teaching, embracing theory and principles of professional nursing and its practice. Each chapter represents a perspective that is unique to the author(s) perception and expertise. The final product is a compilation—a distillation of thought—designed to stimulate further exploration to improve teaching within the nursing profession.

The past decade has been one of considerable ferment and change in nursing and health education. Differences in learner populations (for example, graduate students and registered nurses seeking a baccalaureate degree in nursing, the disadvantaged, the elderly, and persons with chronic or acute physical or mental disorders) dictate the need for different teaching modalities and learning opportunities. The curriculum of a health education program, whether it be for nursing education, staff development, or client education, with its philosophy, purposes, conceptual framework, goals, and expectations for the learner is based on societal needs, mandates, particular philosophical and psychosocial perceptions, and assumptions about humans and the environment—how things are and how they should be. Teaching strategies, learning experiences, and resources are often viewed as separate entities, apart from a curriculum or program of study; however, it is the authors' belief that these are integral components of a curriculum and should be determined at the curriculum development level.

The book contains six chapters. Chapter 1 explores learning theories and principles, types of learning, and forces that influence learning, defining the discipline of teaching and the role of the nurse as teacher. This chapter provides the conceptual framework for the subsequent five chapters that follow.

Chapter 2 focuses on instructional design models and procedures as primary tools for the nurse engaged in establishing effective learning conditions.

Chapter 3 concentrates on factors to consider when determining the direct and indirect (contrived) strategies for creating conditions that influence positive cognitive, affective, and psychomotor learning.

Chapter 4 explores issues related to clinical teaching and learning, focusing on direct supervisory skills, instructional process skills, professional skills, and conditions useful for promoting student learning in the clinical practice setting.

Chapter 5 applies teaching and learning theory and principles to client education, focusing on the teaching role of the nurse and its implications for the selection and use of resources, strategies, and activities to promote health and manage illness.

Chapter 6 concentrates on the significance of the evaluation component of the teaching process, presenting practical guidelines for evaluating teachers, learners, strategies, and programs.

Each chapter includes objectives to establish mind-set and incorporates supportive, relevant research. Summary sections interspersed throughout each chapter, posttests, and application activities sections in each chapter are designed to promote assimilation and transfer of the information presented. Throughout the text, the term client is used when referring to the consumer of nursing care. The term teacher, nurse-teacher, nurse-educator, or instructor is used when referring to the nurse as a teacher of clients, students, or other audience. Similarly, the terms instruction or teaching are used when referring to the professional discipline and intervention of teaching.

We hope this book will be a helpful guide for perspective nurse-teachers, nurse-educators, and practicing nurses. Perhaps if it does nothing more, it will expand the horizons of nurses by offering alternatives that can be used to promote learning based on the individual idiosyncrasies and attributes of students, teachers, and settings.

> No man can reveal to you aught but that which already lies half asleep in the dawning of your knowledge. The teacher who walks in the shadow of the temple, among his followers, gives not of his wisdom but rather of his faith and his lovingness. If he is indeed wise he does not bid you enter the house of his wisdom, but rather leads you to the threshold of your mind. . . . For the vision of one man lends not its wings to another man. And even as each one of you stands alone in God's knowledge, so must each of you be alone in his knowledge of God and in his understanding of the earth. [Kahlil Gibran, *The Prophet*. New York: Alfred A. Knopf, 1973, pp. 62–63.]

The Teaching Process
Theory and Practice in Nursing

1

The Teaching Role of the Professional Nurse

Helen L. Van Hoozer

OBJECTIVES

Upon completion of this chapter, you will be able to:

1. Consider learning theory, types of learning, domains of learning, forces that influence learning, principles and constructs of learning, and conditions for learning to develop a framework for teaching consistent with the role of the professional nurse as a catalyst for learning.
2. Compare constructs, concepts, and principles related to classical and operant conditioning, associationism, Gestalt-field theory, perceptual-existential theory, and humanism.
3. Contrast conditions and constructs associated with incidental learning, signal learning, stimulus-response learning, chaining, verbal association, multiple discrimination, concept learning, principle learning, problem solving, observational learning, and behavior modification.
4. Identify three domains of learning and determine their significance related to the principles and conditions of learning and teaching.
5. Identify internal and external forces that contribute to individual differences and influence learning and teaching.
6. Identify basic principles of learning that serve as guidelines for developing learning experiences.
7. Compare principles of learning related to particular age and developmental levels.
8. Identify responsibilities and competencies of the nurse-teacher as communications-change agent.
9. Apply theories, principles, and conditions for learning when developing teaching plans.

INTRODUCTION

Teaching is one major function of the professional nurse. It is an essential nursing responsibility. Boundless opportunities for teaching exist within all settings in which nurses are employed. Each setting is composed of individuals of varying ages with unique personal attributes, idiosyncrasies, and states of wellness. Nurses must be prepared to assume the responsibility for teaching. What does teaching really involve? Is it simply a skilled intervention or a disciplined process? Can we learn to teach? Do our beliefs, values, attitudes, and behaviors affect what and how we teach? What is learning? How do nurse-teachers promote successful learning? What role should the professional nurse play?

Not only is teaching one of the most important professional nursing responsibilities; it is also one of the most technical and difficult to understand. Like nursing, teaching is a professional discipline that requires prospective practitioners to master a body of theoretical knowledge as a prerequisite to practice. The professional nurse-teacher diagnoses difficulties and strengths, appraises options and solutions, and chooses among them, assuming total responsibility for both strategy and tactics. In contrast, when teaching is viewed only as a skill, expectations are standard diagnosis, correct performance of procedure, and little else. Therefore, a nurse who assumes the responsibility for teaching assumes two professional roles, both of which are grounded in theoretical knowledge.

It follows that the nurse-teacher should develop a self-image compatible with professionalism, an image that subsumes the notion of dedication to the welfare of the client as a unique human being with particular physical and mental attributes, personal needs, and idiosyncrasies, all of which influence learning. A theory of teaching must address factors that predispose the individual to effective learning, the optimal structuring and sequencing of knowledge and skill to facilitate learning, and the nature and pacing of reinforcement to promote transfer of learning and commitment to learning outcomes. The discipline of teaching is therefore concerned with four issues: predispositions, structures, sequences, and consequences. Teaching, then, is an action-oriented, theoretically based process, the purpose of which is to promote learning; it is a highly personal and social phenomenon that involves perception, internal cognitive processing, and outward manifestations that indicate behavioral change. Practical guidelines for teaching can be generated by considering theories, principles, and conditions for learning, types of learning, forces that influence learning, and constructs of change and communication. These are the issues addressed in this chapter.

LEARNING THEORY

Any exploration of the discipline of teaching and the role of the nurse as teacher cannot overlook established theories of learning that have evolved over time. These theories provide the framework for a number of practical principles of learning that guide teaching actions. Learning theory is a study of human behavior. What we do in teaching depends upon what we think people are like. The goals we seek, the things we do, the judgments we make, and even the experiments we are willing to try as teachers are determined by our beliefs about the nature of human beings, their behaviors and capabilities.

Associationism and Behaviorism

The oldest method of analyzing how people learn focused on the theory of association of ideas, stimuli, and responses. Aristotle may have been the first to discover that human beings remember things that are alike, strikingly different, or that occur together in space and time. Centuries later, Thomas Hobbes, John Locke, David Hume, James Mill, Alexander Bain, and others suggested that the mind was formed through the association of experiences and ideas. Not until the turn of the century, however, did learning as a process of association receive experimental study. E. L. Thorndike in the United States and Ivan Pavlov in Russia established a framework for analytical investigation of the process of learning called connectionism, or behaviorism. Thorndike's work is recognized as one of the greatest contributions to the psychology of learning. His experiments with lower animals and later with human subjects revealed that when a subject was presented with a task, a number of exploratory, random, trial-and-error attempts were made prior to learning an appropriate response.

Further, Thorndike found that the learner acquired and remembered responses that had satisfying effects and rejected those that were perceived as annoying or frustrating. A praised response was remembered longer and tended to be repeated because it was satisfying. When faced with a new situation, a learner either refused to react or made random hit-or-miss responses until a successful response was found. If the response was reinforced (rewarded), it tended to be repeated in similar circumstances.

Thorndike's experiments also revealed that mere repetition of a response did not necessarily establish a connection, but that the strength of the connections made as a result of the response depended upon the satisfaction received, readiness for the response, and the degree of belongingness felt after making the response.

Classical Conditioning

A precise picture of the way in which associations can occur was demonstrated by Ivan Pavlov's classical conditioning experiments. Classical conditioning involves the exhibition of a simple reflexlike response when a specific stimulus is presented. It requires the association of two stimuli, with one of them gradually acquiring significance in elicitation of an associated response.

Pavlov's experimental research with dogs involved the association of a neutral conditioning stimulus (a bell) with an unconditioned stimulus (food) that evoked the unconditioned response (salivation). After repeated exposure, the unconditioned stimulus (salivation) was associated with the conditioning stimulus (bell). In other words, after a number of conditioning events, the bell stimulated the salivary response even without the presence of food. Pavlov also found that a primary or secondary *reinforcement* (reward) was a crucial condition for building up and maintaining the conditioned response. Without reinforcement, the response was either not formed or it declined in strength and seemed to be extinguished. The response only appeared to be extinguished, however, because after an interval of time, presentation of the conditioning stimulus evoked the response in even greater magnitude.

When conditioning procedure followed an extinction procedure, reconditioning proceeded at a faster rate than it did in the initial conditioning situation. The opposite was found to be also true. Pavlov inferred from such findings that what was really taking place was learning to respond and not to respond. This discovery led to the principle of partial reinforcement. In fact, subsequent experiments have shown that forgetting is not just caused by the passage of time, but by the interfering effects of other associations that are formed over time. We forget because associations interfere with one another. New learning can interfere with prior learning.

Findings indicate that it is necessary to institute a number of extinction trials on a regular basis to completely and permanently eradicate a conditioned response. Complete behavioral extinction is not often the case in real life, however. We don't often stop doing something just because reinforcement is not received. Usually, behaviors are reinforced intermittently, inconsistently, and spasmodically. Such partial reinforcement results in a behavior being extinguished much more slowly than when every response is reinforced on a consistent basis.

Also derived from classical conditioning are theoretical constructs concerning the tendency to generalize a conditioned response to stimuli that are different from but somewhat similar to the original stimuli and the use of one conditioned response to build up another conditioned response. The latter process illustrates higher-order conditioning and relates to the importance of secondary reinforcement and the acquisition of secondary goals.

Instrumental or Operant Conditioning

Classical conditioning is synonymous with simple signal learning. The value of exploring classical conditioning experiments is that they highlight many of the important features of association learning and introduce more complex kinds of learning, such as instrumental or operant conditioning. Instrumental or operant conditioning involves a response that accomplishes something. It implies that the individual acts upon the environment. The learner actively selects from a repertoire of responses one that will be habitually repeated in a given stimulus situation, provided satisfaction is received from the response. In addition, the behavior of the learner influences whether the reward will be accepted or not. Generally speaking, the acquired response may achieve the negative goal of avoiding fear or punishment, or it may lead to a positive biological goal, such as food or water, or a learned secondary goal. In some cases, it may do both at the same time.

B. F. Skinner's experiments with lower animals revealed four levels of conditioning, all of which are similar in that the learned response is biologically beneficial for the organism. These experimental research efforts have implications for human learning and teaching. A learned response at the lowest level facilitates obtaining a biological reward, such as food or drink, whereas learned response at the highest level involves behavior that has no biological utility but that has in the past been associated with a biologically significant stimulus. Basic features of instrumental learning include drive motivation, general exploratory activity, and goal response. Making a response to receive tokens is an example of secondary reward conditioning. Instrumental conditioning is applied to techniques of behavior modification implemented to change undesirable or inappropriate behaviors. The practice of giving grades or monetary or other tangible rewards based on response can be traced to instrumental or operant conditioning.

As in the case of classical conditioning, instrumental conditioning of response most often occurs gradually over time. Left unused and unrewarded, the response will appear again for a time when the stimulus situation is reinstated. In addition, something similar to sensory or perceptual discrimination does occur in instrumental conditioning, and a response can be generalized to situations that are not exactly the same as the original stimulus; however, the tendency to respond is greater for stimuli that are most similar to the original.

The most significant aspect of Skinner's research is the importance of reinforcement for eliciting behavioral response. Reinforced responses tend to be committed to memory. In operant conditioning, reinforcement is attainment of a goal that satisfies a drive. The strength of a response increases with the number of reinforcements. The shorter the time interval between the response and the reinforcement, the more effective the reinforcement is in building a strong response. Reinforcement is a major condition for learning. Immediate, positive reinforcement should therefore increase the possibility of recurrence of a response. Keeping this factor in view in any consideration of learning is important for teachers. Knowledge of behavior that has been rewarded or has been satisfying to the learner will serve as a tool for predicting future behavioral responses. Also, such knowledge will help in finding ways to change behavior. Viewing learning as a process of reinforcement focuses attention on the effect of the response upon the individual. It alerts teachers to look for need states and past experiences that have led to drive satisfaction.

Conditioned-reflexlike responses do occur in human learning situations. For example, a child becomes conditioned to fear dogs in the following manner: When the child is very young, a dog barks (unconditioned stimulus), which evokes a fear response (unconditioned response). Then any dog (conditioned stimulus) and its bark evokes fear (conditioned response). Eventually, just seeing a dog (conditioned stimulus) evokes fear (conditioned response). The child has learned to fear dogs. If the child gains the attention of significant others when exhibiting fear in the presence of a dog, the response is reinforced. A person's fear of hospitals, doctors, or nurses may be due to operant conditioning.

Conditioning also occurs under structured learning circumstances, even though there is apparently no logical relationship between the ideas and events that are associated. For instance, there appears to be no logical relationship between a person's feeling of inferiority and statistics per se. But if when presented with statistical problems we are made to feel inferior enough times, the activities connected with this subject become linked with emotional responses associated with feelings of inferiority. Finally, just the word *statistics* itself can evoke emotional responses of inferiority.

Associationism is an important aspect of learning and remembering. We learn to associate spoken and written words with objects and persons, pictures with words, letters with sounds, words with ideas and ideas with each other. Automated teaching machines and programed instruction rely heavily upon this theory of learning as does the use of mnemonic devices to help us remember things.

Learning as a Perceptual Process: Gestalt-field Theory

Much of human learning involves a change in the way we perceive the environment. The impetus for this point of view comes from Gestalt-field or cognitive-field theory. Gestaltists contend that learning may be thought of as a change in cognitive structure, a change in the readiness of the individual to perceive objects and events in a new way at a given moment in time. Behavior is seen as a purposive striving toward goals, and the learner ascribes meaning or significance to signs, or cues, that lead to identified goals. Research has shown that interference with response sequences is not sufficient to prevent learners from reaching goals by a new series of responses. To change behavior (learning) in this frame of reference requires that we understand the nature of the individual's perceptual field.

There appears to be no doubt that the senses—sight, hearing, touch, taste, smell—underlie perception and that senses interact during the active perceptual process. The senses involved will depend on the object to be perceived. Perception is dependent on learning and is influenced by individual attributes such as attitudes, emotions, experiences, and expectations, as well as environmental variables. Personal factors such as perceptual style, selective attention and set, motivation, previous experiences with similar cues, and developmental and maturity level will influence cue perception. Perception is therefore a form of discriminating behavior involving overall activity of the person immediately following stimulation of the senses. Perception causes actions that in turn change perception.

One of the most important facts about perception is that it is selective. We do not see everything in our surroundings. In other words, we "choose" those things that are self-enhancing and that provide meaning to our lives. What we assimilate from the environment suits our purposes and fits with our past experiences. What we do, what we learn is thus a product of what is going on in our unique, personal field of awareness. Learning does not really occur until some change takes place in the individual's personal, unique perceptual field. Meanings are formed inside of people and cannot be directly manipulated and controlled.

Because of the personal nature of learning, basic motivation or energized striving toward learning goals comes from within. The natural thrust of motivation can be observed in a very young child. There is almost limitless desire to know and to find out about things. As people enter and progress through formalized education and become increasingly able to make choices and establish goals and objectives, they are given ever decreasing opportunities to search for meaning and make decisions. According to Maslow, sickness results—the sickness of not growing. Kelley calls this "perceptual malnutrition."[1] The task of the teacher is to create conditions and provide situations that stimulate inner motivation. This task calls for teachers who are more than information providers. It requires people who can enter into meaningful and productive relationships. A teacher must be first and foremost a person willing to search for ways in which learners may experience success within a supportive atmosphere. Establishing a warm, accepting, growing, rewarding emotional climate can contribute to successful learning.

For the most part, the teacher's control over learning is limited. A teacher should not be a director or manipulator, but rather one who assists, helping and guiding a growing, living dynamic organism in the process of becoming. To do this efficiently requires skill in creating an environment that promotes exploration and facilitates and encourages the "active" discovery of meaning.

Gestalt, or cognitive, theory enables us to think of learning as a process of patterned organization and understanding. Learning in this sense becomes a perceptual problem-solving process. It is a way of thinking, creating and synthesizing to formulate relationships among experiences. Insightful perceptual changes that lead to problem solving are guided by the internalization and application of steps in a problem-solving process. It is possible to learn a problem-solving attitude, developed by continued experience with solving problems.

Integrated Learning Theory

Within the past quarter of a century, new theories of learning have emerged that synthesize earlier behaviorism, associationism, and Gestalt theories. Perceptual-existential, or third force, psychology and humanism are two schools of thought that provide new perspectives on learning.

Perceptual-Existential Theory. Sidney Jourard, Abraham Maslow, Carl Rogers, Earl Kelley, and Arthur Combs are prominent in the third force movement.[2] This group regards learning as an active process of interaction between the learner and the environment. Learning is dependent upon what the learner does and involves how the individual thinks, feels, and acts. For behavioral change to occur, perceptions must be modified. The learner must be intellectually, physically, socially, and emotionally involved. The learner must act upon or react to a situation in some way. The more actively a situation involves the learner in an experience, the greater its impact upon learning.

Learning is an intense, personal phenomenon that involves exploration, discovery, and striving for personal meaning. Each learner is unique, with a particular hereditary and social background, understanding, skills, values, and attitudes. Individual perceptions are unique responses to the immediate environment. Activities are motivated by a drive to develop, maintain, and enhance self. Learning takes place more readily when the individual attributes, or qualities, and perceptions of the learner are considered.

Learning is regarded as a social phenomenon involving other people. Therefore, the teacher must be a potent social force, arranging experiences that immerse the learner, both personally and socially, in dynamic interactions. The teacher is also viewed as a growing organism, constantly striving for self-fulfillment, whose knowledge, skills, values, attitudes, and feelings are also unique. Such uniqueness will therefore influence teaching behaviors.

When learning is viewed as more than the assimilation of facts and seen as a dynamic search for relevant personal meaning and self-enhancement, the teaching role becomes one of facilitator, helper, and colleague. Activities of the teacher are focused on planning and arranging optimum conditions under which the learner will be free to learn.

The third force teacher is learner-oriented, recognizing and respecting students' needs and potential needs. Learning experiences are designed to motivate and assist the learner to gain the potential for becoming. Verbal and nonverbal communication skills are applied to teaching-learning events.

Humanistic Theory. Humanistic theory adds another dimension to learning theory.[3] This school of thought has evolved from theorists like Maslow, Rogers, and Glasser. According to humanistic theory, motivation for growth toward becoming a self-actualized person is inherent within each of us. As human beings, we are basically responsible for our own behavior, including evaluation of behavior. A person can understand those factors from the past that have contributed to development of a self-identity and can move toward structuring a future, without merely responding to and being controlled by the environment. Self-actualization does not take place in a vacuum. Societal conditions play a significant role in influencing human growth and development. Learning, then, is the process of developing one's full cognitive, affective, and psychomotor potential. The learner is ultimately responsible for learning, even to the extent of defining learning needs and establishing learning goals and objectives.

The teacher's role involves helping the learner to recognize and develop unique potentialities and facilitating the process of individual growth and positive behavior changes through active learner participation. Teacher efforts are directed toward providing means for maintenance and enhancement of the learner as an individual. The focus is not on the teacher and teaching, but on promoting significant self-directed learning initiated by the learner. The teacher's attitudes and behaviors foster self-initiated responsibility for learning and serve as a role model, expressing respect for self and others, empathy, and genuineness.

SUMMARY

Teaching is a professional discipline based on a theoretical body of knowledge. Learning theory attempts to systematically establish constructs and principles to guide the practice of teaching. A number of learning theories have been posed, but as yet psychologists and educators have not been able to agree upon any one of them. Perhaps the best approach to understanding learning and teaching is to combine the essence of each. The theories of associationism, connectionism, classical conditioning, instrumental or operant conditioning, Gestalt-field theory, perceptual-existential theory, and humanism provide a cognitive and affective framework to guide the actions of professional nurses as teachers. It is not a question of Gestalt or behaviorism or humanism. Modern versions of behaviorism, or connectionism, emphasize the objective analysis of behavior and the use of principles of conditioning and associationism. Stimulus-response theory is moving closer to cognitive (Gestalt) theory. There is more interest in predicting the behavior of single individuals as opposed to behavior in terms of group averages.

Human beings are complex, dynamic psychological, biological, and sociocultural beings. As the individual senses the world, interprets it, responds to it, and feels satisfaction or dissatisfaction with results of responses, the body and nervous system are involved. Motives may be conceived in terms of physiological imbalances. Every experience, every act is mediated by neurological events. Learning is associated with changes in the internal state of the individual. This process acknowledges personal biochemical and neurological attributes.

Exploration of learning theory is valuable in that it helps to establish a holistic view of how people learn, internalize principles of learning, and relate these to principles of teaching. Learning is any change in cognitive, psychomotor, or affective behavior that is a result of experiencing. It is made observable through active participation and response to environmental circumstances, and it is dependent upon the personal attributes and idiosyncrasies of the individual. Individuals learn and remember things that are alike, strikingly different, or that occur together in space and time. Actions or responses that are rewarding and satisfying to self will be remembered and repeated. Mere repetition of a behavioral response will not necessarily establish a connection unless the response is seen as self-rewarding. Therefore, the individual must be "ready" to make a particular response and to receive satisfaction. Human beings do not operate in a vacuum. Environmental conditions influence how the individual will respond, as well as which response he or she will choose to make in a given situation.

Learned behaviors do not occur overnight, but gradually over time. Unless a behavior is reinforced, it will tend to disappear for a time. The strength of a particular response increases with the number of positive reinforcements received and the shorter the time interval between the behavior and the reinforcement. Immediate, positive reinforcement tends to increase recurrence of a behavioral response.

Learning is a universal, personal, and sociocultural cognitive, affective, psychomotor phenomenon dependent upon unique attributes and perceptual responses to the environment. The learner must be physically, emotionally, and mentally ready to perceive objects and situations in a way that justifies relatively permanent behavioral change. Learning events must be seen as a means of achieving personal goals that satisfy basic human needs and goals. Both human and nonhuman environmental conditions influence learning.

TYPES OF LEARNING

Psychologists and educators may not agree on particular theories of learning, but it is generally agreed that there are a number of different types of learning and that the more complex forms of learning depend upon those less complex.

Incidental Learning

When we think about learning, we usually recall formalized situations in school settings. Learning is, however, a continual process that occurs from birth to death, every day of our lives, even though we may not be consciously aware of it. Cognitive, affective, and psychomotor changes are learned intentionally, either through self-motivation or under the influence of teachers and structured conditions, or unintentionally (incidentally) through the effects of nature. Regardless of our own or others' intentions, we learn something about things to which we are exposed from day to day.

As human beings, we can acquire new behaviors without being highly motivated or required to make a particular response. Such learned behavior is incidental, or unintended, because of natural forces within the environment. The phenomenon of incidental learning has been investigated. In such studies, subjects have been asked to learn a particular task and then were tested on another, supposedly irrelevant one. Most investigations of this nature indicate that a great deal of incidental learning does take place in formal learning situations. Researchers have tried to isolate specific kinds of stimuli and particular attributes within learning situations to ascertain their effects on incidental learning. For example, Alan Chute studied the effects of color on type of learning and found that the attribute of color within a film helped subjects in the study to learn incidental information, but that it affected learning of task-relevant information differently, depending on the ability of the viewer.[4]

There appears to be no question that incidental learning does occur practically every day of our lives. No one actually structures the learning environment to elicit desired behaviors, but the conditions are there and we attend and respond in some successful manner that reinforces the behavior so that it occurs again under similar circumstances. Incidental learning is not, however, the most efficient, effective, or dependable way to learn because of its random, purposeless nature.

Signal Learning

Signal learning is the least complex kind of learning; it involves a relatively uncomplicated reflexlike response (behavior) to a specific stimulus (condition). The stimulus signals, or triggers, particular behavior. The emotionally pleasant or aversive event precedes the response. At a very basic human level, the body sends out signals indicating the need to sleep, eat, and to be warmer or cooler. We learn to respond to these signals and take action. Recognizing body signals that indicate the onset of illness exemplifies signal learning. For instance, persons with diabetes face the possibility of either hypoglycemia or hyperglycemia; therefore they must be taught to recognize the body signals that indicate these conditions. Body signals indicating hypoglycemia may be slight tingling in the fingertips, a shaky feeling or trembling, irritability, headache, hunger and weakness, double or blurred vision, difficulty in concentrating, confusion when thinking, heart pounding, and a cold, clammy feeling. These signals can all be followed by fainting and even convulsions. The nurse can be instrumental in teaching diabetics to recognize signals that warn of impending illness and the actions that should be taken when they occur.

Through signal learning, we learn emotional responses, such as fear and hope, attitudes, opinions, feelings, and expectations. We respond with fear or pleasure actions to animals, persons, places, or things. We blink at an object flying toward the eye. We jump at loud noises. Pictures of food trigger a salivary response or the act of eating, even though we are not actually hungry. The sound of an alarm clock triggers us to get up in the morning, and the sound of a beeper calls us into action even from a deep sleep. Words also serve as powerful response signals. We react immediately when labeled in a particular manner by someone else. For instance, being labeled *patient* signals particular feelings. Although signal learning is the lowest level of learning, it is the basic link to stimulus-response learning.

Stimulus-Response Learning

Basically stimulus-response learning is goal-directed behavior. It involves making a response to a particular stimulus to obtain an associated reward. The response may achieve the negative goal of avoiding fear or punishment or it may lead to a perceived positive goal.

Stimulus-response learning is observable in the actions of a child responding to phrases like "Play patty cake, clap your hands," or when a child learns to pull a lever to receive a piece of candy. The child may make a variety of responses, including observing, exploring, and touching before discovering the response that leads to the reward (reinforcement), but it is not easy to determine what stimulus controls the action.

The element of reinforcement is essential in both signal learning and stimulus-response learning; however, two different principles are involved. To encourage stimulus-response learning, the reinforcer—the event that increases the likelihood that the response will be repeated in the future—must *follow* the learned response as closely in time as possible. On the other hand, to promote signal learning, the conditioning stimulus should *precede* the response.

In both signal and stimulus-response learning, an acquired response can be extinguished by withholding reinforcement. A conditioned response that has been extinguished may, however, reappear spontaneously after an interval of time following extinction. With repeated extinction trials, the conditioned response may eventually disappear. What is taking place is learning to respond and not to respond to a stimulus. Yet in real life, it is extremely difficult to extinguish conditioned behaviors. People do not often stop doing something just because they don't receive reinforcement. Why? Because rewards and punishments are irregular; hence many of the things we have learned have been learned under conditions of partial reinforcement. If undesirable conditioned responses are to be unlearned or extinguished, then reinforcing every response favors rapid extinction much more than reinforcing only occasionally. In other words, consistency is the key to extinction.

Many of the responses required of nurses in emergency situations are stimulus-response actions. For example, when an individual goes into cardiac arrest, life-saving cardiopulmonary resuscitation measures must be instituted immediately, almost without conscious thought. Nursing students must be taught to respond spontaneously to such life-threatening events. It is the responsibility of the nurse educator to structure conditions for learning that promote achievement of this stimulus-response behavior.

Chaining

Most of human behavior is not just a matter of simple signal or stimulus-response actions. Verbal and nonverbal behavior is organized into chains, or a sequence of events with one response leading to another. The reinforcer for one response becomes the stimulus for the next response. Neither the response nor the stimulus has any behavioral meaning unless both are viewed in relation to each other. Perceptual associations are formed into motor chains, which are a series of actions in a fixed order. Each action depends upon the outcome of the last action and involves perceptual information processing.

Chaining is exemplified by actions such as walking, running, tying a shoelace, driving an automobile, doing a qualitative analysis, explaining a procedure, taking vital signs, writing a computer program, and any number of tasks that require breaking a process down into a series of actions.

Serial, verbal learning represents a mixture of several different kinds of behaviors, including response learning, association learning, and the learning of order. Learning of behavioral chains requires prelearning of the individual associations that make up the chain and any multiple discriminations that may be required to prevent interference among the stimuli in the chain.

Verbal Association

Much of what we learn is verbal, in the sense that we think, speak, and act in terms of symbolic language. After learning what words stand for in the world of objects and events, we learn new things by relating words in new ways or by association.

Verbal association, verbal chaining, or paired-associated learning in its simplest form involves the ability to associate pairs of items, one member of the pair being the stimulus term and the other member being the response term. Examples of this type of learning are naming objects, recalling definitions or sentences verbatim, listing a series of steps in proper sequence for doing a procedure, recognizing and naming a shape, learning the meaning of a chemical symbol, and associating names with pictures.

Verbal association is a multiprocess phenomenon that includes stimulus discrimination, response integration, stimulus selection and coding, association formation, mediation, and organizational processes. Thus, it is far more complex than simple rote learning. First, we must learn to discriminate between stimuli. The more difficult it is to make distinctions between elements, the more the rate of learning is retarded.

Second, we must link appropriate responses to the stimuli so as to recall them. We do not always have to attend to the entire stimulus to be able to discriminate. Redundant or irrelevant information can be ignored. Stimulus selection is frequent and routine. In most cases, we are not even aware that it happens. For instance, to identify a person we need only to see a face, not the entire person. For close friends, we probably only need to see a portion of the face. In general, we select out the most meaningful, familiar, and attention-getting elements to discriminate between stimuli and make verbal associations. This doesn't mean that we fail to perceive other elements that are present; some elements are perceived but not used and some are associated with the response, but to a weaker degree. Overlearning of secondary cues tends to strengthen recall of the associated response. It appears that as we begin to learn a new task, we narrow our attention to some dominant aspect. As we attain mastery, we continue to overlearn, relax our attention, and attend to other cues in the environment.

Verbal association also involves stimulus coding. That is, we often change or transform a stimulus, either overtly or covertly, into a different state or representation in order to make an association. We transform names into acronyms or short-term labels, and words into mental images. Coding does not always improve our ability to learn paired associates, however. If it requires more effort to decode the coding than to make the initial association, then coding will not facilitate learning (or communication).

The formation of new associations and corresponding responses appears to depend either on linkage to associations that have already been internalized or on unintentional or incidental learning situations. Associations can be formed gradually over time or all at once, depending on the circumstances. We also are able to form associations either forward or backward—that is, we can recall the response to a stimulus or given the response, we can associate the stimulus. Backward associations are usually weaker than forward associations.

The learning of verbal associations is not simply receiving or imprinting data, nor is it that a particular stimulus elicits a particular response. Rather, as in a computer, it involves internal organizational processing, storage, and retrieval of information. We cluster information into objective or subjective parts or categories, store these in memory, and recall them when the need arises. More meaningful information is easier to associate and recall because it is more familiar, because more associations have been internalized, because it seems easier to integrate into a functional unit, or because it is less fragmented.

Multiple Discrimination

Mutliple discrimination requires that the individual make two or more individual stimulus-response associations to an equal number of stimuli. The event that most clearly governs multiple discrimination learning is inference. We must be able to perceive or infer differences between objects or events and make complex associations and generalizations. To be able to make multiple discriminations, we must have acquired ability to recall and to symbolically chain objects and events in a fixed order. The ability to select different objects after hearing their names or name different objects shown are examples of multiple discrimination learning.

Concept Learning

If each new learning situation was essentially a matter of conditioning, stimulus-response, or rote learning, we would be overwhelmed by a mass of specifics in a complex world. Fortunately, we are able to learn concepts. Concept learning refers to acquiring a common response, often in the form of a verbal label, to a class of events or objects. It is the act of classifying or systematically organizing stimuli or events that have some attributes or features in common. Concepts are therefore combinations of meanings, values, and symbols.

Concepts can be combined into ideas, facts, principles, or rules to solve problems. For example, as a very young child, we learned to assign the name *two* to collections of any two objects and not to assign it to collections of one or three objects. Later on, we learned that the concept of two was composed of a number of principles or ideas, such that the set of two was formed by joining the sets of one, by taking one member away from the set of three, and so on.

Theoretically, it is not necessary to know words or language to learn a concept. In fact, some concepts are difficult to express in words. A common example is the concept of "love." Most words, however, are used to refer to some common property of objects, and the ability to handle concepts is related to some form of language development. Take for example the word *red.* It is used to label anything having the property of redness.

Concept learning is a complex process involving internal discrimination and generalization based on past experience. It is a personal phenomenon. We learn concepts through trial and error, actual experiential discovery, and by verbal definition. Concepts cannot be learned by words alone, however. A concept that is learned by way of verbally stated principles (definition) only is usually inadequate. Words may even inhibit learning of the concept. To internalize a concept, we must abstract or infer information from actual objects, events, or circumstances and apply it to past personal experience.

How does concept learning compare to paired-associate learning? Paired-associate learning requires that a particular response be learned for a particular stimulus, whereas concept learning involves the learning of a single response for two or more stimuli. A concept can be learned in a rote fashion but for concept learning to have genuinely occurred, the learner must be able to respond to the relevant attributes of the object or event and to ignore irrelevant dimensions. Concept learning, then, involves the ability to discriminate and generalize. When we learned the concept of circle, we most likely encountered a number of circles of different sizes, colors, and other relevant features, which we touched, saw, and may have even tasted. Other shapes were presented, such as triangles, squares, and rectangles, so that we perceived differences. Gradually, we were able to generalize that all objects with the common dimension of "roundness," such that every point was equally distant from the center point, was considered to be a circle. Other concepts are formed based on what we do with members of a class. For example, pizza and ice cream belong to the class of foods. Each has different properties, but we make common responses to both of them depending on life experiences, values, attitudes, and so on.

It is not an easy task to describe how more complex concepts are learned. For example, professional nurse is a concept. Therefore, we should be able to delineate common attributes or qualities that can be observed directly or indirectly that make up the classification. Even more difficult are concepts such as personality, pain, anxiety, compliance, and so forth. The point is that concept learning involves categorizing abstractions through perceptual, cognitive, affective, and even psychomotor processes. The individual attends to some object, event, or circumstance. An impression is sent to the brain through a sensory channel. Impressions are accumulated into meaning and the mental image, or concept, is formed. The initial concept tends to be incomplete. With more experience, however, it becomes more accurate. Perceptual processing and actual sensory experiencing through sight, sound, smell, touch, and taste are crucial factors in concept learning. Reading and listening to spoken words are not concrete sensory experiences; therefore they are not considered to be a part of the basic perceiving process involved in concept learning.

Principle or Rule Learning

Concepts, when learned through verbal definition, are learned through application of principles, rules, or ideas. Principles are combinations of simple concepts. For example, in our previous discussion of the concept of two, the "rules," principles, or ideas are those through which we learn the concept of two—a set of two is formed by joining two sets of one, subtracting one member from three, and so on. A principle is composed of more than one concept.

Principle learning builds upon concepts contained in the principle. We must have learned the concepts contained in the principle before we can learn the principle. The concepts are prerequisites to learning. It is possible to learn principles through extended trial-and-error practice sessions, experiential discovery, or verbal definition. Research indicates, however, that it is advantageous to use the discovery method for principle learning because it promotes retention and transfer. We know a principle has been learned when it can be demonstrated by specific actions that identify its component concepts.

In summary, a principle is composed of a number of related concepts. A communication, usually print or oral, must be made to the learner indicating the sequence of concepts. A principle has been learned when the concepts can be correctly recalled and when the principle can be applied to a problem situation. For instance, "clean to clean equals clean," "sterile to clean equals clean," "sterile to dirty equals contaminated," and "clean to dirty equals contaminated" are principles of asepsis. When the learner can recall the concepts of clean, sterile, dirty, and contaminated and apply the principles correctly in numerous situations under various circumstances when performing medical and surgical aseptic practices, then we know the principles have been learned.

Problem Solving

It is imperative that people develop the capacity to adapt to new situations, to make discriminations, to think creatively and critically, and to make sound, objective judgments to solve problems. Problem solving is the most complex type of learning. It is behavior that involves recalling and selecting principles and concepts in order to generate hypotheses and solve problems in novel ways. Problem solving encompasses behaviors attributed to operant conditioning, chaining, verbal association, multiple discrimination, conceptualizing, generalizing, and applying rules.

Much of what we call human thinking is directed toward solving problems of practical and intellectual significance. Language, thought, and problem-solving processes are significantly related; however, it appears that language is not necessarily essential for the complex mental problem-solving process. Even a person who cannot hear can learn high-level problem-solving behaviors.

Unlike concept learning and paired-associate learning, in which relatively few behavioral alternatives exist, problem-solving tasks allow for many response options. How are such behaviors acquired? Psychologists and educators explain this phenomenon in different ways. According to stimulus-response theory, we try different responses until one is found to be successful in solving a problem. The habits we acquire if successful will be used to solve new problems, provided the new situation is similar. Gestaltists attribute problem solving to a perceptual process that involves perceiving environmental stimuli in new and different ways. According to information processing theory, problem-solving behavior is acquired through certain external and internal conditions. External conditions facilitate receiving stimuli. Internal conditions pertain to the ability to recall learned principles and concepts, selection of those that are relevant to the situation, combining rules and concepts to form new rules, selection of one that may solve the problem, and application of the provisional rule to a specific example to see if it works.

It appears that problem solving can occur without conscious effort. Most of us have experienced such "insightful" happenings. We work hard trying to solve a problem but to no avail and finally turn to other tasks. Unexpectedly, the solution, like a "bolt out of the blue" comes to us in the middle of the night or while walking down the street. Such unconscious problem solving may be due to a period of rest away from the problem situation or to creative thinking processes. Many people report a period of creative thinking, or incubation, when faced with a perplexing problem. Creativity or intellectual inventiveness is applied in many problem situations. It involves reorganizaton of past experiences, learning processes, and acquired knowledge into new and original patterns. Thought processes during creativity revolve around four states of problem solving: preparation, incubation, inspiration, and verification.

Even though it is possible to solve problems through trial and error or conditioned responses and insight, high-level problem solving requires internalizing a process that, when applied systematically, facilitates problem solution. First there is a motive, identification, or recognition phase in which we perceive that there is a problem that we want to do something about. Secondly, we go through a planning phase in which strategies or plans of action are identified. Thirdly, we assess relevant data and determine viable options and generate hypotheses. Next, the hypotheses are tested and relevant data are collected and analyzed. Finally, we reach consensus on a problem solution and take action, again collecting evaluative data to determine to what extent the solution was successful. Much of problem-solving behavior is internal; however, application of the process can be made observable to determine whether learning has occurred and to what degree. The application of assessment skills to make a nursing diagnosis is only one example of many problem-solving behaviors in nursing. In fact, the nursing process is a problem-solving process. Critical and creative thinking and problem solving are crucial attributes of the professional nurse. Consequently, learning experiences should foster this type of learning.

Observation or Imitation Learning

Intellectual, emotional, and social behaviors can be acquired on a vicarious basis through the observation of other people's behavior and its consequences for them. Imitation not only promotes the learning of new behaviors but also strengthens or weakens previously learned responses. Usually we become more inhibited in displaying a behavior when we observe that others experience negative consequences from a behavior. On the other hand, witnessing others being rewarded for a certain behavior may cause us to imitate the behavior. Research suggests that our susceptibility to imitative influences varies with our individual idiosyncrasies, the attributes of the model, and the consequences attached to the modeled behavior. Our ability to learn new behaviors or change old ones simply by observing others underlines the need for the teacher to serve as a motivating model and to actively seek out, organize, develop, and coordinate the activities of others as potential reinforcing agents.

Behavior Modification

If a behavior results in self-satisfaction, we are inclined to repeat it. A problem arises, though, when a learned behavior is not beneficial to self or society. Behaviors can be taught and existing behaviors can be changed or modified using behavior modification techniques.

All behaviors must have a payoff of some kind. Therefore, rewarding a desirable behavior when it is exhibited will increase the likelihood that the behavior will be repeated. First of all, the specific type of response must be identified; then positive reinforcement must be given on a regular basis every time the behavior is exhibited or as often as possible until the desired behavior appears to be acquired, at which time the reward can then be given intermittently. The use of consistent reward is crucial to the behavioral change and the use of inconsistent reward is crucial to maintaining behavior. Timing of the reward is another critical factor. Initially, the reinforcer should come immediately following exhibition of the desired behavior. The delay interval can be lengthened as the individual acquires the behavior.

Rewards can be tangible or intangible. Tangible rewards include such items as raisins, trinkets, points, money, special activities, and so on. Intangible rewards include a smile, wink, physical nearness, touch, attention, verbal or written praise, approval, and encouragement. The nature of the reinforcement used depends on the age, interests, and other attributes of the learner. Tangible rewards should always be accompanied by verbal and nonverbal social rewards so that in time, the social rewards will become more potent reinforcers. A choice of rewards can be especially effective. Verbal feedback on how the person is progressing in acquiring a behavior can also be used as a reward. Successful experiences provide reward in and of themselves.

Initially, it may be impossible to reinforce a behavior because it is not exhibited or observable. In this case, approximations of the desired behavior can be rewarded. Rewarding the first signs of appropriate behavior may induce development of desired behavior patterns.

Peer group praise, recognition, and rejection may have some affect on changing behaviors. Social problem-solving meetings have been found to be an effective method for discussing problems and generating behavioral changes. In addition, studies indicate that approval from a disliked or unpopular peer has greater reward value than does approval from a liked peer.

Contractual agreements that are set up by the learner, the teacher, or both can be effective vehicles for learning. Such contracts are of the nature "you can do this, if you do that." To be effective, the contract must offer a reward that is highly attractive to the learner and that is not obtainable outside the conditions of the contract. Self-contracting demands self-control and initiative.

Certain negative sanctions, if properly used, assist in changing behaviors. Just as giving a reward can facilitate the acquisition or maintenance of behavior, removing a reward can reduce or displace an undesirable behavior. It is desirable to combine extinction with reinforcement techniques. The extinction of behavior is not necessarily permanent. A displaced behavior, if reinforced again, is often easily reinstated. Consistency of extinction and reward techniques is the key.

Particularly troublesome behaviors may require the use of punishment as an intervention to stop behaviors immediately. Research indicates, however, that punishment does not eliminate the response but only slows the rate at which it occurs. The two types of punishment most often used are painful experiences and removal of reinforcers. Both types vary in their effectiveness and side effects that they may promote.

In general, if punishment is used, it should be applied before the behavior is in full force, which is difficult to do. Punishment can result in avoidance behaviors, such as the learner's resorting to sneakiness, faking illness, withdrawal, cheating, and so on. If negative techniques are used, they should be applied in conjunction with positive rewards for appropriate behavior.

The establishment of "rules" of conduct may also facilitate behavioral change. Rules alone, especially when they are imposed, will not usually be effective reinforcers. Giving the learner a voice and choice in establishing rules and selecting rewards may help to enlist cooperation.

SUMMARY

To further understand the phenomenon of learning as a change in behavior, we have explored a number of different but interrelated types of learning. We have established that learning is a continual, dynamic process that occurs under both structured and unstructured circumstances. Different kinds of behavioral change result depending upon environmental conditions called stimuli. These conditions evoke particular responses or behaviors.

Low-level, simple conditioned responses are relatively uncomplicated responses to signals. Classical conditioning or signal learning relates to responding in a reflexlike manner to objects, symbols, persons, places, or events, whereas operant conditioning or stimulus-response learning involves displaying a particular behavior to obtain a reward. When behavior is rewarded, it is strengthened.

In classical conditioning, the emotionally pleasant or unpleasant stimulus precedes and signals the response, but in operant conditioning, the response leads to the reward. Thus, the element of reinforcement is essential in both signal learning and stimulus-response learning. Stimulus-response learning is goal-directed. In most cases, a number of responses will be tried before the appropriate one is learned. Therefore, the ability to discriminate and generalize responses is prerequisite to stimulus-response learning.

Simple, single responses are associated and chained into fixed sequences of ordered actions. Each action depends upon the outcome of the last and the reinforcer for one response becomes the stimulus for the next response. Chaining requires perceptual information processing and involves breaking a process down into a series of decisions and actions. The learning of a behavioral chain, then, is a matter of putting together, in prescribed order, a set of previously learned individual associations.

When we are able to relate a stimulus to a particular response, an association has been developed. Verbal association in its simplest form involves associating words with objects. In order for associations to be established, we must be able to recall previously learned associations, discriminate the stimulus from its surroundings through an information processing and selection process, and link appropriate responses to the significant stimuli. Associations are formed gradually or at the spur of the moment, either forward or backward, and they are more easily formed when information is perceived as meaningful and relevant.

On a higher level, we learn to distinguish or differentially identify two or more physically different stimuli and make multiple discriminations and associations based on previously learned paired associations. We classify and systematically organize stimuli that have common attributes into concepts. Concepts are then combined into ideas, facts, and principles to solve problems.

Concept learning involves the ability to discriminate, generalize, and categorize abstractions. We do this by responding to relevant attributes of objects and events and ignoring irrelevant ones. Concrete, realistic learning experiences facilitate the acquisition of concepts.

Simple concepts are chained into principles or rules. We cannot learn principles unless we have internalized the concepts involved and can recall their meanings. Guided discovery or experiential learning promotes principle learning.

Research has demonstrated that successful learning of concepts and rules is contingent on learner recognition of relevant features in newly encountered instances. Concepts and rules are learned through noticing, labeling, and matching processes. Research with young children suggests that using pictorial cues to focus attention on important features of a concept or rule and specific pretraining on how to use the pictorial information to notice and label relevant rules and concepts facilitate concept formation.

The process of learning and teaching concepts differs significantly from those appropriate for fact, principle, attitude, and skill learning. Acquisition of a concept involves the formation of a mental image of the set of characteristics common to any and all examples of a class. Evidence of conceptualization is the learner's demonstrated ability to consistently distinguish examples from nonexamples by citing the presence or absence of the concept characteristics in individual items. For example, when a child makes the response "horse" to live horses, pictures of horses, horses of different colors and breeds, then generalizing within the class of horses has occurred. The child must also discriminate between the class of horses and other animals; hence dogs, cats, automobiles, and so on are not labeled "horse."

Concept learning differs from principle learning in that principle learning involves acquiring a mental image of the cause-effect process that occurs under certain conditions between examples of two or more concepts. Principle learning is indicated when the learner is able to demonstrate ability to make well-supported and qualified inferences of either cause or effect in new or changed situations.

An attitude is a mental set toward taking some action based on the desirability of anticipated consquences. Evidence of attitude learning is acquired willingness to take or refrain from action based on its consequences. A skill involves proficiency in performing a mental or physical action or set of procedures. Performance is based on the learner's concept of the action, predictions as to the action's effects, and internalization of the procedures through repeated practice. Therefore, concepts cannot be tested by having the learner state facts or perform a skill.

Concepts are learned through generalization and discrimination processes by focusing on several examples and nonexamples of the concept, gathering and verifying information as to the concept-relevant characteristics of each example and nonexample, noting how examples vary and yet are still examples of the concept, noting what is alike about all examples of the concept, noting how nonexamples resemble examples, and how they differ from them, and generalizing about the characteristics that distinguish all examples of the concept from an item that might resemble them in any way. For instance, the visual electrocardiographic patterns of ischemia, injury, and infarction (but not their definitions) can be learned by discriminating between random visual tracings and generalizing among patterns.

Some research indicates that a networking strategy consisting of the formation of mental imagery, a peg-mnemonic memory system, and the use of a hierarchical retrieval memory system (the mental formation of images into a stable cluster of information) is superior to a simple stimulus-response rote learning or incremental learning strategy during a concept learning task.[5]

Problem solving subsumes all other types of learning. The ability to solve problems is essential to becoming fully functioning human beings. In general, problem solving requires the ability to make associations and discriminations and to recall and select multiple concepts and principles to generate and test hypotheses that lead to problem solution. It involves applying creative and critical thinking skills.

Complex intellectual, emotional, and social behaviors can be learned by observing and imitating the actions of others; therefore teachers and peer groups serve as positive or negative reinforcing agents. Behaviors can also be changed through the use of positive or negative tangible and intangible rewards. Consistency must be established, however, and personal preferences must be taken into consideration. It should be remembered that extinction practices, such as punishment, will not eliminate a behavior but only slow its rate of occurrence.

In all types of learning, human language plays an important role, but it is not a mandatory condition for learning. Active sensory involvement of the learner in the learning experience is crucial. In addition, immediate reinforcement is a major condition for most learning. If a particular behavior is satisfying, it will tend to be repeated.

DOMAINS OF LEARNING

Following the early attempt of psychologists to explain learning in terms of one particular all-encompassing theory, and more recently, the emergence of theoretically integrated theories of learning, authorities like Robert Gagné have attempted to delineate and explain specific types of learning. Strong similarities and interrelationships can be seen among these phenomena.

Since the 1950s, educational psychologists like Benjamin Bloom, David Krathwhol,[6] and others, have taken a somewhat different approach. They categorize human behaviors according to cognitive, affective, and psychomotor domains of learning. There is considerable interaction and overlapping among all three domains, however. For instance, the high-level skill of operating a personal computer reflects effective integrated typing movements (psychomotor); the application of strategies, tactics, and knowledge in the form of facts, principles, and concepts (cognitive); and appropriate attitudes, values, and motivation (affective). Nevertheless, hierarchical behavioral categories can be identified for each domain of learning.

The Cognitive Domain

The cognitive domain includes intellectual behaviors that can be attributed to knowledge, comprehension, application, analysis, synthesis, and evaluation. Knowledge represents the lowest level in the cognitive domain and is defined as the remembering of previously learned information. This may involve the recall of information ranging from specific facts to complete theories, but the emphasis is on *recalling* appropriate information. Comprehension is the lowest level of *understanding*. It is the ability to grasp the meaning of information and involves translating data from one form to another by interpreting material and estimating future trends. Application is a higher cognitive level. It refers to the ability to *use* learned information in new and concrete situations. Application requires a higher level of understanding and of transferring of data than comprehension. Behaviors in this category include the application of rules or principles, methods, concepts, laws, and theories.

Analysis behaviors require an understanding of both the content and structure of the information; hence analysis represents a higher intellectual level than comprehension and application. Behaviors involve the ability to *break down* information into its component parts so that its organizational structure can be comprehended. This process includes the identification of parts, analysis of the relationships between parts, and recognition of the organizational principles involved.

Cognitive synthesis refers to the ability to *put parts together* to form a new whole. This may involve the creation of a unique communication, a plan of operations, or a set of abstract relations. Synthesis stresses creative behaviors, with major emphasis on the formation of unique patterns or structures.

Evaluation is the highest level in the cognitive hierarchy. Such behaviors contain elements of all of the other categories and relate to making conscious *value judgments* for a given purpose. Judgments are based on the ability to organize and determine the relevance of information.

The Affective Domain

Attitudes, opinions, beliefs, values, and feelings are among the most important learned responses. Such responses are formed early in life and continue as ever-present behaviors. Although somewhat different in meaning, the terms reflect affective patterns of behavior, which are learned responses to objects, persons, or events. Studies of affective change and persistence indicate that the processes of forming and modifying affect are not much different from other forms of learning: they involve attempts by the individual to achieve desired goals, to find acceptance and self-actualization, and to alleviate frustration. To change such behaviors, it is necessary to establish positive goals and reinforcing conditions and to counteract factors contributing to resistance to change. Teachers, peers, parents, and significant others can serve as role models for affective behavior change.

Attitudes, opinions, beliefs, values, and feelings are predisposing factors to actions. They are internal processes—that is, they are processes that enable a person to interact selectively with the environment. As such, these constructs cannot be directly observed, but they can be inferred from overt behaviors. For example, if we want to know what a person's attitudes about nurses and nursing are, we could observe behaviors that would reflect them. We could observe specific verbal and nonverbal communication behaviors during client interaction, for instance.

The affective domain emphasizes feelings and emotions, such as interests, attitudes, appreciations, and methods of adjustment. Categories within the domain are: receiving, responding, valuing, organization, and development of a value complex.

Receiving represents the lowest level in the affective domain. Behaviors range from simple awareness that a thing exists to selective attention. Receiving refers to the learner's willingness to attend to a particular phenomenon or stimulus.

Responding refers to active participation on the part of the learner. At this level, the learner attends to a particular phenomenon and reacts in some affective manner, such as willingness to respond and satisfaction in responding. Higher levels of the responding category include interests and seeking out the enjoyment of specific events.

Valuing is concerned with the worth or value a learner attaches to an object, event, or behavior. This ranges in degree from the simple acceptance of a value to the more complex level of commitment. Valuing is based on the internalization of a set of specified values, but clues to these values are expressed in overt behavior.

Organizational behaviors are those that reflect the merging of different values, the resolving of conflicts, and the building of an internally consistent value system. The emphasis is on comparing, relating, and synthesizing values.

At the highest level of the affective domain, the individual exhibits behaviors that represent the internalization of a value system. Behavior is pervasive, consistent, and predictable at this level. The major emphasis is on typical or characteristic behaviors of the learner.

The Psychomotor Domain

The psychomotor domain emphasizes motor skills. It includes concomitant cognitive and affective elements, but the demonstration of a motor skill characterized by the acquisition and performance of behaviors that involve coordinated gross- or fine-muscle-movement patterns is the dominant aspect of the response.

The demonstration of a psychomotor skill is the result of reception and analysis of information, decision making, and output actions. In additon, an optimal level of motivation is necessary for performance. Robert Gagné's work on hierarchical types of learning explains psychomotor behavior in terms of chained events or the sequencing of a set of individual stimulus-response behaviors. Chaining occurs when a single stimulus cue triggers an integrated series of responses, in which making a response becomes the stimulus for the next response, and so forth. For learning to occur, each stimulus-response behavior must be executed in proper order and time sequence. Also, each terminal step must be practiced and positively reinforced. Once a chained behavior is learned, it can be generalized to similar circumstances.

According to B. F. Skinner, the effect of reinforcement is crucial to learning a psychomotor skill. His concept of shaping consists of giving reinforcement at each approximation of the desired behavior.

Robert Singer's model of motor behavior emphasizes features taken from information-processing, cybernetic, and adaptive approaches to the study of human behavior.[7] It is Singer's contention that when psychomotor behaviors are acquired, we receive environmental or internal cues to information via auditory, visual, kinesthetic, and tactile sensory neurons, or receptors, which serve as activators for action. These signals are briefly held in sensory stores without regard to feature differentiation and then transmitted to the perceptual mechanism where data are attended to and selectively processed. Some of the input is acted upon and some is immediately transferred to long-term memory to link it to data already in memory. It is in the perceptual mechanism that selected data are recognized and given meaning through association with previously stored information and internal personal attributes such as developmental, structural, and functional capabilities, motivation, personality factors, and individual cognitive style.

The perceptual mechanism achieves recognition of stimuli by analyzing features of incoming stimuli and combining them as a unified whole. Perceptual information is sent to short-term memory, where it is rehearsed and organized for decision making. Short-term memory is where the majority of information processing occurs and decisions are made about movement selection and execution. In addition, short-term memory mechanisms determine which information should be transferred to long-term storage and to the movement generator. The movement generator selects the appropriate musculature to perform the activity, transmits a sequence of efferent neural commands to the chosen muscles, and prepares the short-term memory for sensory consequences of the forthcoming motor act. The effector mechanism, consisting of the muscles that control the extremities, executes the movement response. Feedback is sent to sensory storage, long-term, and short-term memory, where error detection and correction occur.

Apparently, information in short-term memory is rapidly lost when attention or rehearsal is not sustained. With adequate rehearsal, information is sent on to long-term memory, where it is ready to be recalled when needed.

Individual differences in performance can be attributed to differences in the functional capabilities of short-term memory and to the situational context within which the movement must be performed. In order to demonstrate higher-order learning in the form of successful motor performance, the presence of a wide variety of cognitive and perceptual abilities, motor abilities, physical and sensory characteristics, personality attributes, and control mechanisms for emotions is necessary.

Every psychomotor skill reflects the need for varying degrees of physical, cognitive, motor, and emotional involvement. Research on attitude treatment interaction indicates that a person's entering competencies and abilities interact with the manner in which a skill is taught, thus affecting learning outcomes. This varies from person to person.

Elizabeth Simpson developed a taxonomy for the learning of psychomotor behaviors.[8] The taxonomy consists of seven major levels and corresponding sublevels. The seven levels within the classification scheme, beginning with the lowest, are: perception, set, guided response, mechanism, complex overt response, adaptation, and origination. Each level builds upon the preceding one. Perception is the process of becoming aware of objects, qualities, or relationships by way of the sense organs. It is a crucial predisposing condition to performing a motor act and involves auditory, visual, tactile, olfactory, gustatory, and kinesthetic sensory stimulation, cue selection and translation. First, there is impingement of a stimulus on one or more senses. Then cues relevant to the situation are selected to guide action, with irrelevant cues being ignored or discarded. Cues received are given meaning through symbolic translation or insightful perception.

Perceptual processes are followed by the establishment of a preparatory physical, cognitive, and emotional adjustment or readiness "set" for the particular behavior. Under guidance of a model, the behavior begins to develop through imitation or trial and error. This guided response level may be viewed as multiple-response learning, in which the proper response is selected out of varied behavioral options, possibly under the influence of positive or negative reinforcement.

At the mechanism level, the learned response becomes habitual. The learner has achieved a certain confidence and degree of performance proficiency. The act or patterned behavior becomes a part of the internal repertoire of responses to particular stimuli and circumstances. The degree of proficiency progresses to where a person can perform a complex overt response. Response becomes smooth and efficient with minimum expenditure of energy. The behavior is performed without hesitation with a great deal of ease and muscle control.

Adaptation and origination are the two highest levels of psychomotor learning. It is at these levels that we are able to alter motor responses to meet the demands of new situations and create new behaviors from existing understandings, abilities, and skills.

David Merrill contends that psychomotor instruction is designed to enable the learner to exhibit specified psychomotor behavior in response to particular stimulus situations.[9] The acquisition of psychomotor behavior depends upon the basic learning processes of discrimination, generalization, and chaining. Most psychomotor behavior consists of a series of reactions executed in a coordinated manner as if the behavior were a single response. Series of coordinated responses are often combinations of simpler psychomotor responses called psychomotor behavior chains. A major function of instruction for coordinated psychomotor response chains is to promote chaining or internalization of cues by directing the learner's attention to the stimulus cue through prompting mechanisms. When a learner has learned to make some response in the presence of a particular stimulus situation, this same response will occur in the presence of some other stimulus situation that bears some physical or functional similarity to the first stimulus. The more similar the two situations, the greater the probability that the response will occur to both. As the stimuli become less and less similar, the probability of the response occurring decreases.

Most psychomotor tasks require fine discriminations between similar stimulus situations. Promoting stimulus discrimination is one of the primary purposes of psychomotor instruction. The learner who has not yet acquired the behavior is unable to make the required discriminations. The unskilled performer is also often characterized by a failure to change the characteristics of the response when there is a change in the stimulus situation. In psychomotor instruction, learning takes place while the learner is responding, *not* prior to making the response. Instruction must therefore require the student to respond and provide mechanisms for obtaining information concerning adequacy of the response.

For very complex psychomotor chains, the most satisfactory prompting display consists of a combination of verbal commands and demonstration. These prompts *must be eliminated* in the demonstration of the terminal behavior by the learner.

A certain effect of the total stimulus situation is that it serves as a cue for a particular psychomotor response or response chain to occur. Stimulus cues are external to the learner. If future performance of the psychomotor behavior is to occur in the "real world," the cue should be displayed in the same way it will appear in naturally occurring situations.

Practice with appropriate timing, internal and external *immediate* knowledge of results, adequate prompts, and adequate fading of prompts results in high levels of proficiency. If instruction consists solely of reading or listening to a verbal description or viewing and listening to a demonstration, and does not provide opportunity for the learner to practice and receive feedback and knowledge of results, it is not reasonable to assume that the behavior has been acquired. For the teacher, the challenge is to structure the task and guide the learner to take maximum advantage of internal knowledge of results. In a sense, the goal is to make practice self-instructional.

Harrow contends that the psychomotor domain is concerned with manipulative and motor skills, both requiring neuromuscular coordination.[10] Psychomotor behavior connotes mind-movement or voluntary motion, which is observable as voluntary actions or action patterns performed by the learner. Harrow's taxonomy of the psychomotor domain consists of six hierarchically ordered levels of behavior: reflex movements or involuntary responses to stimuli, basic-fundamental movements, perceptual abilities, physical abilities, skilled movements, and non-discursive communication.

Reflex movements are prerequisites to other higher level psychomotor behaviors. They form the basis of all movement behavior, are functional at birth, and develop through maturation. Basic-fundamental movement patterns involve combining reflex movements into movement patterns. This level includes locomotor movements, which involve change in location, such as crawling, creeping, sliding, walking, running, jumping, hopping, rolling, and climbing; nonlocomotor movements, including pushing, pulling, swaying, stooping, stretching, bending, and twisting, which involve staying in one place and moving limbs or portions of the trunk in motion around an axis; and manipulative movements, which are coordinated movements of the extremities.

Perceptual abilities and physical abilities are developed through maturation and learning. The efficiency and degree of skill movement attained is based upon the learner's control of basic or fundamental movements, the degree of efficiency with which stimuli are perceived, and the level of physical ability attained. Efficiently functioning perceptual abilities are essential to develop the affective, cognitive, and psychomotor domains.

Perceptual abilities include kinesthetic discrimination (body awareness, body image, body relationship to surrounding objects in space), visual discrimination (acuity, tracking, memory, figure-ground differentiation, perceptual consistency), auditory discrimination (acuity, tracking, memory), tactile discrimination, and coordinated abilities (eye-hand and eye-foot coordination). Perceptual abilities refer to all the learner's perceptual modalities whereby stimuli are received and carried to the higher brain centers for interpretation. Data are provided, which are then used by brain centers when making a response.

Physical abilities involve endurance, strength, flexibility, agility, reaction-response time, and dexterity. The abilities provide the background for skilled movements. Skilled movements involve economy of movement while perfecting a complex movement and a degree of proficiency or mastery. A learner acquires skill by practicing and attending to a goal to be achieved.

After imitation of a new movement pattern and initial trial-and-error learning, the learner should be able to perform the skill with some degree of confidence and similarity to the original movement. With continued practice and heightened utilization of *feedback* on progress, proficiency attained will be influenced by body structure, body function, acuity of sensory modalities and perceptual abilities, and attitude toward achieving a high degree of efficiency—motivation and aspiration. Activities must be meaningful and worthwhile and match values and interests of the learner, and the learner must be able to realize success.

The development of the learning domain approach to describing learned behaviors has been a major contribution to education. Since its conception in the late 1950s, it has resulted in clarifying the phenomena of teaching and learning, including a more thorough identification and analysis of educational expectations and learning outcomes and evaluation of teaching and learning.

The cognitive, affective, and psychomotor approach to learning can be applied to nursing education and patient teaching. Let us assume that a group of adult learners needs to know how to prevent injury to the lower back. Such learning involves all three domains of learning. At the cognitive level, the learner would identify and recall the structure of the back, including the lumbar, spine, sacrum, lumbosacral junction, coccyx, and disks, and the exact location where injury is likely to occur, as well as causes of low-back injury and principles of good body mechanics to prevent back injury when lifting, standing, and sitting. At the comprehension level, the learner should be able to relate facts about the structure of the back to causes of injury and principles of body mechanics. This would involve such behaviors as distinguishing between examples of good and poor body mechanics. Application behaviors would be applying knowledge of facts and principles to examples of lifting, standing, and sitting. At the analysis level, the learner might analyze an instance of lifting, standing, and sitting to assess the potential for injury or to determine examples of poor body mechanics that could lead to low-back injury. Cognitive synthesis and evaluation would be reflected when the learner is able to exhibit behaviors that indicate integration of all facts and principles for prevention of low-back injury. For example, the learner might create a game about preventing low-back injury and assess its effectiveness in changing behaviors.

Learner behaviors at the lower levels of the affective domain would be reflected by the way the learner attended and responded to the knowledge, concepts, and principles and exhibited sensitivity to the importance of the problem. For instance, the learner might voluntarily point out examples of poor body mechanics that have led to low-back injury. At higher affective levels, internalization of the principles of good body mechanics into the learner's value system would be exhibited if the learner consistently used principles of good body mechanics when lifting, standing, and sitting.

At the lowest levels of the psychomotor domain, the learner would attend to and identify specific body actions that are instituted to prevent injury to the lower back. For example, the learner would focus on identifying the steps involved when lifting a heavy object: standing with the feet approximately 12 to 18 inches apart, with one foot slightly forward, and bending the knees while keeping the back straight as the body is lowered to the object. Moving on up the hierarchy of the psychomotor domain, the learner would practice and perform the sequence of actions until they became habitual and could be performed with confidence and accuracy.

SUMMARY

Human learning can be explained in terms of changes in cognitive, affective, or psychomotor responses to environmental conditions. Thus, we can categorize behaviors according to their primary domain. This is not to say that most behaviors do not involve the interaction of knowing, feeling, and doing, but only that it is possible to isolate behaviors that are more intellectually oriented or skill oriented or feeling oriented. Hierarchical categories have been identified within each of the three domains of learning and each category builds upon the preceding one, flowing from simple to more complex responses. The cognitive domain consists of behaviors related to knowledge, comprehension, application, analysis, synthesis, and evaluation. The affective domain categories—receiving, responding, valuing, organization, and characterization by a value complex—form a continuum for attitudinal behavior from simple awareness and acceptance to internalization as attitudes, beliefs, opinions, values, and feelings, and become a part of an individual's total value system.

Behaviors in the psychomotor domain refer to those involving coordinated use of gross or fine muscles to achieve motor skill performance. Singer's model proposes that psychomotor behaviors are acquired through a process that includes sensory activation, perception, memory storage, and movement generator-effector mechanism. Simpson's proposed hierarchical psychomotor taxonomy consists of perception, set, guided response, mechanism, complex overt response, adaptation, and origination. Harrow looks at attainment of neuromotor behaviors in terms of reflex movements, basic-fundamental movements, perceptual abilities, physical abilities, skilled movements, and nondiscursive communication.

The value of the cognitive, affective, and psychomotor domain approach to learning lies in its practical applicability to teaching and learning, whereby it serves as a mechanism for the establishment of educational expectations and learning outcomes and facilitates evaluation of teaching and learning processes.

FORCES THAT INFLUENCE LEARNING

Behavioral change is a personal phenomenon, in that each individual has unique hereditary and sociocultural background, experiences, needs, understanding, motivation, capabilities, values, attitudes, and emotions. Our personal attributes, past experiences, health status, predispositions, and idiosyncrasies influence what we learn, how we learn it, and to what extent learning will occur under particular circumstances. Therefore, learning is never exactly the same for any two persons or for any one person on different occasions, even under the same conditions. Both internal and external factors influence learning. What are the factors that impinge upon us to help or hinder learning?

Heredity and Environment

The makeup that we inherit through out parents, grandparents, great-grandparents, and so on down the ancestral line determines our *potential* for development and learning. It is assumed that intellectual potential, biophysical structure and function (including body build), disabilities, endocrine function, and other factors that contribute to personality are genetically determined. The final outcome, however, is greatly influenced by what we experience in the way of sociocultural climate and the intellectual nourishment provided through the home, school, community, and overall environment. Intelligence is therefore only one aspect of behavioral potential.

Although there is some disagreement, intelligence can be defined as the general ability of the individual to acquire and retain knowledge from experience, to respond quickly and successfully to a new situation, and to use reasoning powers to solve problems. In the past, it was assumed that general intelligence was an inherited attribute that was not easily changed. Standardized tests, such as the Stanford-Binet scale and Wechsler-Bellevue intelligence scale, were devised to measure an individual's intelligence. The intelligence quotient obtained from a test was used to predict the individual's capacity to learn and ability to adapt to life's tasks. Such tests, however, rely heavily on verbal and mathematical skills, tend to be culturally biased, and are influenced by the motivational state of the individual taking the test, as well as by the attitude and competence of the examiner.

Although traditional intelligence tests may have some predictive validity for achievement potential, they fall far short of indicating fully an individual's intellectual status and potential for learning. This is primarily due to the fact that intellect or cognition is made up of at least fifty factors.[11] Recently, information-processing experts and educators have been investigating intelligence in terms of thinking and learning "skills" that are used in academic and everyday problem-solving situations. The contention is that such skills can be diagnosed, taught, and learned.

The way we react to our endowments is a significant factor in behavior. For example, we can overcome genetic predispositions, physical disabilities, maladjustments, and other handicaps through development of self-acceptance and motivation. In other words, genes give us the potential for development, and a favorable internal and external environment tends to affect this potential positively.

Heredity, environment, and response are inseparably interrelated in every complex human being. Each individual grows and develops physically and mentally at a unique rate. We learn to roll over, sit up, stand, bounce, creep, crawl, walk, talk, read, and achieve various levels of independence and emotional control at different stages in life. Physical and mental growth and development proceeds in an orderly, sequential manner under "normal" circumstances.

Physical maturation influences what can be learned. For instance, if physical maturation has not progressed far enough, no learning—or very little—can occur. A child cannot respond to a face without the physical coordination necessary to fix gaze and the optic apparatus to sort out sensations. Learning to talk is not only dependent upon learning to imitate sounds and to utter them in proper sequence but is also dependent on physiological development.

No informed person would say that what we are is totally determined by heredity or solely due to environmental factors. Research has shown that heredity and environment interact to form a personality. Our inherited genetic makeup determines developmental and growth *potential.* Both heredity and environment affect intellect and learning, although how and to what degree is controversial. Environmental factors significantly influence behavioral change. Enriched, stimulating environments promote learning, whereas impoverished ones usually inhibit learning. Conditions for learning can be structured to increase learning potential.

Growth, Development, and Readiness for Learning

The course of "normal" life is marked by particular developmental levels or stages. Such stages can be thought of as descriptions of competence—the behavior of which one is capable. Fundamental physical attributes and potential intellectual and behavioral developments are established during the prenatal period. Endocrine activity is important during the prenatal phase because the mother and fetus share a common endocrine pool. It is imperative that during this stage of human development, healthful physical and emotional conditions are provided for the fetus through the mother.

At about eight weeks prenatally, the first body movements are exhibited. Between the time of the first movement and the age of 14 or 15 weeks, the fetus develops through maturation almost all the primary reflex movements of different parts of the body. During the remaining five and one-half months, sensory mechanisms develop, movements are refined and integrated and become faster and more powerful. Coordinated reflex movements evolve as various parts of the nervous system develop.

The process of birth marks the beginning of a larger total process of growth and development. When prolonged or difficult birth results in physical injury or deprivation of oxygen, developmental problems that persist long after birth may be incurred. Through birth, the fetus is given the opportunity to gain a better oxygen supply, to develop sense organs, to exercise muscles so they will become more functional, and to develop mentally through exposure to a varied environment.

Postnatal development can be divided into seven primary stages: neonatal, infancy or sensorimotor, childhood or preoperational, preadolescence or concrete operations, adolescence or formal operations, adult or maturity, and senescence. It should be kept in mind that progression through developmental stages will vary from person to person and that age does not necessarily correspond to particular developmental levels.

Roughly, the neonatal period represents the first month of life. Infancy, or the sensorimotor stage, lasts until the second year and is followed by childhood, or the preoperational stage. The stage of concrete operations usually occurs between the ages of 7 and 12, and puberty marks the beginning of adolescence or the formal operations stage, which usually starts at approximately 12 years of age. Adulthood begins at age 20 or when the individual becomes physically mature, and senescence represents the later years of life.

Infancy (Sensorimotor Stage). Infancy, or the sensorimotor stage, is characterized by unstable but rapid patterns of intellectual growth and physical response. Because the infant cannot foresee the consequence of actions, learning is largely achieved through consistent conditioning and trial-and-error processes. The conditioning stimulus is connected to the response by the repetitious recurrence of a conditioning stimulus at or about the same moment as an adequate unconditioned stimulus. The conditioning stimulus will eventually arouse the response. For example, an infant is taught to eat from a spoon by touching the cheek lightly with the spoon to get the child to open the mouth. If the experience is enjoyable and the behavior is socially rewarded through words of encouragement and praise, the child quickly learns to open the mouth and eat from the spoon. Thus, the response is generalized to similar situations.

Conditioning is significant in acquiring adaptive behaviors during infancy (including sleeping, toilet training), acquiring social and emotional responses, exercising curiosity, learning to talk, and developing a concept of self. Early environmental stimulation through concrete "doing" kinds of experiences under conditions of emotional security, safety, belongingness, and love will develop the foundation or substructures essential for later operations.

Early Childhood (Preoperational Stage). The early childhood, or preoperational, stage of development begins around the age of two and proceeds to about the age of seven. The rate of physical growth slows, yet there is a 5 to 10 percent increase in brain weight between the ages of two and four and again at six to eight years of age.

Needs and developmental tasks revolve around adaptation to culture as reflected in family and playmates. It is the period of the development of representational thinking. Thinking no longer pertains only to nearby space, the present moment, and the action in progress as it does in infancy. The child thinks in terms of far-away space, to events outside the immediate perceptual field, to the past, which can be recalled and recounted, and to the future in the form of plans and projects. It is the beginning of concept formation learning. The formation of concepts of reality is dependent upon mental maturity, opportunity for environmental stimulation, and the time and help of interested adults. The learning of concepts such as thick–thin, long–short, round–square, good–bad, empty–full, yesterday–today, and so on is basic to later mental and social development, to logical thought operations, and to subsequent developmental tasks.

Fundamental needs during early childhood include the need for affectionate personal adult interest, safety, and satisfaction of physiological needs. The child responds to a wider variety of emotion-evoking situations, including response to words. Increasing control is exerted over emotions, independence in self-care is achieved, and there is greater awareness of the role and feelings of others. Growth in language and motor skills makes it easier to deal with frustrations and to satisfy needs.

During early childhood, play experiences are sequential in that at about the age of two, the child plays alone. As the child grows older, interest in others is developed and the role of onlooker is assumed. By the age of four, associative and cooperative play occupies the major portion of playtime. This sequential play development indicates that readiness is a basic factor in development.

Preadolescence (Concrete Operations Stage). At about the age of seven or so, there is considerable growth in vocabulary and complexity of sentence structure, logical thinking skills, and concept formation. It is the concrete operations stage of development. Simple and complex quantity problems are no longer problematical. Problems are solved by starting with the real and working toward the possible.

Steady progress is noticed in emotional control with marked individual differences attributed to home and school experiences and socioeconomic factors. The most noteworthy changes of middle childhood occur in social orientation and adjustment. By the end of middle childhood, there is greatly improved ability to function in groups and increased responsiveness to peer expectations. School experiences help to develop cognitive, affective, and psychomotor behaviors. Developing the ability to read, write, and compute are important developmental tasks of childhood.

Again, maturation and readiness are crucial factors during this stage of development. There is another rapid 5 to 10 percent increase in brain weight at the age of 10 to 12 and again at 14 to 16 years of age. Research has shown that learning is related to both biological and psychological growth. Therefore, individual differences must be taken into account and children shouldn't be pressured to learn things that they are not ready to learn. Such pressures will result in frustration, poor attitudes, and even "acting out" or withdrawal behaviors.

Preadolescence, from 7 to about 12 years of age, is characterized by an accelerated growth preceding puberty, perceptible increase in strength and manual dexterity, assertion of independence, teasing of siblings, carelessness of dress, parental conflict, peer identification and affiliation, development of humor, noncommunicativeness with adults, and sexual differentiation and antagonism to persons of the opposite sex. The preadolescent is beginning to learn the concepts of fairness, right and wrong, good and bad, obligation and responsibility, and self-control of pleasure-seeking impulses—the essence of moral conduct and conscience. Previous learning experiences are leaving their accumulation of knowledge, attitudes, and skills that produce more variable behavioral possibilities.

Preadolescents can comprehend cause-and-effect relationships. Logical reasoning powers are becoming more complex, and there is a search for reality and a need for understanding natural phenomena through direct, concrete experience. Preadolescents want to know why and how something happens. Efforts at independence should be praised and respect for privacy and belongings should be shown. Freedom to develop social skills through peer group participation will strengthen identity and self-concept. Failure to be accepted by the peer group may cause some individuals to adopt predelinquent behaviors.

During preadolescence, verbal and nonverbal language shows improvement and clear purpose. The ability to differentiate between absolutes and relatives, between personal and impersonal becomes more pronounced. Efforts to help preadolescents change behavior should attempt to provide direct and vicarious experiences that facilitate the acquisition of meaning, promote autonomy, and foster freedom to explore based on individuality in a loving and caring environment.

Adolescence (Formal Operations Stage). Puberty is the physical index for the onset of adolescence, which is a period of adjustment to cultural demands and transition from childhood to adulthood, or maturity. The adolescent is a product of the interaction of biological heritage and culture; therefore individual differences are expected at this stage of life just as at any other. There is rapid altering of body structure and revision of body image. Physical changes that occur in adolescence stem primarily from altered endocrine functioning. Hormonal changes affect behavior; hence physical and emotional development are closely related. But the view of adolescence as a time of emotional upheaval is subject to question and doubt.

Instead of referring to adolescence as a period of stress and strain, as some do, it is probably more accurate to think of it as a time of emotional lability that is greatly influenced by cultural factors. Emotional patterns, while they are more stabilized than in infancy, early childhood and preadolesence, have not achieved the consistency of adulthood.

Because the adolescent is searching to achieve a self-identity and a sense of worth and a value system, striving for autonomy and emotional independence from parents as well as identification and conformity to peer-group influence can be expected. Adolescence is a time of social expansion and development. A great deal of time is centered around activities, interests, and attitudes of peers. Nearly all adolescents desire acceptance in the eyes of their peers and will frequently go to extremes to gain or maintain acceptance. An awakening interest in human sexuality causes the adolescent to modify social behavior, attitudes, and interests.

The formal operations stage is the period during which new logical thought processes appear based upon earlier development of concrete operations. The stage of formal operations implies that the individual can reason hypothetically in the form of cause–effect relationships. Individuals at this developmental level solve problems by considering what might be possible first. The formal thinker is able to construct hypotheses to account for particular phenomena, deduce from these hypotheses that certain events should occur, and test hypotheses to find out if the events do occur. The formal thinker is able to systematically combine a set of elements to create all possible combinations and to consider only the logical relations between statements while ignoring concrete content. In addition, logically appropriate conclusions can be drawn from invalid premises.

Research indicates that children over the age of 12 can be prompted to use formal operational skills even if they do not spontaneously demonstrate such skills. It is more difficult to teach children under 12 years of age such skills. Cross-cultural studies indicate that even individuals with no formal schooling can think formally when dealing with a familiar topic.

Late adolescence is a period of coming to grips with self and society. It is a period of trying out and settling on methods of relating to others and to the environment. The adolescent must learn through experience the importance of being valued and respected as a person of worth and dignity, of integrity and identity. Many times, this experience is gained through trial and error. The adolescent seeks to develop vocational interests and economic independence. Economic factors within the culture influence options and available opportunities.

A teacher can serve as a role model to help adolescents resolve conflicts in thinking and feeling and plan positive courses of action that will provide for the satisfaction of self-actualizing needs and guidance for achieving maturity.

Adulthood (Maturity). At approximately 20 years of age, the processes of physical growth and maturation slow down; however the drive for cognitive, affective and psychomotor development, and self-actualization continues from adolescence to adulthood, through the adult years and on into senescence.

At the onset of adulthood, physical and mental powers are at their prime, and at this stage of life the individual has the greatest freedom and opportunity to develop behavioral potentials. As individuals mature, the variety of both adjustive and maladjustive behavior manifestations increase. Self-actualizing needs may be expressed in terms of vocations, avocations, community service, family, and social relationships.

Because adults have experienced the world for a given number of years, they have had the opportunity to gain many environmental perceptions and predispositions to objects and events. The sum total of these perceptions forms the past experiences of the individual. Such past experiences are the starting point from which behavioral change must proceed. Adult behavior, including creativity, is probably much more rigid than that of younger persons because it has been formed over a longer period of time. Because of established patterns of behavior and predisposing mental sets, adults may be more resistent to change, especially when beliefs and values remain unchanged. Seeing change as a "threat" causes defensive behavior and even further narrowing and constricting of the perceptual field. Unless the adult can see the personal meaning involved in a behavioral change, it is doubtful that change will occur.

Developmental tasks of adulthood, such as selecting a mate, learning to live with a partner, rearing a family, managing a self-fulfilling life-style, establishing and maintaining a vocation and an economic standard of living, coping with changing societal patterns, and accepting and adjusting to physiological changes, pose adjustment problems that must be resolved through learning new roles, new adjustments, and new modes of conduct. Some adults are flexible enough to face such changes, while others are unable or unwilling to learn and are consequently overwhelmed by problems and are forced into narrow and restricted lives.

During the early years of maturity, emotional concerns tend to be self-centered and primarily involve relationships with others. Studies indicate that between ages 30 and 40, an increase in productivity occurs. Economic worries are dominant at the age of 30 and again at 55. At age 55, loss of work efficiency, health, death, and giving up major ambitions may surface as primary concerns. In the middle-aged years, altered body image and self-image are experienced, yet permanence, stability, commitment, and high-level performance are sought. Middle age is largely concerned with maintenance of self, personal relationships, family, and institutions, yet this is extremely difficult because of rapid and complex changes that appear to be inevitable. Thus, learning to cope with change is critical.

Teachers of adults should gain insight into the individual's past experiences, capabilities, and unsatisfied needs, as well as impinging circumstances, to be able to effectively influence learning. A careful assessment is required to determine level of cognition, psychomotor skill, values, attitudes, and perceived needs in order to establish important, realistic, and relevant goals for learning. Observable positive progress toward meaningful goals can change self-concept and foster motivation for learning.

In addition, adults must be given appropriate time and guidance to acquire new behavior. It must be kept in mind that individual differences during adulthood include differences in rate of learning. As is the case at other stages of development, some adults will learn more slowly or more rapidly than others. The extent to which a person's behavior will change depends on readiness, motivation, perception of need, and mitigating circumstances, such as holding down a job while attempting to acquire more education to keep a job or obtain another.

Senescence. With increased age, a number of changes occur. Aging is not necessarily a declining process; yet generalizations can be made about senescence and development.

Physiological changes do occur as we grow older. The acuity of our senses begins to decline. In the case of vision, the lens of the eye may allow less light to pass through to the retina. The aging retina requires more light to produce the same psychological sensation as in younger years. Changes in the structure of the eyeball and its muscles impair visual acuity, particularly at close range. About one in four persons over the age of 65 has a hearing problem. Overall sensitivity to sound decreases with age, and there is selective loss at high frequencies. In addition, the sense of taste appears to decline. Since sensory experiences are extremely important for psychological well-being and are predisposing factors for learning, teachers of the aged must be constantly alert to sensory problems that can affect behavior.

Beginning in middle age, there is a decrease in height, muscle mass and tone, metabolic rate, cardiac output, renal flow, and slowing of central nervous system reflexes. All endocrine glands decrease production with advance in age. Aging adults must learn to cope with diminishing physical stamina and strive for fitness.

The elderly tend to be somewhat resistant to change and exhibit caution when confronted with a new event or situation. This may be caused by discomfort associated with uncertainty and the expectation or fear of failure. As we grow older, it is also more difficult to unlearn already well-established ways of doing things. Yet contrary to what was once thought, there is little decrease with advancing age in the primary capacity to learn. Behavioral changes as we grow older are a function of perception, set, attention, motivation, physiological state, and the expectations of society and significant others within the immediate environment.

In general, older people learn better when working at their own pace. Consequently, they should not be rushed but should be permitted to proceed at a speed commensurate with their abilities and preferences. This is an important factor to remember when teaching the elderly such things as giving themselves insulin shots, taking medications, caring for their own colostomy dressings, and other self-care tasks.

Studies indicate that older people perform better on concrete tasks that are meaningful and less well on those that are perceived as abstract and more difficult. The presence of irrelevant information and poorly organized information within a learning experience can confuse and inhibit learning. This suggests that providing essential, well-organized information can promote behavioral change in the elderly learner.

In general, aging may lead to impaired memory processes. Memory deficits in the elderly can be attributed to difficulty in retrieving stored information, inhibition that occurs when switching attention from one thing to another, changing mental set or attitude, or "interference" of previously learned information with new information. The use of pictorial cues may be extremely helpful for improving recall. Loss of mental power and capacity has been shown by research to be strongly related to lack of goals and stimulation.

To influence behavioral change, teachers of the elderly need to take into consideration the individual's state of mental and physical health, abilities, disabilities, and idiosyncrasies, allowing individuals to proceed at their own learning rate. Tasks should be made meaningful, simple, concrete, and relevant. Unnecessary, irrelevant information should be avoided and visual cues should be provided.

Physical Factors

An individual at any stage of development is the product of biophysical and environmental factors. Who a person is, what a person does, and what a person becomes can be examined in terms of these interacting forces. Behavior at any given moment is the result of biological, psychological, environmental, and sociocultural factors operating simultaneously. Learning disabilities or potential learning problems may be caused by such internal and external conditions.

Physical or biological disabilities or deviations from the norm can lead to learning problems. Among these are absence of or defects in hearing, speech, eyesight, and other sensory functions; variations in height, weight, muscular strength, or use of extremities; perceived differences in physical appearance, neurological or hormonal dysfunctions, disease, and infection. Long-term, chronic illnesses or other debilitating conditions on a short-term basis will have a profound effect on how an individual perceives a learning experience and the degree of behavioral change that can be achieved.

Recent theory, research, and clinical evidence supports the view that learning is significantly related to brain structure and function. Although there is some controversy, studies indicate that practice and stimulation at the right time will foster learning, particularly among persons with brain injuries or dysfunction.[12]

The final pound of the adult, three-pound brain, which enhances the brain's efficiency and capability, develops between the ages of 2 and 16. This portion of growth involves the development of more remote axon/dendrite extensions throughout the neural network and the formation of an insulating layer (myelin) around axons. Growth occurs in sequences of short periods of rapid growth that create neural networks needed for new cognitive functions, such as speaking and reading. There are also longer periods of practically no growth when the new functions are probably integrated into the total cognitive system. Most normal children experience a rapid 5 to 10 percent increase in brain weight between the approximate ages of 2 to 4, 6 to 8, 10 to 12, and 14 to 16.[13]

Many of the recent findings related to the function of the frontal lobes of the brain in information organization, the encoding role of the cortical hemispheres, the attentional mechanisms, and the influence over perception exerted by the descending reticular system complement recent research in cognitive psychology on memory, motivation, and attention. It appears that the attentional, perceptual, motivational, encoding, and decoding systems and functions of the brain and brainstem are instrumental in the processes of selective attention to and transformation of environmental stimuli and the construction of meaning from experience.[14]

Because of individual differences in brain structure and function, including encoding, storage, arousal, attention, planning, and organizational processes, it seems probable that individuals will differ in regard to how information is received, organized, and transformed. In general, however, research appears to indicate very little relationship between cognitive abilities and the ability to learn motor tasks. Yet, research studies investigating intellectual and motor relationships have indicated higher relationships among young school-age children than among college students. In the near future, such findings may stimulate teachers to move away from the traditional proactive/group/normative approach to a more reactive/individual/diagnostic approach, which focuses on individual learner diagnosis and prescription of the conditions for learning based on assessment findings.[15]

Sociocultural and Emotional Factors. Habits, ideals, aspirations, and responses are extracted from both inherited potential and culture. A population within a particular culture or subculture (poor, elderly, and so on) shares common attributes. These attributes include verbal and nonverbal communication, religion, beliefs about health, values, and even social responses. Culture determines the kinds of experiences provided and influences how the individual perceives, relates, and reacts to the environment. As such, the environment with its objects, events, and personal contacts is a source both of opportunities and limitations that influence the kinds of behavior that can be interpreted and learned by the individual. Membership in a certain social class contributes to the way one behaves, meets needs, selects goals, feels, and responds to people, things, and events. Cultural experiences influence readiness for learning and concern for education in general. For instance, children who come from bookless homes often have difficulty when beginning to read.

Emotional factors, such as stress and anxiety, affect learning. Research indicates that low-anxiety persons improve performance under stressful conditions, whereas those highly anxious do not. This is particularly true when a task is perceived to be fairly complex or difficult, or involves a high degree of psychomotor skill or verbal output. A teacher may not realize the tremendous significance of environmental and cultural factors as they affect the attitudes, adjustments, and behaviors of learners. The assessment of sociocultural and emotional factors is an important part of teaching. If learners are particularly stressed or anxious, the teacher will need to devise ways to decrease anxiety and teach individuals to cope.

Learning Style, Modality Strengths, Cognitive Style, and Learning Preferences

One of the most promising movements in contemporary learning theory is the attention being given to individual differences in learning style, learning preferences, modality strengths, and cognitive style. The movement is based on the principle that individuals vary in regard to the input, processing, and output aspects of learning. Gaining an understanding of these constructs should result in better understanding of both learning and teaching.

Learning Style. Although the concept of learning style has been defined differently, most researchers agree that learning style relates to distinctive behaviors that indicate how a person learns from and adapts to the environment. It encompasses individual preferences for sensory-perceptual and environmental factors that are conducive to learning. Most authorities agree that learning style is not permanent and that it is affected by motivation and interest.

Albert Canfield defines learning style in terms of predispositions and preferences for academic, structural and achievement conditions, content, preferred learning mode and performance expectations.[16] Dunn, Dunn, and Price contend that individuals are affected by environmental, emotional, sociological, and physical preferences such as noise, light, temperature, design, motivation, persistence, responsibility, and perceptual strengths.[17] Anthony Gregorc addresses the element of structure and categorizes distinctive, observable, overt behaviors as concrete-sequential, concrete-random, abstract-sequential, and abstract-random.[18] Preferences for a particular set constitute a learning style, which appears to be both inherited and acquired, yet it can be changed. Gregorc's behavioral analysis suggests that some people operate best in either concrete or abstract situations or both, with sequentially or nonsequentially ordered events or both, in deductive or inductive processing circumstances or both, and in independent or group activity or both. He also contends that the human mind must deal with environmental and physical conditions such as room temperature, humidity, lighting, noise, age, and stage of physical and emotional development.

David Kolb suggests that learning style is a result of hereditary factors, past experience, and the demands of the present environment, which combine to produce individual orientations that give differential emphasis to four basic learning modes postulated in experiential learning theory: concrete experience, reflective observation, abstract conceptualization, and active experimentation.[19]

Authorities on learning style recommend that information obtained from diagnosis through observation, interview, and written tests be used as guides for the development of instructional strategies that match learners with learning tasks and perhaps even with teachers, and be used to design environments conducive to optimum learning. The goal of the learning style movement is to capitalize on strengths and overcome weaknesses.

Cognitive Style. Cognitive style has been defined by Joseph Hill as the unique way an individual searches for meaning.[20] It is reflected in the way qualitative and theoretical symbols are perceived and handled by the individual and involves the ascription of meaning to symbols, a process that is influenced by cultural factors.

Lynna and Floyd Ausburn refer to cognitive style as the psychological dimensions that represent consistencies in an individual's manner of acquiring, storing, processing, and using information.[21] It involves individual differences in cognition, which include perception, thought, memory, imagery, and problem solving. Different factors to be considered in cognitive style include field dependence or independence, scanning, categorizing, conceptualization, simplicity or complexity, reflectivity or impulsivity, risk taking or cautiousness, and visual or kinesthetic preferences. It appears that cognitive style is relatively stable over time and across tasks. Some researchers believe that differences in cognitive style and culture create individual learning styles and that some aspects of cognitive style are particularly resistant to training and change. For example, field independence/field dependence and visual/haptic perceptual attributes appear to be deeply ingrained.

The field independence/field dependence dimension of cognitive style involves the ability to perceive an item that is embedded or disguised within the stimulus field either analytically or globally. It entails the ability to experience items as discrete from their background. The visual/haptic perceptual attribute is concerned with preferences and abilities that allow the individual to deal with information through visual or kinesthetic senses. Preference for one or the other mode results in two presumably quite different approaches to dealing with experiences. Individuals with visual preference prefer to gain and process information through visual means, to convert nonvisual impressions to visual and to retain visual images. On the other hand, haptics, although normally sighted, prefer to rely on kinesthetic and physical means of information reception and processing. Haptics tend to refuse to integrate details and partial impressions, and to internalize nonvisual impressions and experiences kinesthetically rather than convert them to visual form. Thus mental imagery often fails.

It appears that cognitive styles are relatively independent of general ability (IQ), but that there is a relationship. In addition, cognitive styles have been found to be related to several specific types of learning abilities. For instance, when a person is confronted with a problem, stimuli are perceived and processed according to the individual's cognitive style and structure. Then, processed stimuli are used to solve the problem.

Cognitive style mapping seeks to identify strengths and weaknesses through major, minor, and negligible categories. It serves as a basis for developing personalized learning programs, using varied instructional modes to match learners and learning tasks.

Modality Strengths. A modality is any of the sensory channels through which an individual receives and retains information. Thus the three processes of sensation, perception, and memory are involved. A sensation occurs when an object or energy stimulus from the environment impinges on an individual. When we ascribe meaning to a sensation based on short- or long-term memory recall of past experiences, we step into the realm of perception. Overt or covert behavior then follows.

Modality strength is the ability of an individual to perform a relevant task more efficiently through one of the major modalities—auditory, visual, or kinesthetic. It acknowledges both the role of heredity and environment and implies superior functioning within a sensory mode. Modality strength is *not* the same as modality preference. Modality preference refers to an opinion or liking for a particular sensory mode; however, it is usually very difficult to observe one's own behavior objectively. Such judgments tend to be unreliable and inconsistent.

The concept of modality strength is based on the premise that a school-aged child usually has a dominant modality. Through maturation, modalities become integrated in cognitive strategies that transfer information from one modality to another. As a result, it is generally more difficult to identify a single dominant modality in adults. Under stressful conditions, however, an adult will usually resort to a dominant modality. Adults are usually able to process information in whatever mode is presented unless there are extenuating circumstances that prohibit it.

Most people have a secondary modality strength that enhances the dominant one. Mixed modality strengths also occur, with neither the auditory, visual, or kinesthetic sense being clearly dominant. Cognitive maturity and the opportunity to practice in all three modalities may be the principle reasons why mixes occur. For the most part, individuals with mixed modality strengths have an easier time in formal learning situations, because they are able to process in two or three modalities with equal efficiency. Identification of modality strengths of learners should assist teachers to plan learning experiences and design learning environments that help learners to reach their full potential.

Learning Preferences. A few researchers have investigated the concept of learning preferences. This refers to a person's likes and dislikes in regard to particular elements or components within the rubric of learning. The studies that have been done indicate that individuals do have definite opinions about particular modes or methods of learning, such as concrete, tangible learning of practical tasks or abstract, theoretical learning and generating hypotheses, working alone rather than with others, student-structured learning events or teacher-structured learning, the need for organization and direct experience, and preference for drill, recitation, lecture, simulation, discussion, games, and so on. The significance of such findings in relation to achievement of learning outcomes has not yet been clearly established, however.

Implications for Teaching. Research indicates that teachers also have preferences and tend to teach according to their own personal styles, cognitive styles, learning preferences, and modality strengths. The problem is that not all learners will have the same style or preference as that of the teacher, and thus learning may not be effective for all learners. If assessment data on individual learning styles, modality strengths, cognitive styles, and learning preferences are used to guide teaching actions, there should not be preconceived notions about which data will be considered "good" or "bad," but rather what is useful in a particular situation. In addition, information on styles, strengths, and preferences should not pigeonhole learners but should provide avenues to facilitate cognitive, affective, and psychomotor development. Categories should not be considered as limiting factors but as flexible criteria that promote individualized and personalized learning experiences.

Diagnosis of learning styles, modality strengths, cognitive styles, and learning preferences is not yet an exact science. Teachers should be wary of making prescriptions on the results of only one inventory or observation. Data should be used to guide actions that are responsive to the needs and idiosyncrasies of learners to promote motivation for behavioral change and successful learning.

SUMMARY

Both heredity and environment contribute to personality development. As human beings grow, develop and mature, certain patterns of behavior emerge; however, chronological age alone often misrepresents readiness and expectant behavior. Individuals are unique in that progression through so-called life stages varies from person to person. Thus norms of age and developmental levels should be used only as guidelines for considering factors of growth, development, and readiness for learning.

It is during the prenatal period that fundamental physical characteristics, reflex movements, sensory mechanisms, and potential intellectual capabilities develop. Postnatal stages of growth and development begin at birth. Infancy, or the sensorimotor stage, is characterized by rapid, yet unstable patterns of intellectual and physical growth and development. Conditioning experiences are instrumental in establishing behavioral responses.

The early childhood, or preoperational stage, from about the age of two to seven is characterized by increased vocabulary development and representational thought processes including concept formation. Affective responses to significant others and environmental circumstances are refined.

During the concrete operations, or preadolescent stage of development, physical growth and development accelerates. More complex vocabulary and sentence structure is exhibited with refinement of logical thinking skills, concept formation, and attitude and value formation. At the end of the preadolescent stage, establishing identification with a peer group and responsiveness to peer influences, along with development of social skills, is more pronounced.

Adolescence, or the formal operations stage, is characterized by more advanced logical thought processing involving cause-effect relationships and complex problem-solving procedures. It is marked by puberty and altered endocrine functioning, which influences physical, cognitive, affective, psychomotor, and social growth and development. It is a time during which there is a search for independent identity and self-actualization. The individual is gaining experience and knowledge and is interpreting the environment in light of experiences. It is a time for value- and worth-seeking accompanied by increased self-awareness. Hence adolescents tend to attempt emancipation from parental authority and establishment of peer-group attachments.

As individuals mature, the processes of physical growth and maturation decline, but psychological development continues. Early-to-middle adulthood is usually a period of peak physical and mental functioning. Adults seek to establish security, commitment, and productivity while maintaining personal relationships under changing conditions. Physiological and societal changes and pressures during middle age potentiate adjustment problems and inadequate coping behaviors partly because of preestablished rigidity of mind-set formulated through past experiences. For behavioral change to occur, change must be viewed as relevant to personal needs and goals.

Once the individual is past the period of prime functioning, physiological aging processes accelerate. Behavioral changes involve interaction and integration of perception, set, attention, motivation, physiological status, and societal expectations. An individual's unique experiential background can be an asset to learning. On the other hand, abstractness, irrelevant information, and poor organization can inhibit learning.

Throughout all developmental stages, norms must be applied with caution, keeping in mind that as unique human beings, we progress through life at different rates. Developmental norms can, however, establish base-line information to help guide our actions as teachers with respect to a particular age group. Aspects of growth, development, and readiness should be taken into consideration when diagnosing learning needs, establishing learning outcomes, determining teaching actions, and evaluating behavioral changes.

Physical, psychological, and environmental forces interact to affect behavior. Physical or biological disabilities, disease, emotional states, and sociocultural conditions are predisposing forces that may potentiate learning problems and influence readiness for learning. A teacher needs to be cognizant of the role that such factors as defective sensory, neurological, or hormonal functioning; differences in physical appearance and perceived body image; variations in sociocultural background; and emotional stress and anxiety play in learning. A perceptive teacher realizes that diagnosing the individual characteristics of the learner is a prerequisite to any teaching-learning experience.

Individual differences in regard to learning styles, strengths, and preferences are forces that influence learning. Although these constructs are relatively new and lack consistent definition, numerous studies have emerged that verify the value of assessing styles, strengths, and preferences of learners to identify particular attributes that indicate how a person receives, processes, and uses information. The value of diagnosis in these areas lies in the application of assessment data to the practice of teaching, which includes the design, implementation, and evaluation of learning experiences for individuals and groups. The goal is to promote efficient, effective behavioral change.

PRINCIPLES OF LEARNING

Learning theory is often criticized by teachers for being impractical or too difficult to apply to everyday teaching and learning situations. Granted, transition from theory to practice is difficult. A little critical thinking and reflective thought, however, reveals that the study of human learning theory, types of learning, and forces that influence learning can provide guidelines for practice and help teachers establish the conditions necessary for promoting achievement of learning outcomes.

Over the years, theoretical hypotheses about learning and the study of specific forces and conditions that influence learning have resulted in the development of a number of basic principles of learning that have universal applicability. In addition, learning principles have been generated for particular age groups. A teacher who bases decisions on these principles is using the best of all available research to guide professional teaching behavior and has a better chance of interacting effectively with learners than one who is unfamiliar or unwilling to apply theory. The following principles of learning have been supported by empirical evidence and have broad applicability to all types of learners, yet modification based on individual differences and particular circumstances may be warranted.

Basic Principles of Learning

1. If a response is satisfying to self, it will tend to be repeated under similar circumstances.
2. Immediate, positive, tangible, or intangible reinforcement is a major condition for successful behavioral change. Reward is more effective than punishment for changing behavior; however, there should be a slow shift away from extrinsic to intrinsic reward.
3. Negative reinforcement slows down the rate at which a behavior occurs but does not eliminate it.
4. A response is strengthened with multiple and consistent reinforcement. The shorter the time interval between the response and the reinforcement, the more effective is the reinforcement in building a strong response; however, overuse of repetition or reinforcement can lead to loss of interest and will not by itself establish an association or connection.
5. Overlearning (continued, short periods of practice following "mastery") increases memory and improves later performance.
6. The establishment of verbal and nonverbal associations is a critical prerequisite to behavior change.
7. Forgetting occurs because of the interference of new associations with previously acquired ones.
8. Cognitive-perceptual readiness and internal motivation are mandatory conditions for behavioral change. Learning depends on the learner's state of readiness or predisposition toward learning.
9. The ordering of information influences the ease with which learning takes place.
10. Stimulus-response associations and discrimination abilities are prerequisites to chained behaviors; however, a connection or association cannot be established by mere repetition of a response.
11. Active sensory, cognitive, and emotional participation and direct physical involvement in learning are predisposing factors to concept formation.
12. Multiple discrimination and generalization responses facilitate concept formation. The cognitive constructs of perceptual imagery and recognition of features, such as form, spatial arrangement, texture, and so on are prerequisites to concept formation.
13. Perception, concept acquisition, and recall are prerequisites to principle learning.
14. Perception, association, discrimination, concept formation, generalization, recall, and selection responses are prerequisites to problem-solving behaviors.
15. Some cognitive, affective, and psychomotor behaviors can be acquired, strengthened, or weakened by observing and imitating the actions of others.
16. Cognitive knowledge, comprehension, application, analysis, and synthesis responses precede evaluation responses.

17. Affective receiving, responding, valuing, and organization responses are prerequisites to developing general patterns of personal, social, and emotional adjustment.
18. Psychomotor behaviors include affect and cognition. Perceptual awareness, reception, memory, recall, discrimination, association, generalization, chaining, and decision-making responses are prerequisites to acquiring a psychomotor skill.
19. Active, overt, short periods of practice and periods of rest, positive reinforcement, and corrective feedback are crucial conditions for behavioral change. Feedback about performance, which includes why and how, improves learning. If feedback is given too early or too late, it will have little value.
20. Learning can be increased by matching learning activities with the learner's level of development, cognition, abilities, styles, strengths, modalities, and preferences.

Adult and Child Learning Principles

Adults have lived in the world for a number of years; consequently, they have had the opportunity to acquire many perceptions, insights, and relationships from their environment. Past experiences have shaped behavior. Thus, adults are likely to be more rigid than children in thought and action. Throughout life, social behaviors and emotional frameworks consisting of values, attitudes, and tendencies have been established that are consistent with needs and goals. Acquired fears, anxieties, and predispositions toward learning in general will influence attainment of learning outcomes. Predispositions will affect what is learned and how it is learned. In general, adults have decisions to make and problems to solve. They have a great many preoccupations outside the particular learning situation, including job and family concerns. Mental and physical fatigue may decrease motivation, cognition, affect, and skill. Because of the wide range of previous knowledge, skills, motivation, interests, and competencies that adults bring to a learning situation, learning events should be planned on a personal and individual basis.

According to research, adults appear to learn best through experiences in which they apply what is being learned and in formal situations where social interaction takes place. Open and nonthreatening group interaction has been found effective for changing perceptions and affective behaviors through reexamination and rethinking with input from others. Active experiential, sensory learning and accommodation of learning and cognitive styles, modality strengths, and learning preferences maximize transfer and application of learning. Activity learning, with actual hands-on experience, may be of particular importance for adults who possess low scholastic skills. Abstract, word-oriented talk sessions are usually not sufficient for behavior change. Adults tend to dislike jargon they can't comprehend and prefer plain, simple language, at least at first, to understand complex concepts. Individual problem solving and personal investigation are effective means for achieving significant behavior change.

Adults will make a commitment to learning when the goals and objectives are perceived as immediately useful, realistic, important, and relevant to personal, professional, and career needs. They usually want to be originators of their own learning. In other words, adults want to be involved in establishing goals and objectives, content, and activities and participate in evaluation processes. Adults tend to resist learning situations in which they believe there is an attack on competence. Fear of external judgment and failure produces anxiety. Adults need to see the results of their efforts and receive accurate, positive reinforcement and feedback about progress toward goals.

Adult learning is enhanced by individualized and personalized learning events that demonstrate respect, trust, and concern for the individual. It should be remembered that older adults usually require a longer time to achieve learning outcomes. Intelligence and ability to learn remains the same as one grows older, but reaction time decreases. Older adults have greater difficulty in remembering isolated facts; therefore they need to develop mechanisms for remembering. Pictorial cues and highly organized information appear to promote learning, while abstractions, irrelevant information, and poor organization inhibit learning. Most adults prefer a problem-solving approach that utilizes high-level cognitive, affective, and psychomotor behaviors. Change in adults is not an easy process, but behaviors can be modified. If learning outcomes are not accepted or perceived as valid and necessary, however, content will have little meaning, and it is doubtful that behavioral change will occur.

Infants, young children, and youths do not have the physical maturity nor have they had the variety of experiences that adults have had. Consequently, the principles of learning will vary to some extent. Infants and very young children acquire most cognitive, affective, and psychomotor behaviors through simple conditioning, discovery, trial and error, practice, imitation, and association processes. Concepts are learned through direct, real experience with varied examples and nonexamples under simple verbal guidance. According to Jerome Bruner, the growing child first relies strongly on learned action patterns primarily acquired through the manipulation of objects.[22] This is the enactive level. In time, experiences are converted to mental images (ikonic level) and then into symbol systems (language). As children mature and are able to use symbol systems more effectively, they are able to use indirect information and to cumulate information into a cognitive structure that can be acted upon. Thus they go beyond the immediate perceptual environment. Once language becomes a medium for the translation of experience, there is progressive release from immediacy. Internalization of language depends upon interaction with others. Children must acquire ways of representing the recurrent regularities in their environment and they must transcend the present by developing ways of linking past to present to future. It should, however, be remembered that lack of language does not negate the ability to learn.

Many prominent authorities in child development believe that basic changes in level of intellectual functioning are produced by internal equilibriation rather than external reinforcement. Some research indicates that children can acquire and transfer rather advanced, complex problem-solving behaviors through concentrated training over an extended period of time. Ability to solve abstract problems at an early age appears to involve learning to process information by devoting more attention to meaning and classification of an idea suggested by a symbol rather than to the symbol itself. Linking information to personal experience appears to be an important variable in acquiring problem-solving behavior.

Response satisfaction through positive, immediate reinforcement and physical, perceptual, and developmental readiness are essential predisposing factors to behavior change. Young children need to be actively involved (physically, mentally, and socially) in learning. Direct sensory experience within a secure, safe, and caring environment is a critical condition for learning, especially during early childhood. In fact, restricted experience or lack of environmental stimulation may be a more potent factor than lack of language for intellectual development. Although the findings are tentative, it appears that dendritic branches of neurons in the cortex sometimes increase in density in response to stimulating environments. Environmental stimulation and practice at the right time has been found to foster learning in the presence of brain damage or dysfunction.

Like that of adults, the behavior of children of all ages varies with what significant others within the environment permit, encourage, demand, reward, and punish. Yet too much pressure or use of methods that are too offensive for the child's ability will inhibit learning. Individual differences in cognitive style, learning style, modality strengths, and learning preferences can be used to determine the kinds of approaches that can be used to effectively promote behavioral change in children and youth.

SUMMARY

Human learning is a multidimensional phenomenon. It is also a very personal phenomenon. Each person possesses a different package of biophysical attributes, experiences, values, needs, goals, persuasions, ideas, and capabilities, which causes one individual to behave and respond differently from another, even in the same situation. There are basic principles of learning which cut across age and developmental levels. Thus, they can be applied to individuals of all ages. In addition, principles of learning have been established for different age groups based on expected norms during particular phases of life. Nurse-teachers should consider these principles of learning before carrying out teaching actions.

THE TEACHER

A teacher is a potent environmental and social force within the learner's psychological field. It is the teacher's responsibility to structure optimum conditions for learning that involve the learner holistically in learning to promote behavioral change. In order to carry out this responsibility, the informed teacher considers learning theory, forces that influence learning, types and principles of learning in light of each learner's developmental level and existing repertoire of understanding, skills, values, attitudes, abilities, disabilities, preferences, and goals. The teacher who realizes that learning is a personal, observable process influenced by internal factors of growth and developmental readiness, cognition, past experiences, and preferences, as well as external environmental and cultural conditions, realizes that his or her own personal attributes and knowledge will directly affect what is taught as well as how it is taught. Personal values, attitudes, feelings, and understanding about the nature of human beings and the teaching-learning process will be exhibited as observable teaching behaviors.

The Teacher as Change Agent

The professional teacher assumes the role of a change agent. Efforts are directed toward planned change that attempts to modify the cognitive, affective, and psychomotor behaviors of individuals and groups through introduction of knowledge, ideas, and innovations. Therefore, teaching is a dynamic process. The teacher as an agent of change uses a purposeful, systematic decisioning process to cause improvement in a personality. When teaching is viewed as a process of planned change, it becomes more than a skilled intervention. The process involves diagnosis of learner needs and attributes; identification and thorough analysis of subject matter, tasks, conditions, and resources; establishment of goals and learning outcomes; development, validation, and implementation of learning events; and evaluation of teaching and learning processes and products. Through a problem-solving, data-based approach to teaching, the teacher becomes accountable to learners, self, colleagues, and the public, accepting the responsibility for the outcomes of teaching and changing teaching practices based on objective criteria.

The ultimate goal of teaching is the transfer of learning from a learning experience to a similar situation and ultimately to application in real life. The extent of transfer will depend on the teacher's ability to guide the learner to perceive similarities between learning events and their applications. Thus, the teacher focuses on applications, relationships, and methods to stimulate behavioral outcomes that are useful and lasting. Stating meaningful, observable, and measurable behavioral outcomes based on individual needs and types and principles of learning is therefore a major competency of the professional teacher. Learning experiences are determined based on stated outcomes that are compatible with the learner's needs, preferences, strengths, and weaknesses.

It is the teacher's professional responsibility to clearly communicate expectations to promote transfer of learning, but this does not imply that the entire responsibility for establishing objectives lies with the teacher. The teacher must facilitate genuine decision making and responsibility for learning by generating alternatives along with information about consequences, allowing the learner to establish and pursue personal goals and objectives. In this way, the learner's personal involvement, commitment, relevancy, and self-satisfaction are promoted. Even very young children can be given a degree of responsibility for determining personal objectives. For example, a two- or three-year old child may not be able to make a wise decision about whether to drink orange juice or soda pop, but if given a choice between drinking orange juice or tomato juice, it's a different matter. When the child is allowed to participate in decision making and set goals and objectives, learning is personalized and self-satisfying.

The evidence that teachers need to do more to involve learners in establishing learning outcomes is nowhere more evident than at the college or university level. Here we find many students immobilized when asked to set personal learning objectives or course goals. Few college students, even at the graduate level, believe that they have any responsibility to approach a subject area in terms of what they would like to be able to do, know, think about, or explore. It is as if somewhere along the way they have become disassociated from active learning. For them, learning exists *in* their instructors, books, and other instructional materials from which they passively absorb knowledge and then regurgitate it on an examination. Where should the blame be placed?

The Teacher as Communications Agent

Teaching is an interactive communication process; its elements are communicator (teacher and learner), message (elements, structure, content, treatment, code expressed as cognitive, affective, psychomotor behaviors) and receiver (learner and teacher). The teacher structures the circumstances of a learning experience to call forth the desired verbal, nonverbal, auditory, visual, tactile, or kinesthetic responses. The learner selects among stimuli and interprets and transforms information into observable behaviors. The dynamic, interactive flow of verbal and nonverbal messages between the teacher and learner should increase motivation and improve performance. Without feedback, it is impossible to know what message has been received (Fig. 1–1).

The teacher, influenced by internalized beliefs about the nature of human beings and their capabilities, past sociocultural experiences, attitudes, preferences, knowl-

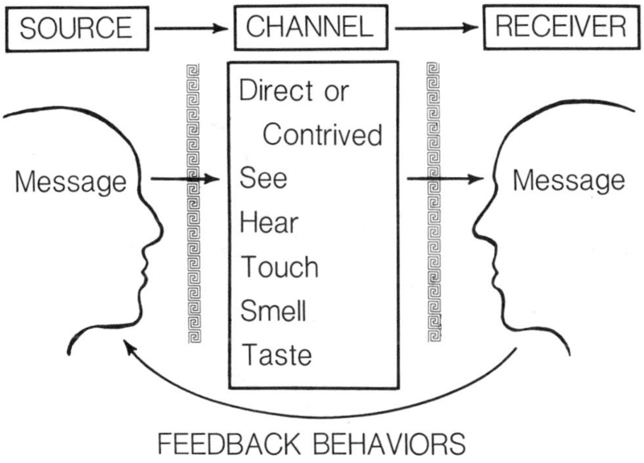

Figure 1–1. Communication process.

edge level, and cognitive style, assesses learning needs and determines constructs, codes, and treatments that compose the message designed to elicit behavioral change in the learner. The message reaches the learner through one or more sensory channels. Sensory messaging strategies used by the teacher may be natural (direct) or contrived (indirect). Natural strategies consist of the verbal and nonverbal messages directly conveyed by the teacher, whereas contrived strategies convey stimuli indirectly. Examples of contrived strategies are books, pictures, video, and computer programs, all of which embody the necessary conditions for learning. More than one sensory messaging channel may be used at one time, and both natural and contrived strategies can be combined to create a total learning experience. The patterning of direct and indirect strategies positively or negatively influences attainment of learning outcomes.

Both the internal and external states of the individual learner play a significant role in what message is received, as well as how it is received and transformed. Internal factors relating to perception, arousal, roles, norms, and attitudes; and external forces such as reinforcement, feedback, practice, temperature, noise, organization of information, priming, and prompting can facilitate or interfere with successful transmission, reception, and transformation of messages. Messages are transformed by the learner through internal processing mechanisms. Transformation of information is the consequence of the dynamic two-way communication process. Consequently, exhibited learner behavior becomes a messaging phenomenon in that these behaviors provide feedback that is used by the teacher to modify successive messages appropriate for the learner. In a dynamic two-way communication situation, the teacher and learner or learner and contrived strategy shift back and forth between source and receiver roles. For example, during direct face-to-face interaction, verbal and nonverbal messages are sent and received by *both* teacher and learner. When messages are conveyed through contrived strategies, mechanisms must be incorporated that provide for two-way interaction and active feedback. If properly designed, programmed instruction and computer-assisted instruction with built-in questions, reinforcement, and feedback exemplify this principle.

The professional teacher creates a supportive, personalized, self-motivated, responsible learning atmosphere through application of a dynamic two-way process of communication and change. The teacher then assumes a facilitator-helper posture. The learner-oriented teacher recognizes and respects the individual's potential and arranges optimum conditions for learning based on individual need. The teacher must have developed not only competencies that enable effective communication of knowledge, but also the ability to communicate verbally and nonverbally, sincere respect for the individual and a willingness to be of assistance.

As an agent of communications and change, the teacher recognizes that human nature makes resistance a normal reaction. This is particularly true of adult learners, but even young children are resistant to change. Resistance is behavior intended to protect one's self from a real or imagined threat to security. Behavior is often defensive in nature, ranging from hostility and aggression to apathy and withdrawal. Individuals tend to resist change when the nature of the change and its effects are not clearly communicated, when individuals are not prepared for the change, when it is not obvious why change is needed, and when the change is imposed without advance consultation. In addition, if information is distorted and change ignores established norms or customs, or if excessive pressure is involved, resistance to change is likely. If insufficient consideration is given to problems that are likely to arise, if there is fear of failure, or if change is seen as inadequate or ineptly managed, there will be resistance.

It is possible for the teacher to overcome resistance to change by establishing an open, interactive learning atmosphere where individuals develop their own understanding of the need for change and are directly and actively involved in making decisions regarding the nature of change and how to accomplish it. The teacher is instrumental in creating a trusting climate conducive to open communication, with interactive feedback to help learners gather facts related to personal learning problems and needs and to bring feelings of resistance to change out in the open.

Good verbal and nonverbal two-way communication is essential to the change process. As change agents, teachers communicate directly or indirectly, both verbally and nonverbally. Verbal and nonverbal feedback is essential to effective two-way communication. Without extensive two-way feedback, the teacher will not know what effect the message has had on the learner's behavior, nor will the teacher know how to achieve better communication the next time.

Half the process of direct communication involves active listening on the part of both the teacher and the learner. Active listening denotes the ability to understand, comprehend, and retain the message that has been sent, and it requires the development of nonverbal attending skills and verbal responding skills, which involve paying attention and responding. The nonverbal cues that indicate that the listener is attending are primarily physical and include facing the other person, leaning toward the person, maintaining good eye contact, being relaxed, and reflecting attention through facial expressions. Approximately 90 percent of a communicated message is composed of nonverbal cues that contribute to interpretation of the message. Nonverbal feedback cues include voice inflection, tone, and pitch, gesturing, facial expression, touching, and even the clothes, objects, and so on that compose the environment. Verbal evaluative, interpretive, supportive, and probing responses provide information about how a message is being interpreted. Body language and spoken language are dependent upon each other. Spoken language alone will not convey the full meaning of what a person is saying. Congruity between verbal and nonverbal messages helps the teacher to create clear, meaningful communication that facilitiates behavioral change.

Written or oral questioning is one of the most valuable communication-and-change skills of the teacher. Questioning strategies can play a vital role in facilitating learning outcomes; however they need to be carefully planned and used. Bloom's taxonomy of the cognitive domain can serve as a guide for planning questioning strategies. Questions at the knowledge level emphasize recall of facts. Words such as *what, who, when, which,* and *how* exemplify low-level questions designed to elicit a specific response. Such low-level questions should be used sparingly. Questions at the comprehensive level reflect translation, interpretation, and extrapolation. Translation focuses on the learner's ability to translate or paraphrase a message.

The emphasis is on employing knowledge to understand particular information. At the interpretation level, the learner is directed to derive the essential meaning of a message. Extrapolation questions ask the learner to translate, infer, and expand information. At the analysis level, questioning strategies stress relationships between elements, profuse interrelationships, and compositions. Questions at the synthesis level should facilitate convergent and divergent thinking. The learner is encouraged to reorganize information from multiple sources and formulate a "new" whole. At the evaluation level, questions require the learner to use internal and external criteria to make judgments and evaluate the extent to which particulars are accurate, effective, economical, or satisfying.

Researchers have found that placing emphasis on higher cognitive questions rather than recall-oriented recitation or "fact" questioning generally produces better learning. Despite this evidence, most teachers do not emphasize higher cognitive questioning and they do not focus on improving responses that are given, such as pursuing clarity, plausibility, and accuracy through redirection, probing, and providing explanations that clarify and correct the response. Teachers should both acknowledge the learner's response and build on it to improve learning by applying prompting and priming questions to stimulate independent thinking.[23]

Consideration of the complex art of questioning is particularly relevant to the discussion strategy of teaching and learning. Because discussion involves exchange among students as well as between teacher and students, questions should solicit student opinions and thoughts, not just "right" answers. Players in a discussion are disposed to examine and to be responsive to different points of view with the intention of developing their knowledge, understanding, and judgment on the topic under review. Reasonableness, peaceableness, orderliness, truthfulness, freedom, equality, and respect are presuppositions for effective discussion and the teacher as the discussion leader must subscribe to these conditions. Otherwise, discussion is merely recitation. In this sense, techniques of questioning are secondary to establishing a climate conducive to open discussion, yet appropriate high-level questions that encourage learners to ask questions and voice opinions should be asked. It is important to wait two to three seconds after asking a question to encourage participation and to insert periods of deliberate silence to allow learners to think and respond. Central questions to be brought out in the discussion should be planned and written out prior to the discussion. As Dillon notes, "To conceive an educative question requires thought; to formulate it requires labor; and to pose it, tact."[24] Dillon goes on to say that "a single well-formulated question is sufficient for an hour's discussion."

When teachers communicate messages visually through graphic or pictorial images, retention, recall, and transfer of learning should be enhanced. Inappropriate use of visuals or gimmicks may actually inhibit learning, however. In fact, research indicates that in general, people remember 10 percent of what they hear, but when appropriate visuals are added to verbalization, retention increases to approximately 50 percent.[25] At least 70 percent of the sensory perception reaching the brain comes via the visual sense.

Visualization is a mental act. It is an integral part of thought. We imagine, dream, explore, organize thoughts, make value judgements, and solve problems by visualizing. It is important to remember that visualization skills vary according to individual aptitude and habit. They are therefore an element of one's cognitive style and directly influence learning and teaching style. When considering whether to visualize a message and what type of visual to use, the teacher needs to assess learner characteristics, the type of message to be conveyed, the conditions for learning, and the expected behavioral outcome. Francis Dwyer, a leader in the field of visual communications, has generated a number of guidelines that can be used by teachers when developing and using visuals to communicate.[26] He contends that specific individual differences such as age, IQ, prior experience, cultural background, and reading comprehension appear to determine the effectiveness of different types of visualization. For example, individuals exposed to new messages would most likely profit from line drawings, whereas learners more familiar with content would profit from more realistic visual images. Too much realistic detail, however, may lead to negative motivation or even impede understanding and achievement of outcomes. On the other hand, oversimplification or editing of realistic detail may reduce or eliminate important elements that are prerequisite to learning. If complex visuals are used, the learner needs adequate time to make perceptual discriminations.

Varied methods of visual cuing can be used to increase interest and enthusiasm for learning; however, too many or too few cues can adversely affect learning. For instance, constant repetition of a single type of cue may cause learners to lose interest. It has been found that the judicious use of color as a cuing mechanism is a useful instructional variable for prompting achievement.

When messages are conveyed through the visual modality, visual testing rather than verbal testing provides a more reliable and valid assessment of learner achievement. In general, no single type of visual can be identified as being most effective for promoting learning, but pictures may lead to better learning than visually presented words in some cases.

The Professional Nurse-Teacher

The role of the professional nurse as teacher is unique because of the diverse nature of the nursing profession and the learner population. Teaching is usually only one of the functional responsibilities of the community or occupational health nurse, school nurse, nurse clinician, or nurse practitioner. Even when the nurse is employed as an educator of undergraduate or graduate nursing students or a nursing staff, obligations may include primary care nursing. The kinds of learners that nurses teach vary in age, developmental level, and health status. The teaching function of the professional nurse usually involves groups as well as individuals. It is therefore essential that the nurse-teacher be able to apply knowledge of the individual learner to groups of learners. The nurse-teacher must be alert to common group needs, yet sensitive to individual needs. Depending on the employment setting, learners may be nursing students, well or ill clients, practicing nurses and nursing assistants, teachers and other public or private school personnel, or the general public. In any case, the unique nature of the learner, including physical and emotional state, age, social and cultural background, experience, developmental level, and so on, is of primary concern. Predisposing problems, worries, and environmental conditions influence the teaching strategies used by the nurse. For example, the chronically ill client may not be able to concentrate on learning because of physical or emotional problems or worries. If the teaching-learning setting is the home, the nature of the environment itself, such as daily routine, lack of space or equipment, or uncooperative family members may impose barriers to learning. Learning will be difficult, if not impossible, when there are serious blocks in communication between nurse and learner owing to age, culture, or emotional or physical factors.

The nurse as communications-change agent considers learning theory, forces that affect learning, and learning principles to determine the appropriate conditions for learning that guide the development of learning experiences. By actively involving the learner in the process, the nurse-teacher assists the learner to attain relevant learning outcomes. The professional nurse-teacher realizes that the more the learner is actively involved in learning, the more will be achieved and that learning is largely affected by the appropriateness of the processes and strategies employed and the degree to which the learner is prepared to learn a new task.

The nurse-teacher employs teaching strategies based on the characteristics of the learner, attributes of strategies, conditions for learning, and the expected outcomes. Through active involvement in the process, learners develop new knowledge, skills, and insights that help them to develop their human potential and maintain well-being. By directly or indirectly eliciting cognitive, affective, and psychomotor responses through natural and contrived strategies, a nurse can be a potent social force for influencing change that is beneficial to self and society.

The nurse-teacher recognizes that the total learning environment, which includes teacher behaviors and teaching style, will affect achievement of expected outcomes. Therefore, the nurse-teacher-learner relationship is a critical variable. The attitude and behavior of the nurse-teacher serve as a role model for the learner. The nurse-teacher creates an atmosphere of empathy, respect, warmth, and genuineness to minimize threat and promote the positive change that is characteristic of self-actualization.

The nurse-teacher diagnoses learning problems and needs; analyzes content and tasks; assesses learner characteristics; establishes goals and learning outcomes; identifies, selects, and designs teaching strategies, activities, and materials; structures helping relationships; creates environments conducive to learning; and validates, implements, and evaluates learning outcomes, teaching-learning processes, and products. Thus, the nurse assumes professional teaching status consistent with a philosophy of teaching and learning dedicated to data-based decision making and accountability for the outcomes of teaching and learning.

SUMMARY

Competencies of the teaching professional include structuring supportive conditions for learning to maximize transfer of learning, establishing measurable learning outcomes, effectively communicating expectations and consequences, providing active involvement in learning, and facilitating two-way communication with dynamic, interactive feedback mechanisms. Such actions facilitate reception and transformation of intended messages that are exhibited as observable behaviors.

As a change agent, the teacher recognizes that change takes time, is achieved in stages and that resistance to change is inevitable, but that such resistance can be overcome by establishing an open climate of verbal and nonverbal two-way communication and personal involvement. Communicating for change involves applying active nonverbal attending skills and verbal responding skills, using well-planned written and oral questioning techniques and visualizing messages graphically or pictorially to prompt retention, recall, and transfer.

The nurse-teacher accepts professional responsibility and leadership as a communications-change agent within practice and academic settings, all of which are composed of diverse individuals and learner groups. Therefore, the nurse-teacher develops a philosophy of learning and teaching, assesses, plans, sets objectives, intervenes, and evaluates to bring about effective, successful learning.

The nurse-teacher serves as learner advocate and accepts full professional resonsibility and accountability for the consequences of teaching, including openness and willingness to evaluate self and change teaching behaviors to accommodate the predispositions and idiosyncrasies of the learner, while at the same time possessing a high degree of professionalism, skill, and knowledge.

SELECTED RESEARCH ON TEACHING

Research on teaching deals with a subset of the conditions under which learning occurs in an individual owing to the efforts of a teacher. The current trend is to isolate and analyze well-defined components of teaching that can be taught, practiced, evaluated, predicted, controlled, and understood. In this regard, teaching effectiveness has recently been viewed as mastery of a repertoire of competencies and the ability to use these competencies in professional decision making. Barak Rosenshine's review of fifty process-product studies presents evidence that at least some aspects of teacher behavior (teaching style or dimensions of classroom climate) are related to student achievement.[27] The patterns of behavior identified as distinguishing effective teachers include clarity of presentation, variability of learning activities, directness and enthusiasm, task-oriented or businesslike teacher behavior, use of positive, constructive criticism in the learning situation, the teacher's acknowledgment and encouragement of ideas, student opportunity to use a variety of types of prompting mechanisms, content presented, and the use of structured comments at the start of and during a learning experience.

Methodology of research on teaching effectiveness appears to involve three variables: measures of teaching effectiveness based on student learning, measures of teacher behavior derived from systematic observation of classroom interaction, and information about the teacher's intentions or purpose. There is some indication that a formal, direct teaching model with its behavior-analytic, detail-specific, teacher-directed, large-group and narrow-questioning approach is more effective for obtaining gains in basic skills. On the other hand, the more open model of teaching that focuses attention on inquiry, choice, individualized work, and exploration and discovery appears to be more suitable for achieving intuitive and creative learning outcomes, independence, curiosity, and favorable attitudes toward learning. In addition, research indicates that some individuals do better in a more open, flexible learning environment while others do better in a more direct and structured environment because of differences in learning style, cognitive style, modality strengths, and learning preferences.[28]

Research to date suggests that variables such as a strong focus on learning with encouragement and concern for individual success, systematic selection of learning strategies and events that include provision for small and large group interaction, questioning, and controlled practice in teacher-led groups are usually associated with amount of content, amount of time actually engaged in learning, and attainment of learning outcomes.

Avoidance of negative affect appears to be important for learning, as is teacher direction, establishment of objectives, and selection of activities, but with some degree of individual involvement and choice. The amount of learner freedom that is most functional for both learning tasks and thinking depends on the complexity of the learning task and the characteristics of the learner. More complex tasks may warrant a somewhat greater degree of freedom.

In general, research indicates that learners who are actively involved in learning for the greatest amount of time will achieve more than those who are less involved. In addition, differences in degree of involvement are highly related to learner characteristics, such as motivation to change. All studies reviewed appear to share one underlying principle—if teaching processes and procedures elicit learner behavior, learner involvement is likely to increase. In contrast, if the conditions of teaching shift learner attention from the main foci of the learning task or if instruction is misleading or disturbing, then active learning time is likely to decrease. Thus, instructional conditions, including explanations and directions for learning, have the potential to alter learner involvement and hence achievement of learning outcomes. Participative learning is largely affected by two sets of conditions: the appropriateness of teaching methods and procedures and the degree to which learners are prepared for acquiring the learning outcome—attainment of prerequisite knowledge, skills, and interest.

Much evidence supports the powerful contribution of feedback and corrective procedures to learning effectiveness and student performance.[29] Thorndike suggested that knowledge of results improved performance only when the learner was motivated, when knowledge of results was informative, and when the learner was helped to correct mistakes. Bruner in *Toward a Theory of Instruction* emphasizes that learning depends upon giving knowledge of results at a time when it can be used for correction.[30] Feedback and correction involve (1) the establishment of a realistic standard of performance; (2) the gathering of relevant and valid evidence to provide information about achievement of the standard; and (3) the use of corrective learning opportunities to facilitate attainment of the preset standard. Establishing performance standards alone will not improve learning and teaching unless feedback and corrective procedures are also involved. Providing specific and informative feedback is necessary, but it has little effect on learning unless learners are given opportunities to correct difficulties and reach preset standards. Research indicates that feedback and corrective procedures related to an "appropriate" standard (learning outcome) help most learners, regardless of intelligence or aptitude, to learn. As learners realize that they are capable of mastering the standard, they develop greater self-confidence in their ability to learn and greater interest in the subject matter. The literature indicates that if learners are deprived of standards, feedback, and correction, most will accumulate errors and achieve much less than might be expected. If only one of the three components is used by teachers, learning can improve only to a small degree for a few. Each of the components must be clearly involved and related to each other.[31]

Performance standards set the criterion for judging learning and teaching. James Block found that higher standards resulted in higher cognitive outcomes.[32] Those with higher standards performed better on knowledge of learning materials, application to new situations, and retention of knowledge. But if standards were too high, learner attitudes and interest decreased. Most researchers do not regard 100 percent mastery of subject matter as a necessary or appropriate standard of achievement.

Research indicates that learners who are given information about instructional objectives prior to learning will remember information better than those who are not told. Specific behavioral objectives have the greatest effect on learning. Melton emphasizes that if objectives are too general or ambiguous, or are extremely difficult, knowing the objectives will have little effect on learning.[33] If learners are not interested in the objectives or if they are already highly motivated to learn, advance knowledge of objectives will do little to enhance learning. Objectives are also more effective when they emphasize the same things emphasized in the teaching strategy. Objectives guide teachers in thinking about and planning learning experiences and help to select and develop methods and materials that are likely to produce intended learning. When conveyed prior to instruction, objectives function as orienting stimuli and cues to learning. They focus students' attention on relevant information and processes and help determine study habits, organization, and information processing. When learners are told specifically what is to be expected of them through objectives, they are likely to make the expectations their standards of learning.[34]

Timing is a crucial variable for the effective use of feedback. Feedback should be provided when learning and teaching improvement is still possible. When feedback is given at the end of a semester or "grading" period, it has little value. Errors have accumulated, learners usually become less motivated, and it is more difficult to unlearn acquired associations over time. In addition, the teacher cannot now use obtained feedback to alter teaching procedures and materials.[35]

Much research has focused on the relationship between instructional cues—the stimuli that convey the content to be learned and directions for what to do and how to do it—and attainment of learning outcomes. Questions, visuals, objectives, and practice experiences are instructional cues or messages that can be used by teachers to improve learning. Each type of cue has its own function and specific purpose at various stages in the learning process. For example, inserting questions in instructional materials can enhance learning through selective attention and active concentrated learning time.[36] Research demonstrates that recall of information from learning materials is greatly enhanced if appropriate visuals accompany verbal material. Several recent studies reveal that a variety of instructional materials, particularly visual and manipulative, can contribute to learning. Demonstrations, illustrations, and other visual communications are effective instructional cues; however, they must be informative, clear, and simple, and must activate desired behaviors.[37]

A study by Levin demonstrated that practice on a limited, narrow set of homogeneous problems developed a learner's ability to apply knowledge only in a narrow range of problems, whereas practice with a set of varied heterogeneous problems developed a learner's ability to apply rules to a broad range of new situations.[38]

A recent study conducted by David Jonassen indicates strong predictive relationships between personality variables (specifically, Jungian type indicators), cognitive styles, individual learning styles, and teaching styles of preservice teachers.[39] Preferences for learning, which are usually experientially and culturally influenced, appear to determine how teachers choose to teach. For example, those who prefer to assign readings tend to prefer to read themselves. Those who prefer to visualize teachings do not learn well from listening only. Visualizers avoid categorical, rule-oriented modes of thought, opting for a more holistic approach to instruction. Such findings are consistent with brain hemisphericity studies. Teachers who prefer direct experiences, such as laboratory or simulation events, are more tactile and prefer direct, participative involvement in learning.

SUMMARY

Researchers have begun to focus on the alterable characteristics of learners and teachers and their interrelationships. Greater interest is being given to causal relationships between student achievement and interest in learning, use of teaching time, and essential conditions for learning, such as establishing mental set, facilitating cognitive closure, involving learners in planning in addition to learning, providing for repetition and distributed practice, and controlling the amount of information and rate of presentation. Careful selection and sensitive use of alternative teaching strategies, resources, and materials can reduce individual differences in achievement of learning outcomes. Varying stimuli, appropriate sequencing, and organization of information, timing of transition from one activity to another, rational performance standards, and use of corrective feedback and positive reinforcement can be effective means for matching or adapting learning opportunities to individual learners, either in group or independent learning situations.[40] Successful, effective teaching appears to depend also on the teacher's willingness to change and correct procedures through formal and informal self-evaluation, positive and sensitive acceptance of learner's responses and capabilities for learning, and confidence in professional teaching ability.

POSTTEST

TRUE OR FALSE

1. A professional nurse-teacher exhibits empathy, respect, and genuine concern for learners as unique human beings by establishing a learning environment conducive to self-actualization and well-being through application of a two-way interactive communications-change process, actively involving the learner in assessment, planning, intervention, and evaluation processes. *True False*
2. When teaching a psychomotor skill, such as self-administration of medication to an adult or child, the nurse-teacher utilizes trial-and-error learning with repeated practice and positive reinforcement. *True False*
3. Intermittent verbal or nonverbal feedback with corrective measures based on diagnosis of learning and cognitive style is the most effective means of changing behaviors. *True False*
4. Retention and transfer of learning that is dependent upon lifelike learning experiences and active involvement in learning is the ultimate goal of professional teaching. *True False*
5. Because of the incongruity and confusion among established and emerging theories of learning, the professional nurse-teacher must assume the responsibility for evaluating the constructs and principles of each and adopt one as a basic philosophy that will serve as a framework for teaching actions and behaviors. *True False*
6. A nurse-teacher who teaches the concept of burns would use abstract written or oral verbal associations and multiple discriminations rather than other sensory communication modalities. *True False*
7. Simple learned responses attributed to classical or operant conditioning and associationism most often occur on the spur of the moment or through incidental or insightful learning episodes. *True False*
8. Sally, aged two, has moderate brain dysfunction. It is not likely that environmental and physical stimulation and practice will stimulate behavioral change. *True False*
9. Instrumental conditioning or stimulus-response learning implies that the individual acts upon the environment to attain a perceived goal that is important to self; thus, this construct is like Gestalt-field learning theory in this regard. *True False*
10. Psychomotor learning takes place as the learner is actually responding, not prior to making the response while watching, listening to, or reading about steps involved in the skill. *True False*

11. The intelligence quotient obtained using the Stanford-Binet scale validly and reliably indicates an individual's total intellectual capacity, developmental level, and behavioral capabilities during life stages. *True False*

12. Norms and patterns relative to age and developmental level should be used by teachers to help diagnose individual readiness for learning, to assess learning needs, to establish learning outcomes, to determine teaching actions, and to evaluate behavioral change. *True False*

13. A person's learning style is permanent and relates to distinctive observable behaviors that indicate how information is acquired and processed, whereas modality strength refers to the teacher's use of auditory, visual, or kinesthetic sensory and cognitive preferences for teaching. *True False*

14. The primary value of diagnosing learning styles, cognitive styles, modality strengths, and learning experiences relates to the teacher's use of such subjective data to plan, develop, and evaluate learning experiences. *True False*

15. Some authorities contend that children from the age of two on can be expected to assume some degree of responsibility for establishing personal learning objectives, that they rely strongly upon learned action patterns primarily acquired through manipulation of objects, and that they can be taught complex problem-solving behaviors through concentrated learning over time. *True False*

16. The primary role of the nurse-teacher is standard diagnosis, correct performance of procedure, and dissemination of information. *True False*

MULTIPLE TRUE/FALSE

Mark each statement or item as you would a traditional true-or-false question. Which of the following statements reflect positive principles of learning?

17. Readiness for learning is the sum of all genetic attributes and prior experiences and includes the learner's developmental and maturity level, sociocultural background, and perception of need for behavioral change. *True False*

18. Learning is a continual, dynamic personal and social phenomenon synonymous with the acquisition of new thoughts, feelings, and actions. *True False*

19. Both intrinsic and extrinsic motivation for growth toward becoming self-actualized are the teacher's responsibility. *True False*

20. Relatively immediate feedback, reinforcement, and satisfaction with response are necessary conditions for learning that tend to help the learner acquire, remember, and repeat responses. *True False*

21. Continual, repeated practice of a response will ensure acquisition and transfer of a behavior. *True False*

22. Discrimination, generalization, and association abilities are prerequisite to signal learning, stimulus-response learning, psychomotor, concept, principle, and problem-solving behaviors. *True False*

Students are asked to write the names of ten important components of an IV infusion system as they view and compare the components illustrated on slides. Sometimes more than one item is pictured on a slide. This is an example of which of the following?

23. Multiple discrimination. *True False*
24. Problem solving. *True False*
25. Rule using or principle learning. *True False*
26. Concept learning. *True False*
27. Verbal association. *True False*

Jane exhibits nervous eye twitching when speaking before a large group. It is most likely that her behavior may be attributed to which of the following?

28. Gestalt-field learning theory. *True False*
29. Classical conditioning or signal learning. *True False*
30. Instrumental conditioning. *True False*
31. Behavior modification. *True False*
32. Stimulus-response learning. *True False*

A nurse-teacher hands out a case study depicting a high-level managerial/leadership situation, appoints a group leader, and asks the small group of seven senior nursing students to collectively analyze the situation, identify the dysfunctional aspect, consider circumstances and alternatives for action, establish long- and short-term goals, and arrive at a group consensus on ways to alleviate the problem. The group interaction is recorded on videotape. Following group consensus, the teacher discusses the case study with the group, replays the recording, and points out strengths and weaknesses of leader behavior and group interaction. Positive suggestions are given. The teacher also models positive leader behavior. Which of the following constructs are being depicted and applied in this teaching-learning experience?

33. Application of basic principles of adult learning. *True False*
34. Modeling as a negative reinforcer. *True False*
35. Observation learning. *True False*
36. Cognitive and affective learning. *True False*

37. Principles of psychomotor and rote learning. *True False*

38. Use of immediate sensory feedback, correction, and positive reinforcement principles. *True False*

39. Active, overt learner participation with social interaction. *True False*

40. Concrete, realistic application of concepts and principles to promote problem solving. *True False*

Danyelle, aged 32, is obese because of compulsive eating habits. It would be best to use constructs from which of the following types of learning to help her redirect her eating habits and get her weight under control?

41. Signal learning. *True False*

42. Stimulus-response learning. *True False*

43. Chaining. *True False*

44. Behavior modification. *True False*

Mr. Johnson, aged 68, has chronic obstructive pulmonary disease. He needs to use a held-held nebulizer for inhalation therapy at home. Which of the following factors and conditions will be most beneficial for achievement of the learning outcome and positively influence transfer of learning?

45. Diagnosis of Mr. Johnson's cognitive, perceptual, and neuromotor abilities and his level of internal motivation and interest in learning to use the nebulizer. *True False*

46. Using limited intermittent practice and negative reinforcement while visually demonstrating steps involved in using the nebulizer. *True False*

47. The nurse's use of simple, clear, well-organized verbal directions and explanations with visual demonstration and actual hands-on practice, giving positive reinforcement and feedback on progress using the nebulizer, in a nonthreatening manner. *True False*

48. The degree of satisfaction Mr. Johnson experiences from use of the nebulizer at home and periodic follow-up evaluative home visits by the nurse. *True False*

POSTTEST ANSWER KEY

1. True
2. False
3. False
4. True
5. False
6. False
7. False
8. False
9. True

10. True
11. False
12. True
13. False
14. False
15. True
16. False
17. True
18. True
19. False
20. True
21. False
22. True
23. True
24. False
25. False
26. False
27. True
28. False
29. True
30. False
31. False
32. False
33. True
34. False
35. True
36. True
37. False
38. True
39. True
40. True
41. True
42. True
43. False
44. True
45. True
46. False
47. True
48. True

SUGGESTED APPLICATION ACTIVITIES

1. Debate the issue ''Nurse-teacher: Humanist or behaviorist.''
2. Interview a nurse-teacher and observe actual teaching-learning situations to determine his or her philosophy of teaching and learning.
3. Choose a particular topic to be taught to a group or individual. Determine which of the eleven types of learning would apply to the topic and give specific examples of each type.
4. Analyze actual teaching events, determine types of learning taking place, and the conditions created by the nurse-teacher to promote learning.
5. Select one of the types of learning, such as concept learning, principle learning, or problem solving. Design a specific teaching-learning situation and explain methods and strategies for promoting learning of this type.
6. Analyze a specific subject matter or task and determine which learning domain(s) would apply. Justify your decisions giving specific examples of particular content for identified domains. Then develop specific objectives for the domain(s).
7. Design a research study that would investigate the influence of particular hereditary, environmental, and cultural factors on learning.
8. Conduct a literature search and review the literature on the effects of heredity and environment on learning. Write a research paper, drawing conclusions based on the review.
9. Develop a tool, or use one that has been developed, to gather data on one individual over a period of time to validate patterns of behavior and ability relevant to age and developmental level. Draw inferences and relate findings to learning principles and implications for teaching.
10. Assess an individual with a physical or emotional disability and explain how

the disability may affect learning. Describe the conditions that will need to be provided by the nurse-teacher to facilitate a particular learning experience for this person.

11. Obtain a validated instrument designed to assess learning style, modality strengths, cognitive style, or learning preferences. Administer the instrument to two or more persons to obtain data on individual styles, strengths, and weaknesses. Explain your findings.
12. Observe at least one teaching-learning event involving an adult, a very young child, and an adolescent. Gather data that reflects learning principles used by the nurse-teacher for each individual. Analyze and compare data. Draw inferences and conclusions based on findings.
13. Select one of the following situations and develop a plan for teaching. Include a discussion of the implications for teaching, the learning principles you would apply, and the forces that may influence learning within the situation.
    a. You are a nurse-educator in an academic setting. Your assignment is to teach a class on the legal, ethical, and professional aspects of nursing. There are 70 students in your class: 50 percent of the students have had a two-hour course called "The Nurse: Negligence and Malpractice;" 60 students have had a basic introduction to charting and its legal implications; 10 students are registered nurses employed part-time.
    b. You are the inservice director in a large hospital. You have determined that the staff needs to either become certified or recertified as basic rescuers according to the standards of the American Heart Association. There are approximately 100 nurses who will need training or review within six weeks to meet requirements for certification. The average nurse's age is 35. The majority are female RNs from three-year schools of nursing. Each staff nurse works a full eight-hour day, sometimes longer. The majority are married and have children.
    c. You are the coordinator of a regional continuing nursing education conference on aging. The conference is for practicing nurses and other health professionals interested in helping individuals cope with aging. You are responsible for planning the educational program as well as delivering portions of the content.
    d. You are a staff nurse and are responsible for teaching a 19-year-old boy how to walk using crutches. The client broke his leg playing football. He attends the local university, lives with a roommate off campus, and has never used crutches before.
    e. You are employed by the local visiting nurses' association and are to teach colostomy self-care to a 25-year-old female client. She lives in a small apartment with her three small children, aged two, three, and six, and is on welfare. She has a high school education.
14. Start improving instruction by developing a computerized diagnostic and learning-style profile for a particular student population. Collect data for input using diagnostic, aptitude, achievement, and sociometric tests; anecdotal records, at-

titude scales, learning and cognitive style inventories, interest inventories, conferences, questionnaires, and observations. Code the items in relation to the objectives, activities, and materials for a given subject. Program the computer to produce both individual and group profiles to match student learning difficulties to specific objectives. Suggest relevant activities, related materials, and evaluation tests, and formulate teaching plans using student profiles.

REFERENCES

1. Perceiving Behaving Becoming: A New Focus for Education. In AW Coombs (ed), ASCD 1962 yearbook. Washington, D.C., Association for Supervision and Curriculum Development, 1962, p. 89.
2. Pugh E: Dynamics of Teaching-Learning Interaction. Nursing Forum 15:47–58, 1976.
3. King VG, Gerwig NA: Humanizing Nursing Education. Wakefield, MA, Nursing Resources, 1981, pp. 1–5.
4. Chute AG: Effect of Color and Monochrome Versions of a Film on Incidental and Task-Relevant Learning. Educational Communications and Technology Journal 28:10–24, 1980.
5. Canelos J, Taylor W, Altschuld J: Networking vs. Role Learning Strategies in Concept Acquisition. Educational Communications and Technology Journal 30:141–149, 1982.
6. Gronlund NE: Stating Behavioral Objectives for Classroom Instruction. ed 2. New York, Macmillan, Inc., 1978, pp. 26–31.
7. Singer RN: Motor Learning and Human Performance: An Application to Motor Skills and Movement Behaviors, ed 3. New York, Macmillan, Inc., 1980, pp. 131–177.
8. Gronlund NE: Stating Behavioral Objectives, for Classroom Instruction, ed 2. New York, Macmillan, Inc., 1978, pp. 32–34.
9. Merrill MD: Psychomotor and Memorization Behavior: Paradigms for Psychomotor Instruction. In MD Merrill (ed), Instructional Design: Readings. Englewood Cliffs, N.J., Prentice-Hall, Inc., 1971, pp. 196–214.
10. Harrow AJ: A Taxonomy of the Psychomotor Domain: A Guidebook for Developing Behavioral Objectives. New York, David McKay Co., Inc., 1972.
11. Guilford JP: Intelligence Has Three Facets. In HF Clarizio, RC Craig, WA Mehrens (eds), Contemporary Issues in Educational Psychology. Boston, Allyn & Bacon, Inc., 1970, pp. 351–363.
12. Chall JS: Educational Implications of Recent Brain Research. Educational Leadership 39:11, 1981.
13. Sylvester R: Educational Implications of Recent Brain Research. Educational Leadership 39:7–10, 1981.
14. Wittrock MC: Educational Implications of Recent Brain Research. Educational Leadership 39:12–15, 1981.
15. Sylvester R: Educational Implications of Recent Brain Research. Educational Leadership 39:9, 1981.
16. Canfield AA: Canfield Learning Styles Inventory. Rochester, MI, Humanics Media, 1970.
17. Dunn R, De Bello T, et al.: Learning Style Researchers Define Differences Differently. Educational Leadership 38:372–375, 1981.
18. Gregorc AF: Learning/Teaching Styles: Potent Forces Behind Them. Educational Leadership 36:234–236, 1979.

19. Dunn R, De Bello T, et al.: Learning Style Researchers Define Differences Differently. Educational Leadership 38:375, 1981.
20. Ibid.
21. Ausburn LJ, Ausburn FB: Cognitive Styles: Some Information and Implications for Instructional Design. Educational Communications and Technology Journal 26:337–354, 1978.
22. Bruner J: The Course of Cognitive Growth. In HF Clarizio, RC Craig, WA Mehrens (eds), Contemporary Issues in Educational Psychology. Boston, Allyn & Bacon, Inc., 1970, pp. 297–313.
23. Gall M: Synthesis of Research on Teachers' Questioning. Educational Leadership 42:40–47, 1984.
24. Dillon JT: Research on Questioning and Discussion. Educational Leadership 42:55, 1984.
25. How to be an Effective Presenter. St. Paul, MN, Visual Products Division/3M, 1978, p. 4.
26. Dwyer FM: Behavioral Approach to Visual Communication, Instructional Communications and Technology Report (No. 11). Washington D.C., Association for Educational Communications and Technology, 1980.
27. Peterson PL, Walberg HJ (eds): Research on Teaching: Concepts, Findings and Implications. Berkeley, CA, McCutchan Publishing Corp., 1979, p. 15.
28. Ibid., p. 16–67.
29. Levin T, Long R: Effective Instruction. Alexandria, VA, The Association for Supervision and Curriculum Development, 1981, p. 17.
30. Bruner J: Toward a Theory of Instruction. Cambridge, MA, Harvard University Press, 1966.
31. Levin T, Long R: Effective Instruction. Alexandria, VA, The Association for Supervision and Curriculum Development, 1981, pp. 22–23.
32. Block JH: The Effects of Various Levels of Performance on Selected Cognitive, Affective and Time Variables. Unpublished doctoral dissertation, University of Chicago, 1970.
33. Melton RF: Resolution of Conflicting Claims Concerning the Effect of Behavioral Objectives on Student Learning. Review of Educational Research 48:291–302, 1978.
34. Levin T, Long R: Effective Instruction. Alexandria, VA, The Association for Supervision and Curriculum Development, 1981, pp. 27–28.
35. de Tornyay R, Thompson MA: Strategies for Teaching Nursing, ed 2. New York, John Wiley & Sons, Inc., 1982, pp. 10–11.
36. Levin T, Long R: Effective Instruction. Alexandria, VA, The Association for Supervision and Curriculum Development, 1981, pp. 26–27.
37. Ibid., pp. 32–33.
38. Levin T: Instruction Which Enables Students to Develop Higher Mental Processes. In BH Choppin, NT Postlesthwaite (eds), Evaluation in Education: An International Review Series. Elmsford, N.Y., Pergamon Press, 1979.
39. Jonassen DH: Personality and Cognitive Style Predictors of Teaching Style Preferences: An Exploratory Study. In M Simonson, E Hooper (eds), Proceedings of Selected Research Paper Presentations at the 1981 Convention of the American Association for Educational Communications and Technology. Ames, IA, Iowa State University, 1981, pp. 233–259.
40. Gage NL: An Analytical Approach to Research on Instructional Methods. In HF Clarizio, RC Craig, WA Mehrens (eds), Contemporary Issues in Educational Psychology. Boston, Allyn & Bacon, Inc., 1970, pp. 67–81.

BIBLIOGRAPHY

Anderson RC, Faust GW: Educational Psychology: The Science of Instruction and Learning. New York, Dodd, Mead & Co., 1973.

Bantock GH: Education, Culture and the Emotions. Bloomington, IN, Indiana University Press, 1968.

Bany MA, Johnson LV: Educational Social Psychology. New York, Macmillan, Inc., 1975.

Barbe WB, Milone MN: What We Know About Modality Strengths. Educational Leadership 38:378–380, 1981.

Barbe WB, Swassing RH: Teaching Through Modality Strengths: Concepts and Practices. Columbus, OH, Zaner-Bloser, Inc., 1979.

Barclay JR: Foundations of Counseling Strategies. New York, John Wiley & Sons, Inc., 1971.

Bateman BD: The Essentials of Teaching. San Rafael, CA, Dimensions Publishing Co., 1971.

Bernhard LA, Walsh M: Leadership: The Key to the Professionalization of Nursing. New York, McGraw-Hill Book Co., 1981.

Bigge ML: Learning Theories for Teachers. New York, Harper & Row, Publishers, Inc., 1982.

Blair GM, Jones RS, Simpson RH: Educational Psychology, ed 2. New York, Macmillan Inc., 1963.

Burnside IM (ed): Nursing and the Aged. New York, McGraw-Hill Book Co., 1976.

Canelos J, Taylor W, Altschuld J: Networking vs. Role Learning Strategies in Concept Acquisition. Educational Communications and Technology Journal 30:141–149, 1982.

Carter SL: The Nurse Educator: Humanist or Behaviorist? Nursing Outlook 26:554–557, 1978.

Clifford MM: Practicing Educational Psychology. Boston, Houghton Mifflin Co., 1981.

Clarizio HF, Craig RC, Mehrens WA (eds): Contemporary Issues in Educational Psychology. Boston, Allyn & Bacon, Inc., 1970.

Combs AW (ed): Perceiving Behaving Becoming: A New Focus for Education, 1962 ASCD Yearbook. Washington, D.C., Association for Supervision and Curriculum Development, 1962.

Davis DD, Schwimmer PC: Style—A Manner of Thinking. Educational Leadership 38:376–377, 1981.

Davis RH, Alexander LT, Yelon SL: Learning System Design: An Approach to the Improvement of Instruction. New York, McGraw-Hill Book Co., 1974.

Day MC: Thinking at Piaget's Stage of Formal Operations. Educational Leadership 39:44–47, 1981.

De Tornayay R, Thompson MA: Strategies for Teaching Nursing, ed 2. New York, John Wiley & Sons, Inc., 1971.

Dropkin S, Full H, Swartz E: Contemporary American Education, ed 2. New York, Macmillan Inc., 1970.

Ehrenberg SD: Concept Learning: How to Make It Happen in the Classroom. Educational Leadership 39:36–43, 1981.

Frantz R: Selecting Media for Patient Education. Topics in Clinical Nursing 2:77–85, 1980.

Glasser W: Reality Therapy. New York, Harper & Row, Publishers, Inc., 1965

Green CP: Teaching Strategies for the Process of Planned Change. The Journal of Continuing Education in Nursing 14:16–23, 1983.

Gronlund NE: Stating Behavioral Objectives for Classroom Instruction, ed 2. New York, Macmillan Inc., 1978.

Guinee KK: Teaching and Learning in Nursing. New York, Macmillan Inc., 1978.

Harrow AJ: A Taxonomy of the Psychomotor Domain: A Guidebook for Developing Behavioral Objectives. New York, David McKay Co., Inc., 1972.

Hergenhahn BR: An Introduction to Theories of Learning. ed 2. Englewood Cliffs, NJ, Prentice-Hall, Inc., 1982.

Hill, HE: Communication Research and Instructional Technology. Educational Communications and Technology Journal 26:47–53, 1978.

Hill W: Contemporary Developments Within Stimulus-Response Learning Theory, National Society for the Study of Education Yearbook, 63. Chicago, The University of Chicago Press, 1964, pp. 27–53.

Hitt WD: Two Models of Man. American Psychologist 24:651–665, 1969.

Horrocks JE: The Psychology of Adolescence: Behavior and Development, ed 2. Boston, Houghton Mifflin Co., 1962.

Huckabay LMD: Conditions of Learning and Instruction in Nursing: Modularized. St. Louis, C.V. Mosby Co., 1980.

Hunkins FP: Questioning Strategies and Techniques. Boston, Allyn & Bacon, Inc., 1972.

King VG, Gerwig NA: Humanizing Nursing Education. Wakefield, MA, Nursing Resources, 1981.

Knopke HJ, Diekelmann NL: Approaches to Teaching in the Health Sciences. Reading, MA, Addison-Wesley Publishing Co., 1978.

Knopke HJ, Diekelmann NL (eds): Approaches to Teaching Primary Health Care. St. Louis, C.V. Mosby Co., 1981.

Lancaster J, Lancaster W: The Nurse as a Change Agent. St. Louis, C.V. Mosby Co., 1982.

Leddy S, Pepper J: Conceptual Basis of Professional Nursing. Philadelphia: J.B. Lippincott, 1985.

Levin T, Long R: Effective Instruction. Alexandria, VA, The Association for Supervision and Curriculum Development, 1981.

Maslow AH: Toward a Psychology of Being, ed 2. New York, D. Van Nostrand Co., 1968.

McKeachie WJ: Teaching Tips: A Guidebook for the Beginning College Teacher, ed 7. Lexington, MA, D.C. Heath & Co., 1978.

Mechner F: Complex Cognitive Behavior: The Teaching of Concepts and Chains. In DM Merrill (ed), Instructional Design: Readings. Englewood Cliffs, NJ, Prentice-Hall, Inc., 1971.

Munn HE Jr, Metzger N: Effective Communication in Health Care. Rockville, MD, Aspen Systems Corp., 1981.

Owen SV, Froman RD, Moscow H: Psychology: An Introduction, ed 2. Boston, Little, Brown & Company, 1981.

Peterson PL, Walberg HJ: Research on Teaching: Concepts, Findings and Implications. Berkeley, CA, McCutchan Publishing Corp., 1979.

Pohl ML: The Teaching Function of the Nursing Practitioner, ed 2. Dubuque, IA, Wm. C. Brown Co., Publishers, 1973.

Poteet JA: Behavior Modification: A Practical Guide for Teachers. Minneapolis, MN, Burgess Publishing Co., 1973.

Pugh E: Dynamics of Teaching-Learning Interaction, Nursing Forum 15:47–58, 1976.

Schmeck RR: Improving Learning by Improving Thinking, Educational Leadership 38:384–385, 1981.

Singer RN: Motor Learning and Human Performance: An Application to Motor Skills and Movement Behaviors, ed 3. New York, Macmillan, Inc., 1980.

Singer RN (ed): The Psychomotor Domain Movement Behaviors. Philadelphia, Lea & Febiger, 1972.

Skinner BF: The Technology of Teaching. New York, Appleton-Century-Crofts, 1968.
Sless D: Learning and Visual Communication. New York, John Wiley & Sons, Inc., 1981.
Smeltzer CH: Psychological Evaluations in Nursing. New York, Macmillan, Inc., 1965.
Smith JM, Lusterman DD: The Teacher as Learning Facilitator: Psychology and the Educational Process. Belmont, CA, Wadsworth Publishing Co., 1979.
Sprott RL (ed): Age, Learning Ability and Intelligence. New York, Van Nostrand Reinhold Co., 1980.
Sternberg RJ: Intelligence as Thinking and Learning Skills. Educational Leadership 39:18–20, 1981.
Tennyson RD: Pictorial Support and Specific Instructions as Design Variables for Children's Concept and Rule Using. Educational Communications and Technology Journal 26:291–299, 1982.
Verduin JR Jr, Miller HG, Greer CE: Adults Teaching Adults: Principles and Strategies. Austin, TX, Learning Concepts Inc., 1977.
Wood FH, Thompson SR: Guidelines for Better Staff Development. Educational Leadership 37:374–378, 1980.

2

Systematic Planning for Teaching and Learning

Barry D. Bratton

OBJECTIVES

Upon completion of this chapter, you will be able to:

1. Distinguish between instruction and education.
2. Compare the nursing process and the instructional design process.
3. Describe basic procedures in designing instruction.
4. Distinguish between "systematic" and "systemic" approaches to designing instruction.
5. Describe the essential characteristics of each of the following instructional design models:
   a. Kemp
   b. Davis, Alexander, and Yelon
   c. Briggs
   d. Dick and Carey
6. Compare and contrast the four instructional design models.
7. Apply instructional design procedures to nursing and client education.

INTRODUCTION

Throughout much of history, teaching has been thought of as an art. Some individuals were blessed with this gift whereas others were not. Often, too, the quality of a person's teaching was judged in terms of one's ability to communicate information to learners through lecture. Individuals who were known to possess a strong intellectual grasp of a body of knowledge and who could stand before a group of learners and expound in an interesting and thought-provoking way were considered master teachers.

While this view of teaching still has its supporters, the trend today has shifted away from the art of teaching and toward a science of instruction. The emphasis now is on *learning* and how best to ensure that it occurs during instruction. Teaching is seen as the means to help individuals learn. The term most often given to the processes of systematically planning, developing, implementing, and evaluating experiences that promote learning is instructional development.

There is a distinction between instruction and education. *Instruction* is viewed as a purposeful and directed activity during which learners interact with a teacher or teacher-prepared materials. In such situations, for example a classroom, both the learner and the teacher overtly or tacitly acknowledge that the goal is learning, that both are expected to work toward that goal, and that one or both is accountable for the learning that occurs. Both also recognize and accept that the teacher is directing or controlling the learning environment. Finally, in instructional situations there is the mutual understanding that the learner will be evaluated in terms of the expected outcomes. The evaluation results can serve as one source of information about the teacher's effectiveness. Teaching nursing students aseptic techniques, which they are expected to later demonstrate to the instructor for evaluation purposes, is an example of an instructional activity.

Education, on the other hand, is conceived as a broader notion in which learning occurs as a result of a person living and exploring in the world. Educational experiences are not necessarily structured and can occur while reading a book, hearing a talk, watching television, browsing in a museum, or talking with people. It is very difficult to define expected learning outcomes or to evaluate the results of an educational activity. Giving a talk to clients in the obstetrics ward about the birthing process would be considered an educational activity. Neither the listeners nor the speaker feel accountable for any learning that does or does not take place.

The content of this chapter focuses only on instruction. While it is true that many instructional development concepts and practices can be applied to educational activities, it is frequently impossible to know if educational goals are met or if any learning has occurred.

COMPARISON OF THE NURSING PROCESS AND THE INSTRUCTIONAL DEVELOPMENT PROCESS

Instructional development, like the nursing process, is a problem-solving endeavor. Both involve assessment, planning, implementation, and evaluation. The nursing process ideally results in better client care and, hopefully, client wellness. The instructional development process ideally creates effective instruction that results in learning. While the focus of this chapter is the application of instructional development to nursing education, the same process can be used in medical education, dental education, allied health education, and in fact, to any discipline or field where instruction occurs. Table 2–1 shows the relationship of the nursing process and the instructional development process to a general problem-solving process. Note the components in each approach.

During the nursing process, the professional nurse recognizes the client's needs, gathers relevant information about the client, develops a nursing care plan, imple-

TABLE 2–1. COMPARISON OF PROBLEM-SOLVING PROCESS, NURSING PROCESS, AND INSTRUCTIONAL DEVELOPMENT PROCESS

General Problem-Solving Process	Nursing Process	Instructional Development Process
1. Diagnose a general problem area.	1. Diagnose client needs.	1. Diagnose learner needs.
2. Collect relevant data.	2. Gather information about the client.	2. Collect information about the learner.
3. Develop a potential solution.	3. Develop a nursing plan.	3. Develop an instructional plan.
4. Implement the solution.	4. Implement the nursing plan.	4. Implement the instructional plan.
5. Evaluate the solution.	5. Evaluate the effects of the nursing intervention.	5. Evaluate the effects of the instructional intervention.
6. Decide if the solution is adequate.	6. Decide if the intervention is adequate.	6. Decide if the intervention is adequate.
7. Recycle through the process.	7. Recycle through the process.	7. Recycle through the process.

ments the plan, evaluates the intervention, and makes further decisions based on the evaluation. Similarly, the instructional development process asks the nurse-educator to recognize the goals of the educational program and the learner's needs, gather relevant information about the learner, develop an instructional plan, implement the plan, evaluate the intervention, and make further decisions based on the evaluation data.

In this chapter, the terms *design, development, implementation,* and *evaluation* will be used to explain the general process of creating effective instruction. As the terms are defined, refer to Table 2–1.

Design

The term *design* is used at times as an action verb, for example, "The instructors *designed* the course outline." Other times it is used as a noun, for example, "The instructors used the course *design* to develop the instructional materials." In the first case, design is equated with the cognitive activity of thinking and planning. It means taking into account all the relevant factors as one formulates an instructional intervention. The bulk of this chapter will present the factors that are typically taken into consideration when designing (planning) instruction. In the second case, design refers to the tangible results of the planning. It is the framework, or superstructure, of the instruction. The design frequently consists of the learner objectives, the instructional activities, and the evaluation methods that will be used during the instruction. This chapter will focus on design as a planning activity, because careful planning is requisite to carrying out quality instruction.

Development

The term *development* refers to the process of acquiring or creating the instructional and evaluation materials stipulated in the design. Here, lectures might be written, films previewed and selected, discussion questions prepared, self-instructional materials created, and test items drafted.

Implementation

Implementation refers to the actual delivery of the instruction. The form of the implementation is obviously dictated by the decisions made in the design and development phases. If, for example, the instruction were designed for hospitalized clients using the institution's closed-circuit television system, implementation would occur when the live or videotaped materials were broadcast. If the instruction were designed for delivery as a live lecture in a classroom setting, implementation would occur when the lecture was presented.

Evaluation

The term *evaluation* connotes the gathering of information and making subsequent decisions based on the data. Evaluation can occur both during the implementation phase, when the teacher seeks feedback from the learners about the clarity of the instruction, as well as at the conclusion, when test information is used to assign grades. Evaluation data are also gathered at the end of instruction to help the teacher determine if the current design and delivery are adequate or should be modified. Chapter 6 of this text is devoted to the topic of evaluation.

SUMMARY

Teaching has one primary goal—to bring about learning. The processes of systematically planning, developing, implementing, and evaluating experiences designed by teachers to promote learning is called instructional development. It can be compared to the nursing process in that both are problem-solving processes. Careful planning or design is requisite to the effective development, implementation, and evaluation of instruction.

BASIC PROCEDURES IN DESIGNING INSTRUCTION

Numerous guidelines, or models, have been created that describe ways for designing (planning) instruction. Forty such models were identified by Andrews and Goodson.[1] The differences among the models frequently reflect an emphasis on a particular component or the unique settings for which they were developed. Nearly all models, however, share some common assumptions: (1) the teacher bears equal responsibility with the learners for the learning that occurs during instruction; (2) planning will help the teacher meet this responsibility; (3) the teacher's primary role is to facilitate learning rather than functioning solely as a dispenser of information; (4) learners should be informed at the beginning of instruction of what they are expected to know or do at the end of instruction; (5) the teacher should be adept at using a variety of teaching methods to help learners master the content; and (6) evaluation data should be collected to provide feedback to the teacher so that instruction can be improved.

In addition, most models suggest the following components are crucial to consider when planning effective instruction: instructional objectives, subject content, instructional strategies, and evaluation methods. The key here is not the order in which the components are planned, but that each component is considered in relation to the others. The rationale for this is that decisions regarding one component affect and are affected by decisions about the other components. In other words, all the components are interrelated, and whereas the teacher might focus on only one at a time during planning, the potential impact of a decision about one component on each of the others must be kept in mind. Each of these four components are discussed, followed by an in-depth examination of several specific models or guides for designing instruction.

Instructional Objectives

Two types of instructional objectives should be planned. One type is the teaching objectives, the other is the learning objectives. The difference is more than just semantics. The former focuses on what the teacher wishes to accomplish during the period of instruction. For example, the nurse-educator may wish to demonstrate a procedure, discuss important cause-effect relationships, or instill a positive attitude. The notion of teaching objectives has been widely accepted for many years.

The concept of learning objectives, on the other hand, is relatively new. Learning objectives focus on what the learner should be able to do, know, or feel after the instruction is completed. In other words, learning objectives are the mirror-image of the teaching objectives in that they are stated from the learner's perspective. The following is an example of a teaching objective and a learning objective.

Teaching objective: The teacher will discuss shock and the appropriate nursing care.

Learning objective: The learner will be able to list the common types of shock, the causes of shock, the signs and symptoms of shock, and the appropriate nursing interventions.

Notice how much more specifically the learning objective is stated. Such specificity can only result when the teacher thinks carefully about what the learners should accomplish. Note, too, that by thinking in terms of the learner, the teacher also describes the content that must be presented. The rationale behind designing learning objectives is that learning is acquired more readily if (a) teachers plan their instruction with the learner's point of view in mind, and (b) the learners are informed at the beginning what is expected of them.

Learning objectives can be classified into three types: cognitive, affective, and psychomotor. Cognitive objectives are those that are concerned with internal mental processes like recalling, naming, or explaining. Bloom developed a classification scheme for various levels of cognitive activity.[2] This taxonomy proceeds from basic knowledge to higher levels of learning: (1) knowledge level—example: define, list, recall, name; (2) comprehension level—example: classify, explain, describe, discuss; (3) application level—example: solve, apply, use, illustrate; (4) analysis level—example: distinguish, calculate, compare, contrast; (5) synthesis level—example: formulate, design, manage, plan; and (6) evaluation level—example: judge, assess, predict, choose. Here is an example of a cognitive objective at the knowledge level: The at-risk client will name three reasons for avoiding foods high in cholesterol. An example at the synthesis level might be: The nursing student will formulate a nursing care plan for a new patient with juvenile diabetes.

Affective objectives focus on instilling attitudes, beliefs, and feelings in learners. This type of objective has not been as extensively researched as the cognitive type, perhaps because some educators argue that it is more important for teachers to concentrate on knowledge and skills. Others disagree and hold that some outcomes of instruction can only be expressed in affective terms, for example, that nurses will voluntarily participate in continuing professional education programs. The act of volunteering suggests that one has a positive attitude. It is generally felt that teachers can teach affective objectives by showing their learners, students and clients, positive role models to emulate.[3] Here is an example of an affective learning objective: The client will choose to eat only foods that are low in cholesterol. Another example is: Nursing students will establish their own routine of reading current journals in their field.

The third type of objective is the psychomotor objective. This type refers to physical skills such as giving injections, starting an intravenous infusion system, or changing a dressing. Objectives in the psychomotor domain are probably the easiest of the three types of objectives for educators to state, because they are readily observable. An example of a psychomotor objective is: The nursing student will dress appropriately for surgery while maintaining a sterile field.

Subject Content

All educators face two fundamental decisions about the content or information to be taught: what specifically to teach and how to organize the content for presentation to learners.

The nursing setting frequently influences what is taught. For example, for a client education program in a primary care setting, the nurse-educator may have a great deal of freedom in determining what information is most appropriate for a client or group of clients and how best to organize the information. This is often not the case in academic nursing institutions where accreditation guidelines, licensure requirements, institutional norms, and historical precedent all exert influence (and sometimes dictate) what is taught. In such an environment, the nurse-educator's choice may be limited to organizing the content for teaching purposes.

Two techniques that can be used to help determine what content should be included in instruction are called task description and content analysis. A *task description,* as the term implies, is a description of how a task is actually performed. The technique can be used to describe both overt action tasks (such as surgical gloving) or covert action tasks (like computing drug dosages). Listing all the steps in a task has two benefits. First, nurse-educators (like most teachers in all fields) are often master performers who practice their profession so automatically that they are unaware of the individual steps involved. By creating a detailed description of an important task, one can be sure to include all the critical steps when teaching others. Secondly, once the description is complete, it can be analyzed to determine which of the steps are absolutely fundamental for adequate performance and which are desirable but not necessarily essential. The following portion of a task description for the overt actions in administering intradermal injections developed by Margaret Rankin might easily become the organizational structure for teaching the procedure.[4]

1. Withdraws into syringe 0.1 to 0.2 cc sterile normal saline to simulate usual medication, maintaining sterile technique.
2. Selects a site on medial aspect of anterior surface of patient's forearm (2 inches above the wrist and 2 inches below the elbow).
3. Cleanses site with an alcohol swab.
4. Allows site to air dry.
5. Pulls anterior skin taut with the thumb and forefingers of the nondominant hand.
6. Uses the dominant hand to rest the barrel of the syringe almost parallel to the skin surface.
7. Inserts the needle into the skin, with the bevel up, just until the bevel is no longer visible (1/16 to 1/8 inch) at no more than 5- to 10-degree angle.
8. Injects medication slowly to form a bleb.

Frequently, subject matter does not have an action component, that is, the action is not visible. The content is a collection of facts, concepts, and principles that the learner must acquire and understand. Two examples of this type of content are: (1) the concept of the nursing process and (2) the history of the nursing profession. In cases such as these, a *content analysis* may be helpful in organizing the subject matter. Simply stated, a content analysis entails examining the subject matter for its fundamental underlying facts, concepts, and principles. Figure 2–1 contains an example of a content analysis of the Cori cycle.[5] Notice that visualizing the concept promotes learning and makes it a useful teaching aid. The nursing process can be visualized in a similar manner.

If the teacher is unable to construct a task or content analysis in a particular subject based on personal experience, other sources from which to glean relevant information are textbooks, journals, mediated programs, and observations or interviews with skilled experts.

Obviously these procedures require time to complete, and it is unrealistic to

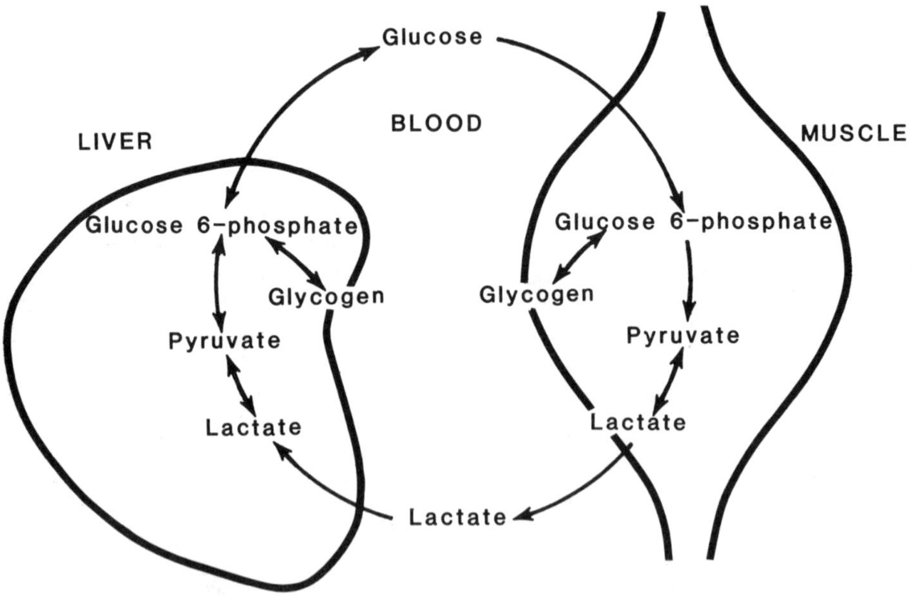

Figure 2-1. Content analysis of the cori cycle. (*From Ortin J, Neuhaus O: Human Biochemistry. St. Louis, C.V. Mosby Co, 1982.*)

expect nurse-educators to use them regularly for all teaching programs. When the instructor is uncertain what information to present to learners, however, task and content analyses can provide insight into selecting and organizing content.

Unfortunately, there are no explicit guidelines for organizing the presentation of content to learners. The present state of knowledge in this area indicates that there is no one best method. The important concepts from a teaching perspective are that the presentation is organized in some fashion and that the organizational principle is made known to the learners. For example, the content might be organized in the following ways: beginning to end, to demonstrate a procedure; simple to complex, when explaining a biological or social phenomenon; historically, to describe the evolution of nursing roles; or concrete to abstract, when presenting the nursing process.

Instructional Strategies

For many years, prior to the emergence of instructional design as a field of professional study, educators in all fields and professions wanted to know the answer to the same question, "What's the best way to teach?" Teachers wanted to know, for example, whether the lecture method or the discussion method was best or if using slides and films would enhance teaching and learning. Concerns such as these reflected the notion that there must be one or perhaps several teaching strategies that were more effective than others. Such is not the case. Neither experience nor research has shown that there is one best teaching method for all situations. Does this imply that because there is no single best way to teach that any strategy will do? Not at all!

Because professional educators today are placing more emphasis on the learning process and how to facilitate it rather than on the art of teaching, it has come to be understood that there is no one perfect teaching method for all situations. Rather, educators are becoming aware that the choice of teaching strategies must take into account the instructional objectives, the characteristics of the learners, the resources available, and the subject content. The implication is that educators in all the professions, including nursing, should be knowledgeable about and competent in using a broad range of strategies that can be used effectively in one-to-one, small-group, and large-group instruction. It also means that nurse-educators should be competent not only in traditional teaching roles, such as lecturer, discussion leader, clinical instructor, or demonstration guide, but also in employing contemporary and emerging technologies (slides, films, overhead transparencies, video and computer programs, teleconferencing, and so on) for instructional purposes. Chapter 3 focuses on factors that influence selection of instructional strategies.

Evaluation Methods

Choosing the appropriate evaluation method, like selecting the suitable teaching strategy, is based on a number of factors. The major question that the nurse-educator should ask is: what is the purpose of the evaluation? It may be to determine what knowledge, skills, or attitudes the learner has acquired as a result of the instruction. A related purpose may be to assign grades to learners. In other situations, it may be to find out how effective you, the nurse-educator, are and to receive feedback on how you can improve. Or, the purpose may be to evaluate an entire program or intervention, not only in terms of its effectiveness, but also in terms of its cost and time requirements. Each of these purposes calls for skills and approaches that nurse-educators should be familiar with.

Some other factors that affect the choice of evaluation methods are the time available to do the evaluation, the setting in which the evaluation will occur, the characteristics of the client or learner, and the resources available to conduct the evaluation. In fact, because the authors of this book consider evaluation so important, Chapter 6 is devoted exclusively to this topic. As a preface to Chapter 6 and to other sections of this book where evaluation is mentioned, several prominent evaluation ideas relating to the design of instruction are briefly presented here.

One important evaluation concept is needs assessment. This refers to a process for determining what information or skills clients or learners possess at present as opposed to what they should ideally have. A discrepancy between the current and the ideal can become the core subject matter for a course, workshop, presentation, clinical experience, or curriculum. Another is materials evaluation. Here the nurse-educator previews instructional materials to determine which, if any, might be useful for a particular program. A third is teacher evaluation. In this instance, a teacher seeks information from learners and perhaps from teaching colleagues about one's effectiveness and areas for improvement. Finally, there is program evaluation. Here information is collected about the quality of a program, perhaps a continuing nursing education conference, a wellness program, or an academic curriculum. The purpose is to determine the overall worthiness of the program.

When the goal of the evaluation effort is to improve something, it is called formative evaluation. For example, the instructor who has created a prototype computer-assisted learning module might observe several students as they use the new program to see where improvements can be made in its effectiveness and appeal. Summative evaluation, on the other hand, generally connotes the collection of data to make a final decision. For instance, test scores are frequently used to determine grades, admission data are ranked to determine who is admitted to college, and faculty members evaluate textbooks to select them for courses.

Each of these concepts related to evaluation, in addition to factors associated with test construction and questionnaire design, are discussed in Chapter 6.

SUMMARY

A number of guidelines, or models, for designing instruction have been developed by educators. They share a number of common philosophical assumptions and at least four common planning elements: objectives, content, instructional strategies, and learner evaluation. Note the philosophical orientation and the attention given to these planning elements in each of the four instructional design models presented in the next section.

COMPARISON OF INSTRUCTIONAL DESIGN MODELS

The preceding section has provided an overview of the basic factors generally taken into consideration when designing instruction. In this section we will examine four specific models or approaches to instructional design. These models were selected because they were created by prominent experts in the field of instructional design and they have been widely disseminated and used by educators in all professions, including nursing education. While each espouses a unique approach to designing instruction, you will also note similarities across the four models. Nurses will find these models, and their individual elements, useful as they plan their teaching activities.

It is important, first, however, to briefly discuss the terms *systems* and the *systematic design of instruction*. Health professionals are familiar with the concept of systems as it applies to the functioning of the human body. When the various parts of the total body system work in harmony, we generally observe a healthy, well-functioning person; however, when one of the body's subsystems—for example, the cardiovascular subsystem—malfunctions, the effects are evident in other subsystems. In other words, the total body system is composed of many subsystems, all of which must work in harmony to maintain the total system. Systems concepts are

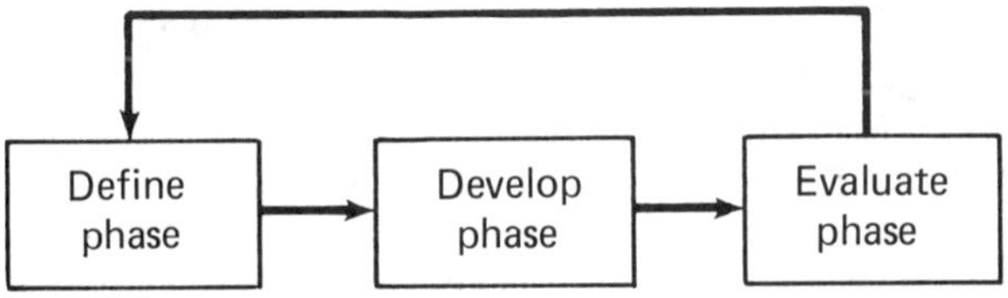

Figure 2-2. A systematic model for designing instruction.

also used in other fields, such as architecture, art, engineering, sociology, and education.

An awareness of systems concepts is important to understanding and using instructional design techniques because the literature in this field is replete with phrases like "the systematic design of instruction," and "the systems approach to instruction." It is unfortunate that some authors treat the two terms as synonyms, and thereby create confusion in the uninformed reader's mind. For example, some theorists envision their models as recipes, which if diligently followed, produce expected and consistent results, i.e., learning. In their way of thinking, the process is systematic, procedural, and invariant. All steps in the process are completed in a prescribed order. Should the desired outcome not be achieved, they advocate the planning process be repeated from the beginning to locate and modify the step or steps that interfered with the final results.

Figure 2–2 shows an example of *the systematic design of instruction.* The nurse-educator first defines what should be taught and learned, then develops the appropriate teaching method, and lastly creates the evaluation procedures. Only after all three phases have been considered is the initial planning in the two previous phases reconsidered.

Others maintain that the design process is a dynamic, interactive one that cannot be reduced to a simple procedure or recipe. Davis, Alexander, and Yelon represent this position when they label the process as "iterative and interactive" and describe it in these words:

> All decisions made in one phase of the process have implications for the decisions made in the other phases. . . . The designer must continually look back to what he has already done and ahead to what remains to be done in order to consider the impact of each decision . . . [6]

Figure 2–3 illustrates *the systemic approach to instructional design.* In this model, the nurse-educator is encouraged to think of all the activities as interrelated;

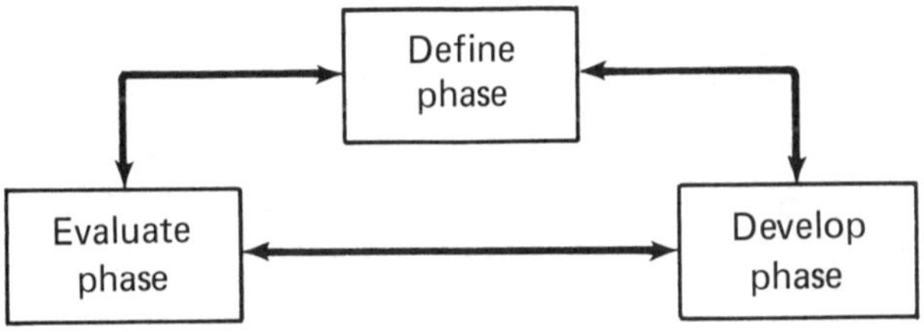

Figure 2-3. A systemic model for designing instruction.

thus it matters little if one begins first considering a teaching method, creating the evaluation, or selecting the content to be learned. Because the process is cyclical and interactive, each phase will be considered and perhaps modified several times as tentative decisions are made and changes made in the other phases.

The difference of opinion among professional educators about the systematic versus the systemic nature of the instructional design process continues. Examples of both points of view are represented in the following descriptions of several design models.

Kemp Model for Instructional Design

Jerrold Kemp developed an instructional design model based on the *systemic* approach that can be applied to most educational or training situations.[7] The model is shown graphically in Figure 2–4.

Notice that the Kemp model consists of nine parts and a revision (feedback) component. Note, too, the graphic representation communicates that there is no one starting or ending point. The author reinforces this notion by emphasizing the interdependence among the elements, suggesting that planning decisions in one area affect decisions in others, and arguing the sequence and order for planning rightfully lies in the hands of the educator.

Goals, Topics, General Purposes. During this phase, the teacher considers the broad educational goals of the institution or organization. This is important because the

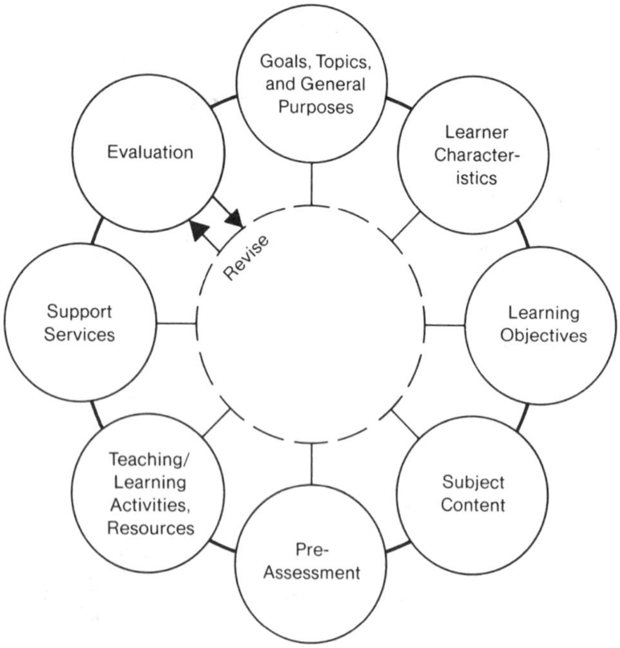

Figure 2-4. Kemp model for instructional design. (*From Kemp J: Instructional Design, ed 2. Belmont, CA, Fearon Publishers, Inc., 1977.*)

goals of an academic nursing program in a university setting are different from the goals of an associate degree program in a community college setting, and both of these differ markedly from a client education program in a hospital, community, or home environment.

In cases where the goals are not known by the teacher, they can sometimes be surmised from the present curriculum, the subject matter being taught, and the nature of the learners. In some instances, educational goals must reflect accreditation and licensure guidelines. The current ideas expressed in prominent textbooks and journals can also influence the goals of a program. Societal health care needs are a prominent force in nursing education and client care.

The nurse-educator must select the major topics of content. The selection, to a great degree, is influenced by the overall program goals. The topics for an academic course on the subject of nursing diagnosis, for example, might include assessment, diagnostic strategies, scope of practice, legal and ethical implications, and future directions. For a one-day community health workshop on smoking, the topics might be limited to such areas as societal influences on smoking, effects of smoking on the body systems, and techniques for reducing and eliminating smoking behaviors.

The selection of instructional topics influences and is influenced by the purpose of the instruction. Stating a general purpose provides a starting point for future instructional design decisions. The purpose is an expression of what you, the teacher, want to accomplish. For example, you might wish the learners to acquire a skill, master a procedure, understand the importance of a topic, or develop a positive attitude toward a subject.

Learner Characteristics. In this phase the teacher considers the relevant characteristics of the learners. Factors such as age, attention span, socioeconomic background, sex, vocational interests, attitudes, emotional level, as well as academic factors such as achievement and aptitude scores, reading level, motivational level toward the content, and previous grades are taken into account.

In addition, Kemp suggests that the impact of the learning setting should be considered. This includes the physical environment (number of learners, furniture arrangement, noise and temperature level, and so on) and the emotional environment (learner expectations, teacher style, group personality, and so forth).

Learning Objectives. During this phase of planning, the teacher considers what knowledge, skills, and attitudes the learners will or should possess at the conclusion of the instruction. It is generally accepted that the types of learning that occur in formal instructional settings fall into these categories: cognitive learning, psychomotor learning, and affective learning. Kemp draws upon the works of Bloom[8], Kibler,[9] and Krathwohl[10] to explain these categories of learning.

Cognitive learning, according to Bloom, is associated with several mental abilities: (1) to store and retrieve from memory selected facts and ideas, (2) to restate information in one's own words, (3) to apply or use this information in new situations, (4) to explain the relationship among the various facts and ideas that make up a body of knowledge, (5) to relate new ideas and facts together to form a larger understanding of a body of knowledge, and (6) to make evaluations or judgments in new situations using all the preceding abilities.

Psychomotor learning, according to Kibler, is associated with such physical activities as these: gross body movements, finely coordinated body movements, nonverbal communication movements, and speech behavior movements.

Krathwohl contends that affective learning is associated with attitudinal and value expressions: actively attending to an event, reacting to an event, accepting an event, and applying value judgments to an event.

Kemp advocates that educators use the behavioral orientation when specifying desired learner outcomes. He suggests that when formulating objectives educators ask themselves what they want the learner to do at the conclusion of the instruction. Here is an objective expressed in the classic behavioral format: Students will label the wave forms of the ECG on five rhythm strips with 100% accuracy.[11] The following objective violates the behavioral format: Students will know parasitology. In this example, it is unclear what the students are expected to learn.

Kemp also draws on educational psychologists Bloom and Gagné[12] to suggest that the stated behavioral learning objectives should be organized according to a hierarchical order of learning, namely, fact learning, concept learning, principle learning, and problem solving. Kemp also advocates that the learners be informed of the objectives. He acknowledges that it is more difficult to write objectives for the higher learning levels, that not all learning outcomes can be easily specified in behavioral terms, and that they may be modified by the teacher as the planning/design process proceeds.

Subject Content. During this phase, the educator plans the organizational structure of the subject matter. Kemp points out that the organization may take one of a number of forms, such as known to unknown, beginning to end, easy to difficult, or concrete to abstract. It should be obvious that the choice of an organizational pattern is influenced by the type of objectives and the learner characteristics.

A specific technique for ensuring all the pertinent information to complete a specific skill, such as using a piece of equipment properly, is called task analysis. This procedure simply entails listing each discrete step in the execution of the skill or procedure. There are several reasons why a task analysis can be valuable. One, the educator may be so familiar with a procedure that significant steps or checks are unconsciously omitted during the explanation. Second, the activity may uncover steps that the educator needs to learn more about prior to the teaching session. Third, the steps listed during the task analysis process can form the content of the instruction. Fourth, the steps suggest one pattern for organizing and presenting the instruction. Another advantage may be that the subject content becomes visible and may be a useful learning tool for the students or clients.

Preassessment. During this phase the instructor plans how to determine if the learners possess the necessary background preparation for the content and how much they know about the subject prior to the instruction. Kemp advocates the educator use preassessment techniques. This means determining how much the learners know and don't know about the content before the actual instruction begins. One form of preassessment, called *prerequisite testing,* reveals to the teacher if the learners have the necessary background and prerequisites to grasp the new content. A second form, called *pretesting,* lets the teacher know how much the learners already know about the content. By asking selected questions, either verbally or in written form prior to or immediately at the start of instruction, the nurse-educator has information to decide what is the appropriate level to begin.

Teaching/Learning Activities and Resources. During this phase, the instructor plans what instructional methods (teaching and learning activities) and instructional resources will be most appropriate to help learners achieve the objectives. Since there is no accepted formula for matching instructional methods to objectives or content, as Kemp points out, competent educators must be familiar with various methods including self-instructional techniques. This means the educator not only plans in terms of what he or she does during the instruction but also what the student will be doing—hence, the term teaching/learning activities. Nurse-educators, therefore, should be familiar with and use not only psychological principles that promote learning in traditional teaching formats, such as lecture, demonstration, and discussion, but also a range of approaches to individualizing instruction.

Self-instructional strategies include self-learning modules, which can be films, videotapes, sound-slide programs, computer programs, printed programmed instruction units, and so on. Other strategies that are partially self-instructional and partially teacher-led include the Personalized System of Instruction,[13] the Audio-Tutorial System,[14] and Guided Design.[15]

Support Services. Scheduling facilities, arranging for audiovisual or practice equipment and health care supplies, getting the approval of administrators, acquiring funding, receiving the cooperation of colleagues—all of these essential support services must be included in planning. Sometimes the planning requires only arranging for handouts and tests to be duplicated. In other cases, it may necessitate the scheduling of rooms, equipment, projectionists, print materials, requesting adequate funds, and meeting with administrators and teaching colleagues. As all experienced educators have learned, the best ideas can be ruined by failure to plan for the necessary administrative, collegial, and technical support.

Evaluation. Kemp raises several evaluation issues that should be decided when planning instruction. What is the purpose of the evaluation: to measure the students' level of knowledge, to assess their skills or attitudes, to evaluate the teacher, to evaluate the overall course or educational program? How will the evaluation data be collected: paper/pencil tests, checklists, interviews, rating scales, questionnaires? If traditional tests are to be administered, what types of questions will be used: true/false, matching, multiple-choice, essay? If other means are to be used, what questions or items will be included on the checklist, interview form, rating scale, or questionnaire? How will the learners be judged: in terms of each other's performance (called grading on the curve or norm-referenced evaluation) or in terms of accomplishment of the stated objectives (called performance or criterion-referenced evaluation)?

Because the instructional design process is not foolproof, and instructional programs are seldom perfect, Kemp urges educators to plan for formative and summative evaluation. Formative evaluation data provide feedback to the teacher about the quality of the instruction itself. Formative evaluation is particularly useful when implementing new or modified instruction. The purpose is to provide insights to the educator on ways to improve the instruction further. Summative evaluation, on the other hand, is the gathering of information to assess the overall effectiveness of a new instructional program relative to a similar or perhaps prior program or to some established goal. The purpose here is to make a judgment about the success of the new program. (*See* Chapter 6 for further discussion).

Davis, Alexander, and Yelon Model for Instructional Design

Robert Davis, Lawrence Alexander, and Stephen Yelon[16] offer an approach to designing instruction that emphasizes learning principles within the design plan. Their major ideas are as follows:

1. Describe the current status of the instructional environment.
2. Derive and write the objectives.
3. Plan the evaluation.
4. Describe and analyze the tasks.
5. Incorporate principles of human learning and motivation.

While visually the model appears to be systematic and procedural, this is not the case. It is an example of the *systemic* approach. Recall that these authors referred to the design process as "iterative and interactive" and emphasize the cyclical nature of their model.

Describe the Current Status of the Instructional Environment. Here, the larger environment (for example, the nursing school, the hospital, the social service agency, the home) in which the instruction is to occur is examined to note changes underway, resources available to draw upon, and constraints that must be reckoned with. Interestingly, the authors cite the recent changes in nursing curricula based on new emerging roles for nurses as an example of how the environment, in this case the health field, does influence instructional programs. They also point out that potential resources in the teaching environment should be noted, for example, the availability of teaching assistants, laboratory monitors, instructional software, audiovisual hardware, classroom equipment, laboratories, client education areas, and specialists who consult with instructors about instructional design and teaching matters. Constraints are identified in terms of insufficient time to cover a topic adequately, restrictions on innovative teaching because of curricular demands, lack of personnel, space, or funds, numbers of learners, and traditional philosophies held by administrators.

The authors mention four instructional problems that students frequently encounter: unclear directions about what to study or why it's important, disorganized or trivial content, poor teaching methods (often reflected in a lack of motivation and interest), and unfair testing procedures. When teachers observe any of these problems in their own situations, they might consider examining their teaching in light of instructional design procedures.

Derive and Write the Objectives. In most cases, the educator decides what is to be taught and frames the content in terms of expected learning outcomes, or objectives. Davis, Alexander, and Yelon take a behavioral perspective toward stating learner objectives, but they provide one insight that would seem to be of interest to nurse educators. This is the notion of the "referent situation," that is, a typical situation outside of the classroom or laboratory where learners would be likely to use the content and the behaviors stated in the objective. Examples of referent situations are later courses in the curriculum, on-the-job activities, and general experiences in life. These authors believe that objectives ought not to be trivial or based solely on instructor interests or historical precedent but should have some potential utility at some point in the learner's life. Equally important, they advocate that the learners be informed of the referent situations the instructor has in mind. To assist teachers in devising and stating clear learning objectives, the authors created a guide for this purpose, which is presented in Figure 2–5.

Plan the Evaluation. Davis, Alexander, and Yelon feel instructors should plan to collect evaluation data at three points in time: prior to or at the beginning of the actual instruction, during the instruction, and at the end of the instruction.

Learners are evaluated prior to the instruction to determine if they possess the prerequisite knowledge or skill the instructor anticipated. Gathering these data tells the teacher how many of the learners possess the desired information and behaviors. The instructor then has several options: (1) to provide a brief review for students who studied the material previously but have forgotten it; (2) to provide remedial instruction at first and reduce the overall amount of regular instruction planned; (3) to permit only those who possess the entry behaviors to participate; (4) after informing all the learners of the evaluation results and the implications for their progress through the planned instruction, to let them individually decide if they wish to continue; or (5) to ignore the evaluation results and continue with the instruction as planned. The first three options seem most practical. The last one makes little sense from the instructional design perspective.

During the instruction, evaluation data are collected for two purposes: to provide feedback to the learner as he or she proceeds through the experience and to provide feedback to the instructor. In many instances, the same evaluation can serve both purposes. For example, testing (written, oral, and demonstration) provides feedback data that can be informative to the students and to the instructor. In-class exercises, homework assignments, and periodic student interviews can be helpful. A particular technique to provide feedback to the educator is the "periodic postclass questionnaire," which is simply a brief written questionnaire given at preplanned times during the training session or when the instructor feels that something is wrong.

Step I: Write a General Goal

Part A. Notes: What should students get from my course? ______

They should ______

Part B. Check: Did you state an outcome (not how to achieve the outcome)?

Yes ____ No ____

Step II: State a Referent Situation

Part A. Notes: Where will students use what they have learned? ______

______

Part B. Check: Is the goal important to the student in the referent situation?

Yes ____ No ____

Step III: Write a Referent Situation Test

Part A. Notes: If I could observe a student in the referent situation, how would I know whether he had achieved the goal? ______

Conditions: ______

Behavior: He would ______

Standards: So that ______

Part B. Checks: Do these conditions occur in the referent situation?

Yes ____ No ____

Is this behavior required in the referent situation?

Yes ____ No ____

Are these the standards used to judge performance in the referent situation?

Yes ____ No ____

Step IV: Write the Objective

Part A. Notes: How will I test students at the end of instruction?

Conditions: Given ______

Such as: ______

Aids or restrictions: ______

Test Behavior:

The student will ______

Standards (Use one or more of the following):

Time limit: ____ Speed: ____ Accuracy: ______

According to: ______

So well that: ______

Part B. Checks: Do the conditions closely approximate conditions in Step III?

Yes ____ No ____

Do the conditions affect performance? Yes ____ No ____

Is performance in behavioral terms? Yes ____ No ____

Is behavior a close approximation of behavior in Step III?

Yes ____ No ____

Do standards closely approximate standards in Step III?

Yes ____ No ____

Step V: Write Lower Limit of Performance Stability

Part A. Notes: On final test, how many chances will a student be given to show that he has achieved the objective? ______

______

What proportion of times must he succeed (e.g., 9/10)? ____

Part B.	Checks:	Is this proportion of successes needed in the referent situation?
		Yes ____ No ____
		Is this proportion of successes needed for retention?
		Yes ____ No ____
Step VI:	Check Your Objectives for Clarity	
Part A.	Notes:	Rewrite your objective here:
		Conditions: ____________________
		Behavior: ____________________
		Standards: ____________________
		Limits: ____________________
Part B.	Check:	If two of your colleagues looked at the above objective and a student's performance, could they agree whether or not the standards and limits had been achieved?
		Yes ____ No ____

Figure 2-5. Guide for Deriving and Writing Learning Objectives. (*From Davis RH, Alexander LT, Yelon SL: Learning System Design. New York, McGraw-Hill Book Co., 1974.*)

The questionnaire might ask the learners what they like best and least about the instruction, what changes they would suggest, and what concerns they have about the content.

At the end of instruction, the desired outcomes are evaluated in terms of student achievement and course effectiveness. Achievement is typically measured by formal testing that covers the course or unit objectives. The effectiveness of a course can be measured by the proportion of students who achieved the planned objectives and by learner opinions on the final periodic questionnaire at the end of instruction. In addition, students can provide feedback about the instructional strategies by emphasizing which ones to retain in the future and which to revise. The authors discuss many of the same concepts regarding test characteristics, design, and interpretation presented in Chapter 6.

Describe and Analyze Tasks. The authors advocate that instructors consider using techniques called task description and task analysis. The former was discussed earlier in this chapter with the example of the administration of intradermal injections. It is simply a description of how a task is performed. A task analysis, on the other hand, is a study of the task description by the instructor to identify the necessary learner entry characteristics, the types of learning involved to master the steps, and the special steps or conditions, if any, involved in performing the task. Ideally, the results of the analysis should yield prerequisite entry behaviors as well as the underlying concepts, principles, and skills that must be taught for learners to be able to perform the task.

Incorporate Principles of Human Learning and Motivation. Davis, Alexander, and Yelon, all learning psychologists, advocate that the instructor plan to incorporate principles of student learning and motivation into the instructional strategy. An explanation of these nine principles, derived from psychological experimentation and research, is presented in Table 2–2. Using these principles should result in effective learning and a positive attitude by the learners.

Briggs Model of Instructional Design

Leslie Briggs has edited a book that contains a model with similarities to others in this chapter. Presented below, the model describes a process for instructional design in traditional classroom situations.[17] A brief study of this model should reveal that many elements are similar to those in previous models.

1. Identify goals.
2. Organize the course.
3. Write objectives.
4. Prepare assessments of learner performance.
5. Analyze objectives.
6. Design instructional strategy.
7. Design lessons.
8. Design formative evaluation.

Identify Goals. On the surface, this element of the Briggs model would appear to be no different from the corresponding element in the Kemp model. Actually, there is a major difference. It will be recalled from the Kemp model that instructional goals are drawn from existing institutional documents, for example, curriculum guides, course and workshop descriptions, or accreditation guidelines. In other words, Kemp assumes the goals of the instruction are present in existing documents, and one job of the instructor is to locate them.

According to Briggs, however, the goals for instruction should be based on needs, where a need is defined as the discrepancy between the present state of affairs and the desired state of affairs. Stated differently, a need is the difference between the way things are and the way they ought to be. Suppose a goal for a baccalaureate degree in nursing is that all graduates will be able to write a nursing care plan; however, an evaluation of the senior class uncovers the fact that only 60 percent of them are able to do this at the acceptable standard. This discrepancy, or gap in performance, is labeled a "need." A potential learning need exists anytime there is a discrepancy between what a learner ought to know or be able to do and what the learner does know or can do. When learning needs are traced to a lack of skill or knowledge, they then can become the goals of the instruction.

TABLE 2-2. PRINCIPLES OF LEARNING AND MOTIVATION

Number	Principle
1	Students are more likely to be motivated to learn things that are meaningful to them. The instructor should relate the content to the learners' past experience or show its potential usefulness in their future.
2	Students are more likely to learn something new if they have all the prerequisites. The instructor should first analyze the instruction to determine the prerequisite knowledge and skills that are assumed; second, gather information from the learners to ascertain if they possess the prerequisites; and, third, teach the prerequisites to those who lack them.
3	Learners are more likely to acquire new behaviors if they are presented with a model performance to watch and imitate. Modeling is particularly effective in teaching technical procedures as well as social and professional roles. For example, effective instructors do not lecture about how to handle communication with problem patients; they demonstrate proper behaviors via live in-class role-plays or through appropriate media programs.
4	Students are more likely to learn if the presentation is structured so that the instructor's messages are open to the student. Give the learners written information about your objectives, course requirements, evaluation procedures, etc. Ask for feedback periodically. Use aural and video communications to get the subject across.
5	Students are more likely to learn if their attention is attracted by relatively novel presentations. Vary what the learner regularly sees and hears during instruction. Use a variety of instructional strategies, e.g., discussion, role-play, case study, self-instruction materials, lecture, demonstration, audiovisual presentations, etc.
6	Students are more likely to learn if they take an active part in the practice geared to reach the objective. Too often teaching means an active instructor and passive learners. Students should be actively involved—either overtly or covertly. During lectures, occasionally ask questions or pose a problem relevant to the content to stimulate the learners to think about the subject. Consider using various instructional strategies as mentioned in principle 5.
7	Students are more likely to learn if the practice is scheduled in short sessions distributed over time. This principle is self-explanatory. Discourage students from cramming or practicing new skills for extended periods.
8	Students are more likely to learn if the instructional prompts are withdrawn gradually. When students are first learning a new skill or concept, provide hints—for example, mnemonics—to assist them. As they gain confidence and skill, gradually reduce the prompts and hints.
9	Students are more likely to continue learning if the instructional conditions are made pleasant. Try to create a pleasant learning situation by controlling environmental factors like temperature and noise. Model enthusiasm and respect for the content and the learners. Give the learners feedback regarding their performance during the instruction as well as at the conclusion.

From Davis RH, Alexander LT, Yelon SL: Learning System Design. New York, McGraw-Hill Book Co., 1974.

When needs are uncovered, the alternatives are to: (1) ignore them, (2) reduce the stated goal to match the actual state of affairs, or (3) try to raise the current performance to match the desired goal. When the last option is selected, the inappropriate or missing performance should be studied to determine the cause. The cause may be a lack of incentive or motivation to perform, negative consequences for performing, a lack of knowledge or skill, or some combination of these. Only when the cause is traced to a deficiency in knowledge or skill is instructional design the appropriate solution. (Readers interested in solutions to other types of performance problems might examine two references listed in the bibliography, Mager and Pipe: *Analyzing Performance Problems*, and Gilbert: *Human Competence*.)

Briggs recommends that those individuals involved in needs assessment represent as many constituencies as are affected. In the case of nursing education, the group might consist of representatives of the faculty, students, administration, graduates, and practitioners. In hospital staff development, a committe of employees, administrators, and perhaps community representatives might be the best. With regard to client education programs, those involved would surely include the client educators, the practitioners, other involved members of the health care team, and perhaps client representatives.

How does one do a needs assessment? Briggs suggests a four-step process. First, the group should identify a range of desirable goals for a particular educational program. This might be accomplished through structured brainstorming sessions, surveys, or questionnaires. The purpose is to state the desirable goals in measurable terms with performance criteria. Second, rank the goals in some numerical way that represents the group consensus as to what goals are most important. Third, measure actual learner performance against these goals to determine if any discrepancies appear. Use the performance criteria specified in step one to help determine if significant discrepancies exist. Some ways to measure actual performance are paper-and-pencil tests, simulations, and performance ratings. Fourth, if discrepancies are detected, the group must determine if they are significant and, if so, which are most serious. The result is a list of identified needs ranked in order of importance. The final decision of the group is to determine which needs (discrepancies) to attack first. One criterion to consider is cost—what is the cost if the need is not addressed and what is it if it is. Costs can be thought of in terms of money, personnel, work, prestige, and so forth. Other cost considerations include the number of learners involved, the estimated time to correct the need, and the overall severity of the need. Once specific needs are identified and their etiologies are traced to a lack of knowledge or skill, the needs become goals and instructional design can begin.

Organize the Course. Briggs uses the term *course* as a reference to the total planned instruction, which may be as brief as a workshop or as long as a college semester. He acknowledges there is little research evidence to guide the instructor in organizing a course, but suggests that several options be considered. One way is to organize it around the needs uncovered during the needs assessment process. Another is to base it on broad goals stated in behavioral terms. A third is to build it around lifelong objectives—those cognitive, affective, and psychomotor skills that will aid the learner throughout life. A fourth method is to develop specific end-of-course objectives, prepare the final examinations, and then build the course content around these. Fifth, the course might be divided into units, an arbitrary delineation based on specific competencies to be mastered or content topics to be learned. The sixth method is to base the course entirely on lists of behavioral objectives, which are sequenced to lead the learner through increasingly more difficult material.

Write Objectives. Briggs is unique among the authors of instructional design models presented in this chapter in that he eschews the behavioral approach in favor of a cognitive orientation.[18] The major difference is that this approach does not focus exclusively on behavior. Rather, it emphasizes five domains of "learning capabilities" that a student can acquire during instruction. Table 2-3 contains the domains, the prescribed action verb for each, and nursing examples. Note there are five major categories of capabilities, with one category broken into four subsets, to create an overall list of nine capabilities and nine action verbs matched to the capabilities. By focusing on the capabilities, the educator can select from a range of behaviors that would be acceptable indicators of a particular capability.

This approach provides the nurse-educator with an alternative to the traditional behavioral way of formulating instructional objectives. It also encourages the instructor to think not only of discrete behaviors but also the higher-order mental processing that is often required for many nursing concepts, principles, and skills.

TABLE 2-3. RELATIONSHIP OF LEARNING DOMAINS AND COGNITIVE CAPABILITY VERBS

Learner Domain	Capability Verbs	Examples
Intellectual Domain		
a. Discrimination	Discriminate	Discriminates, by matching the appropriate disease process with the abnormal lab values.
b. Concrete concept	Identify	Identifies, by naming, the four basic food groups.
c. Refined concept	Classify	Classifies, by using a definition, the concept "family."
d. Rule using	Demonstrate	Demonstrates, by solving written examples, calculation of drug dosages.
e. Problem solving	Generate	Generates, by synthesizing pertinent data, a list of nursing diagnoses.
Cognitive strategy domain	Originate	Originates a solution to the stress of parenting by applying principles of anticipatory guidance.
Informative domain	State	States orally the major steps in performing a newborn assessment.
Motor skill domain	Execute	Executes insertion of a urethral catheter, using sterile technique.
Attitude domain	Choose	Chooses to pursue employment in a hospice with terminally ill clients.

From Briggs L (ed): Instructional Design. Englewood Cliffs, NJ, Educational Technology Publications, 1979.

Prepare Learner Assessments. Like all the previous authors of models, Briggs advocates that the evaluation items and the learner objectives should be highly congruent. For this reason he suggests that the assessment methods and procedures be created soon after specifying the course objectives.

Analyze the Objectives. All educators face a similar dilemma: what to teach and how best to teach it. The answers can be found in a thorough analysis of the objectives. Specifically, three types of analyses are suggested. One is called information-processing analysis, which is best suited for understanding procedural tasks, for example, surgical gloving techniques. The instructor who employs this method observes himself or herself or a competent colleague performing the task and notes all the discrete steps that are performed. Flow charts are sometimes useful when the procedures are very complex. A second technique for analyzing objectives is to examine them in light of an accepted taxonomy of learning. (See Bloom, Hastings, Madaus: *Handbook on Formative and Summative Evaluation of Student Learning*, and Gagné: *The Conditions of Learning,* in the bibliography.) Unfortunately, there are no specific guidelines for matching the objectives to specific components of taxonomies. The third method is labeled learning task analysis. Here the educator looks for the prerequisite skills that are assumed by the objective. Once the prerequisite skills are identified, they are sequenced in terms of what the learner must recall from previous learning and what new skills the learner must acquire through the instruction. Prerequisite skills may be classified as either essential or supportive if new learning is to occur. Essential prerequisites, as the name implies, are those that the learner must possess in order to learn the new objectives. For example, the ability to subtract is one essential prerequisite to learning the skill of long division. Supportive prerequisites, on the other hand, are skills that may assist the learner to master new learning objectives. For instance, a positive attitude toward oneself and others may help the nursing student learn effective communication skills more easily.

Regardless of which technique is used, the desired result of the analysis of the objectives is a better understanding of what prior skills must first be mastered and a categorization of the new learning into one of the five domains.

Design Instructional Strategy. The intent of this activity is to arrive at the most effective sequence of instructional techniques to move the learner toward accomplishing the desired objectives. This is accomplished by first identifying the enabling objectives (essential and enabling prerequisites) for each major learning objective and then deciding in what order to teach them. The next task is to select the teaching activities, called events of instruction, to help the learners acquire the desired learned capability and to perform it at an acceptable level. These steps or events have been labeled by Gagné and Briggs as follows: (1) gain the learners attention; (2) inform the learner of the objective; (3) stimulate the learner to recall relevant prerequisite learnings; (4) present the new material; (5) provide learning guidance; (6) elicit the performance from the learner; (7) provide feedback about the performance to the learner; repeat step 6 if necessary; (8) assess the final performance; and (9) enhance the learner's retention and transfer.[19]

These events may be prompted by the teacher directly, by the group activities planned by the teacher, or by the instructional materials selected or developed by the instructor.

Thus, the instructional strategy consists of, first, the sequencing of instruction for each objective and, second, selecting the instructional events to be used to help the learner master objectives.

Design Lessons. Briggs outlines six steps in planning an individual lesson: (1) identify the objectives, (2) list the desired activities for each instructional event, (3) select the most appropriate media, (4) select the most appropriate materials, (5) analyze the materials and activities for the events of instruction they supply, and (6) plan other means for the remaining events of instruction. He also points out that while the instructor can (and often does) carry out all of these steps, some can be accomplished through the selection of appropriate mediated materials and learner-centered activities. Well-designed instructional media (for instance, a sound-slide program) can present the stimulus materials, guide the learning, elicit the performance, and provide feedback to the learner.

It must be realized, of course, that the mediated materials are simply an extension of the instructor. It is the instructor who either selects or creates instructional materials because they provide the appropriate events of instruction equal to or better than the live teacher.

Design Formative Evaluation. The ideas presented by Briggs on this component of the instructional design process are similar to those described in Chapter 6.

Dick and Carey Model of Instructional Design

Walter Dick and Lou Carey created a specific model for designing self-instructional programs or modules.[20] The authors define a module as a self-contained unit that has the following characteristics: (a) an integrated theme, (b) objectives, (c) content information, (d) learning activities, and (e) tests. It typically serves as one part of a larger course, training program, or curriculum. A self-instructional module on foot care for the diabetic patient, for instance, might consist of a teacher's guide, a patient's manual, a videorecording that demonstrates the correct procedures, and an evaluation component. Well-designed modules do not simply ask the learner to passively read or observe materials, but rather the learner works interactively with them. The learner is required to perform appropriate learning tasks and there is some type of evaluation/feedback strategy. The onus is on the creator of self-instructional modules to demonstrate that they in fact teach and result in behavioral changes. Therefore, modules must be validated, that is, tested to insure that they produce learning. Dick and Carey caution educators who wish to design self-instructional modules to have a firm grasp of the content, to select a topic that can

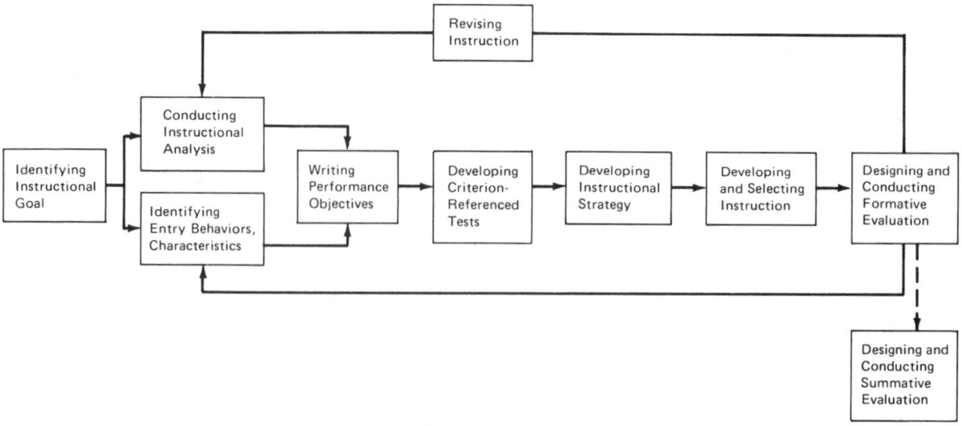

Figure 2-6. The Dick and Carey systems approach model for designing instruction. *(From Dick W, Carey L: The Systematic Design of Instruction, ed 2. Glenview, IL, Scott, Foresman, & Co., 1985.)*

be taught in a reasonable amount of time (several hours), and to have learners available to provide feedback to them during the evaluation phase. This model of instructional design is presented in Figure 2-6.

Identifying Instructional Goals. The goals for a module can be derived from existing documents, like curriculum guides and job descriptions, through communication with colleagues, students and clients, and from observations in the classroom and clinic. The goal should be stated at the beginning of the module and should clearly describe what the learner will be able to know, do, or feel after completing it.

Conducting Instructional Analysis. The purpose of this element is to insure that the educator identifies all the relevant skills and subskills that are essential if the learner is to achieve the goal. For content that is primarily procedural (for example, making a bed), the most effective way for the educator to analyze it fully is to walk through the task slowly, noting each step and decision in the sequence. Another method is to observe and interview experts as they complete the task. A third but less desirable option is to use descriptions prepared by others. Care must be taken not to accept such descriptions on face value. Though experts may have prepared the descriptions, it does not mean that they will be useful to new learners. Many of us have felt the frustration of trying to assemble a toy or appliance by following the written directions of some "expert" who did not understand the instructional design process! An example of a procedural analysis appeared earlier in this chapter in the task description for administering intradermal injections.

For activities that are not procedural in nature, Dick and Carey favor a hierarchical approach. Here one identifies the critical subskills a learner must master

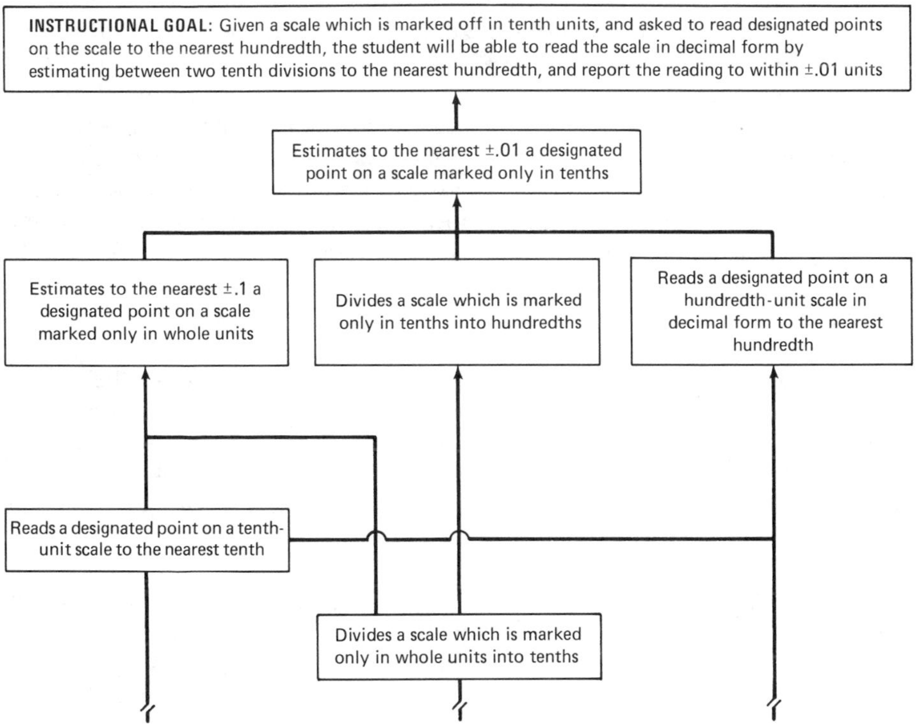
INSTRUCTIONAL GOAL: Given a scale which is marked off in tenth units, and asked to read designated points on the scale to the nearest hundredth, the student will be able to read the scale in decimal form by estimating between two tenth divisions to the nearest hundredth, and report the reading to within ±.01 units
Estimates to the nearest ±.01 a designated point on a scale marked only in tenths
Estimates to the nearest ±.1 a designated point on a scale marked only in whole units
Divides a scale which is marked only in tenths into hundredths
Reads a designated point on a hundredth-unit scale in decimal form to the nearest hundredth
Reads a designated point on a tenth-unit scale to the nearest tenth
Divides a scale which is marked only in whole units into tenths

Figure 2-7. Portion of a hierarchical analysis for reading a scale. *(From Dick W, Carey L: The Systematic Design of Instruction, ed 2. Glenview, IL, Scott, Foresman & Co., 1985.)*

to achieve the desired higher-level skill. Figure 2–7 shows an example of the subordinate concepts and skills learners must process in order to read a scale, which is the goal of one section of a module.

Notice in Figure 2–7 that the authors not only listed the fundamental intellectual skills necessary to read a scale but also arranged them in relationship to each other. Specifically, the more elementary skills are listed at the bottom and the more sophisticated near the top. A content analysis such as this not only reveals the essential information that must be presented to the learner but also gives the teacher insight into what ideas or skills should be taught first, second, third, and so forth to help the learner grasp the overall objective.

Dick and Carey stress the importance of a thorough analysis because the instruction will be delivered in a self-learning mode and therefore must be as clear as possible. They suggest the educator discuss the analysis with knowledgeable colleagues or professional instructional designers to help insure its accuracy.

Identifying Entry Behaviors and Characteristics. Learners bring to instructional training situations a culmination of their past learning and experiences. These are referred to by Dick and Carey as entry behaviors. In addition, the learners have other general characteristics that influence their learning, such as age, maturity level, general intellectual ability, and preferred learning style. All of these factors should be taken into account by the nurse-educator so that the self-instructional module begins at the optimal level and teaches in a motivating and interesting way. Educators sometimes err by overestimating or underestimating the learner's entry behaviors about a subject. These erroneous assumptions can result in learner frustration and poor performance because the instruction is either too advanced or too elementary. To determine the entry behaviors of a group, selected learners can be interviewed and tested. Otherwise, the designer can only estimate the entry level, build the module, and plan to revise it later.

Writing Performance Objectives. Like Kemp, Dick and Carey favor the behavioral approach to writing performance objectives. They do acknowledge, however, the worthiness of the "learned capabilities" approach advocated by Briggs. The objectives are based on a combination of the goals, the instructional analysis, the assumed learner characteristics, the difficulty of the subject matter, and the time estimated to complete the module.

Developing Criterion-Referenced Tests. The tests that accompany the instructional materials are designed with two purposes in mind: (1) to evaluate the learner's progress through the module and (2) to provide feedback to the educator-designer about the effectiveness of the module. The tests are objective-referenced, meaning they are based on the objectives of the module.

The authors believe four types of tests should be planned: an entry test, a pretest, an embedded test, and a posttest. An *entry test* measures the knowledge and skill levels the educator sets as prerequisites for studying the module. The learner must perform adequately on the entry test in order to study the module. Those who do not pass the entry test would be directed to other learning experiences.

A *pretest* determines how much of the content contained in the module is already known by the learner. If the learner has already mastered the content, it is not necessary to study the module. On the other hand, poor performance on the pretest indicates the learner will benefit from studying the module. Pretest questions are drawn from the content in the module as well as derived from the overall objectives.

It should be noted that the entry test and the pretest need not be two physically separate tests. Questions focusing on both areas can be intermingled in the same test form. The educator, however, must be aware of which items represent each area when the test results are calculated.

The third type of test is the *embedded test*. This is not a single test. Rather, it is a series of questions placed strategically at points throughout the module. Embedded tests serve two functions: to inform the learner about his or her progress and to provide feedback to the educator about the teaching effectiveness of the modular materials and activities.

The fourth test, called the *posttest,* is identical to, or an alternative form of, the pretest. Its main purpose is to measure how well the learners met the module's objectives. The posttest results tell the learner if the objectives were met or if further study is required, while they give the module designer an indicator of its effectiveness.

Procedures for writing test items, evaluating test items and constructing various types of tests are described more fully in Chapter 6.

Developing an Instructional Strategy. In traditional instruction, the text material (books, articles, handouts) serve primarily as sources of information, whereas the instructor defines the objectives, motivates the learners, presents supplemental information, administers the tests, and so on. With self-instruction, these same teaching activities are all designed into the module.

Self-instructional modules (or modular instruction) typically consist of several components or instructional strategies.

Preinstructional Activities. The goal here is to motivate the student to want to use the module. Some learners may be self-motivated, of course, but others may require encouragement. The preinstructional strategies should describe how the learners will be able to use the information when they have successfully completed the module. The prospective learner might be told how the information within the module can affect his or her professional career or life-style. Some learners may be motivated by knowing how much knowledge they already possess based on the pretest scores.

Information Presentation. This component deals with how much information to include in the module and in what order to present it. Unfortunately, there are no reliable guidelines for planning how extensive the content should be. A common error is to present too much information. Certainly the characteristics of the learners, the objectives, and the time available for studying should be taken into account. Beyond that, the educator can solicit the opinions of colleagues and professional instructional designers who have had experience with this type of teaching strategy. Ultimately, the feedback received from the learners and the posttest performances will give some clue as to the appropriate amount of information. In terms of sequencing the instruction, there are no rules, only heuristics. Procedures are usually taught from beginning to end; however, teaching the final step first and then working backwards can also be effective. Hierarchical learning is best achieved if the prerequisites and subordinate skills are taught first, followed by the progressively more complex higher-order skills.

Student Participation. Designing instruction with the intent of involving the learners is crucial. Passive learning in self-instructional modules will often cause the learners, with the exception of the most highly motivated, to abandon the exercise. The educator who creates self-instructional modules builds in opportunities for the learner to practice (overtly or covertly) and to receive feedback. The learner might be directed at some point in the module to observe a procedure, watch a film, interview a client, or answer questions placed within the module. The principles of learning and motivation advocated by Davis, Alexander, and Yelon[21] can be readily applied to designing the learning activities that are incorporated within the instructional package.

Testing. Testing occurs throughout a module, beginning with the entry tests and ending with the posttest. The critical feature seems to be that the learner is given feedback after each test. Learner performance on the tests also provides feedback to the educator as to what portions of the module may need revisions and improvements.

Follow-through Activities. Follow-through activities include materials or recommendations for further study of the content. For learners who performed above a specified level on the posttest, enrichment study may be recommended. For those whose performance was lacking, remedial study activities can be suggested.

Developing Instructional Materials. Dick and Carey recommended that the educator plan to develop four types of materials: (1) learner materials that contain the goals, objectives, content to be learned, and participation activities (these can take the form of written documents and/or mediated materials, such as video, slide, or computer programs); (2) learner manuals, which provide the rationale for the module and directions on how to use the materials; (3) testing materials that include the entry test, pretest, embedded tests, and posttest; and (4) instructor guides for educators who wish to use the module. The guide describes the overall module, discusses how it can be used, and contains copies of all necessary print materials.

Designing and Conducting Formative Evaluation. Formative evaluation is the process of collecting information to revise and improve instructional modules to make them as effective as possible. Typically, such evaluation involves three phases. The first is one-to-one evaluation in which the educator who designed the module asks individual volunteer learners (who have similar characteristics to the target learner group) to work through draft versions of the materials and tests. The learners are encouraged to tell the educator when they find the directions unclear or are unsure of what to do next. The educator notes where the learners make errors and omissions. Also during this phase, the educator-designer may ask colleagues and other content experts to check the subject matter contained in the module for accuracy and timeliness.

During the second phase, the designer meets with a small group of students who are representative of the target group and administers the modular components as they would be used in an actual situation. The designer notes general and specific problems the learners encounter. Later, the students are interviewed to determine their attitude toward the module and to gather their suggestions for revision and improvement.

The third phase of the recommended evaluation process is a field trial. Here the designer observes another instructor using the module with an actual learner group. Again, any problems are noted and corrections made.

Revising Instructional Materials. Based on the data collected during the formative evaluation phases, decisions are made regarding the content of the materials and the instructional procedures used. For example, pretest and posttest scores are compared, embedded tests are studied to determine if the learners had difficulties working through the materials, and information gathered during learner interviews are reviewed. All of this information is used to make decisions about revising the materials. Extensive modifications may mean that another field test is advisable.

Summative Evaluation and Grading. Summative evaluation is the process of collecting information for the purpose of determining the worth of the instructional module. Ideally, the unit can be used by instructors who were not involved in the design or formative evaluation phases. Pretest and posttest data are again collected, but this time the reason for doing so is to demonstrate the effectiveness of the module. Sometimes the module can be compared with another form of instruction or some attribute of the module can be studied.

SUMMARY

Four models for designing instruction have been described. Each is unique in terms of the overall approach as well as specific phases within it. All, however, exhibit some common characteristics: goals, objectives, presentation techniques, feedback, and evaluation. These models can be used when planning traditional classroom instruction, clinical and laboratory exercises, client education, and continuing nursing education programs. The competent instructor stays current with new developments in instructional design and applies those procedures that apply to the situation at hand. It therefore behooves health care educators not only to be competent in their disciplines but also to be aware of developments in instructional design approaches and their application to foster learning.

IMPLICATIONS FOR RESEARCH

There are many opportunities for research in the area of instructional design. Needs assessment studies could be conducted at theoretical and applied levels. Investigations of learner characteristics, in particular, learning styles of nursing students, nursing practitioners, and clients may be fruitful, as outlined by Ostmoe, et al.[22] While the effects of learning objectives alone have been the object of extensive research efforts,[23] their contribution within the overall design process is not clear. Similarly, individual teaching methods have been researched,[24] but not within the context of instructional systems.

The advent of computer-assisted instruction and interactive video and audio technologies provides a wealth of opportunities for developing and testing new instructional approaches. Many questions about developing and incorporating computerized strategies into the nursing curriculum remain.

A particular area ripe for concerted research is continuing education in nursing and all professional fields. While the area of testing has received much attention from researchers, the broader concept of evaluation, particularly as it applies to developing and assessing the effectiveness and efficiency of instructional options, has not been investigated thoroughly.

Different types of research designs are needed. The experimental approach has received the most attention in the past, but survey, descriptive, and ethnographic studies may also be helpful.

The field of instructional design is evolving and growing. While many of the ideas discussed in this chapter will likely withstand the test of time, new concepts and techniques will surely emerge and change the way we currently view instruction and the teaching/learning process. Nursing educators who possess a firm grasp of instructional design processes will be on the forefront of these advances.

POSTTEST

1. Explain the similarities between the nursing process and the instructional development process.
2. Define the following terms as they relate to teaching: design; development; implementation; evaluation.
3. List at least four assumptions about teaching and learning inherent in most instructional design models.
4. List the five components that are considered crucial when designing (planning) effective instruction.
5. What is the difference between learning objectives and teaching objectives?
6. List the three categories of learning objectives and describe each of them.
7. What is the rationale for planning (designing) instruction in terms of learning objectives?
8. What do the techniques of task description and task analysis have in common?
9. List at least three ways information might be organized for instructional purposes.
10. Why is it important for nurse-educators to be knowledgeable about a variety of teaching strategies?
11. Explain the purposes of formative and summative evaluation.
12. How do the systematic and systemic philosophies for designing instruction differ?

13. List the steps in the Kemp model.
14. List the steps in the Davis, Alexander, and Yelon model.
15. List the steps in the Briggs model.
16. List the steps in the Dick and Carey model.
17. What features do each of the above four models have in common?

POSTTEST ANSWER KEY

1. Each is an example of the general problem-solving process. Specifically, each calls for the initial diagnosis of need, the gathering of further information, the development, implementation, and evaluation of a plan of action, the assessment of the effectiveness of the action, and recycling through the process if necessary.
2. *Design:* Planning the instruction

   Development: Creating or acquiring the instructional materials (lecture outlines, handouts, tests, films, slides, modules, computer programs, and so on)

   Implementation: Delivery of the instruction via either live or mediated (contrived) formats

   Evaluation: Gathering data for the purpose of determining the effectiveness of the instruction.
3. a. The teacher bears equal responsibility with the students for the learning that occurs during instruction.
   b. Planning will help the teacher meet this responsibility.
   c. The teacher's primary role is to facilitate learning rather than functioning solely as a dispenser of information.
   d. The learners should be informed at the beginning of the instruction of what they are expected to know and/or be able to do at the end of the instruction.
   e. The teacher should be adept at using a variety of teaching methods to help learners master the content.
   f. Evaluation data should be collected to provide feedback that the teacher can use to improve instruction.
4. Instructional objectives, subject content, instructional strategies, evaluation methods.
5. Learning objectives are stated in terms of what the learner should know, do, or feel following the instruction. Teaching objectives, on the other hand, focus on what the teacher wishes to accomplish during the instruction. The learning objectives and the teaching objectives should complement each other.
6. The three categories of objectives are: cognitive, affective, and psychomotor.

Cognitive objectives focus on mental processes like remembering facts, comparing and contrasting different viewpoints, synthesizing new information, and so forth. Affective objectives deal with feelings, beliefs, and attitudes. Psychomotor objectives are concerned with skills, like giving injections, making a bed, drawing blood, and so on.

7. Learning is more likely to occur when the instruction is presented in terms of the learning objectives and the learners are aware of what is expected of them.
8. Both are methods nurse-educators can use to determine the appropriate information (subject content) to include in an instructional program.
9. Information (subject content) might be organized in the following ways: (1) beginning to end, (2) simple to complex, (3) historically, and (4) concrete to abstract.
10. Teaching strategies provide the conditions for learning. The combination of the instructional objectives, the characteristics of the learner(s), subject content, the resources available, the setting, and so on influence the selection of teaching strategies most appropriate for a given situation. Therefore, nurse-educators should be not only knowledgeable about a variety of teaching strategies but also adept at using them.
11. Formative evaluation, as it applies to instruction, is the gathering of information to determine the effectiveness of a teaching strategy or technique to ascertain how it might be improved. Summative evaluation, on the other hand, usually connotes the gathering of information to pass judgment or make a final decision.
12. The systematic philosophy of designing instruction views the process as procedural and lockstep; all steps in the process are completed in a prescribed sequence. The systemic philosophy, on the other hand, sees the design process as an interactive and dynamic one and believes that it matters little where one begins or ends but that all the elements within the process are addressed at some point during the planning process.
13. The steps in the Kemp model are:
    a. Goals, topics, general purposes
    b. Learner characteristics
    c. Learning objectives
    d. Subject content
    e. Preassessment of learners
    f. Teaching/learning activities and resources
    g. Support services
    h. Evaluation
14. The steps in the Davis, Alexander, and Yelon model are:
    a. Describe the current status of the instructional environment
    b. Derive and write objectives
    c. Plan the evaluation
    d. Describe and analyze the tasks
    e. Incorporate principles of human learning and motivation

15. The steps in the Briggs model are:
    a. Identify goals
    b. Organize the course
    c. Write objectives
    d. Prepare learner assessments
    e. Analyze objectives
    f. Design instructional strategy
    g. Design lessons
    h. Design formative evaluations
16. The steps in the Dick and Carey model are:
    a. Identifying instructional goals
    b. Conducting instructional analysis
    c. Identifying entry behaviors and characteristics
    d. Writing performance objectives
    e. Developing criterion-referenced tests
    f. Developing an instructional strategy
    g. Developing the instructional materials
    h. Designing and conducting the formative evaluation
    i. Revising the instructional materials
    j. Summative evaluation and grading
17. All of the models emphasize goals, objectives, instructional strategies, and evaluation.

SUGGESTED APPLICATION ACTIVITIES

1. Regularly peruse selected journals in nursing, related fields, and education that deal with instructional design issues. Some suggestions are: *The Journal of Nursing Education, Nurse Educator, Journal of Medical Education, Journal of Instructional Development,* and *Educational Technology*.
2. Create a plan for a brief unit of instruction (no more than several hours) using one of the models described in this chapter. Show the plan to a colleague for feedback.
3. After you fully develop an instructional unit following instructional design procedures, try it out in an actual situation and gather the evaluation data. Determine if the unit is effective.
4. Become familiar with several of the instructional strategies discussed in this chapter and try using them in your teaching.
5. Select one element in the instructional design process (for example, needs assessment, objectives, learner characteristics, instructional strategies) that interests you and gather in-depth information about it from journals and texts.

6. Systematically compare and contrast the instructional design models presented in this chapter to highlight the distinctive features of each.
7. Read some of the interesting references in the bibliography at the end of this chapter.
8. Attend presentations and conferences, or take a course that focuses on topics relevant to the design of instruction.
9. Plan a research project dealing with some aspect of instructional design in nursing.
10. Choose a topic and write at least five behavioral objectives for each of the three learning domains. Construct a grid to see what level each of your objectives fits. Refer to relevant references in the bibliography to explore writing objectives.
11. Select a topic and write a task description, content analysis, and task analysis.
12. Discuss the topics of education and instruction.

REFERENCES

1. Andrews D, Goodson L: Comparative Analysis of Models of Instructional Design, Journal of Instructional Development 53: 2–16, 1980.
2. Bloom BS, et al.: Cognitive Domain, Taxonomy of Educational Objectives, Handbook 1. New York, David McKay Co., Inc. 1956.
3. Eisner E: Instructional Expressive Objectives: Their Formulation and Use in Curriculum. In J Popham (ed), Instructional Objectives: An Analyses of Emerging Issues. Chicago, Rand McNally Co., 1969.
4. Rankin MA: Administering Intradermal Injections. Unpublished paper, The University of Iowa, 1984 p. 4.
5. Ortin J, Neuhaus O: Human Biochemistry. St. Louis, C.V. Mosby Co., 1982, p. 670.
6. Davis RH, Alexander LT, Yelon SL: Learning System Design. New York, McGraw-Hill Book Co., 1974, p. 313.
7. Kemp J: Instructional Design, ed 2. Belmont, CA, Fearon Publishers, Inc., 1977, p. 9.
8. Bloom BS, et al.: Cognitive Domain, Taxonomy of Educational Objectives, Handbook 1. New York, David McKay Co., Inc., 1956.
9. Kibler R, Barker L, Miles D: Behavioral Objectives and Instruction. Boston, Allyn & Bacon, Inc. 1970.
10. Krathwohl D, et al.: Affective Domain, Taxonomy of Educational Objectives. Handbook 2. New York, David McKay Co., Inc. 1964.
11. Mager R: Preparing Instructional Objectives, ed 2. Belmont, CA, Fearon Publishers, Inc., 1975.
12. Gagné R: The Conditions of Learning, ed 4. New York, Holt, Rinehart & Winston, 1985.
13. Keller F, Gilmore S: The Keller Plan Book. Menlo Park, CA, W.A. Benjamin, Inc., 1974.
14. Postlethwaite SN, Novak J, Murray H: The Audio-Tutorial Approach to Learning. Minneapolis, MN, Burgess Publishing Co., 1972.
15. Wales C, Stager R: The Guided Design Approach. Englewood, Cliffs, NJ, Educational Technology Publications, 1978.
16. Davis RH, Alexander LT, Yelon SL: Learning System Design. New York, McGraw-Hill Book Co., 1974, pp. 23–24.

17. Briggs L (ed): Instructional Design. Englewood Cliffs, NJ, Educational Technology Publications, 1979, p. 12.
18. Gagné R, Briggs L: Principles of Instructional Design, ed 2. New York, Holt, Rinehart & Winston, 1979.
19. Ibid.
20. Dick W, Carey L: The Systematic Design of Instruction, ed 2. Glenview, IL, Scott, Foresman & Co., 1985, pp. 2–3.
21. Davis RH, Alexander LT, Yelon, SL: Learning System Design. New York, McGraw-Hill Book Co., 1974, pp. 197–218.
22. Ostmoe PM, et al.: Learning Style Preferences and Selection of Learning Strategies: Considerations and Implications for Nurse Educators. Journal of Nursing Education 23: 27–30, 1984.
23. Briggs L (ed): Instructional Design. Englewood Cliffs, NJ, Educational Technology Publications, 1979.
24. Kemp J: Instructional Design. ed 2. Belmont, CA, Fearon Publishers, Inc., 1977.

BIBLIOGRAPHY

Andrews, D, Goodson L: Comparative Analysis of Models of Instructional Design. Journal of Instructional Development 3: 2–16, 1980.

Banathy B: Instructional Systems. Belmont, CA, Fearon Publishers, Inc., 1968.

Bloom BS, Hastings J, Madaus G: Handbook on Formative and Summative Evaluation of Student Learning. New York, McGraw-Hill Book Co., 1971.

Bloom BS, et al.: Cognitive Domain, Taxonomy of Educational Objectives, Handbook 1. New York, David McKay Co., Inc., 1956.

Briggs, L (ed): Instructional Design. Englewood Cliffs, NJ, Educational Technology Publications, 1979.

Davis, RH, Alexander LT, Yelon SL: Learning System Design. New York, McGraw-Hill Book Co., 1974.

Dick W, Carey L: The Systematic Design of Instruction, ed 2. Glenview, IL: Scott, Foresman & Co., 1985.

Eisner E: Instructional Expressive Objectives: Their Formulation and Use in Curriculum. In J Popham (ed), Instructional Objectives: An Analysis of Emerging Issues. Chicago, Rand McNally & Co., 1969.

Foley R, Smilansky J: Teaching Techniques: A Handbook for Health Professionals. New York, McGraw-Hill Book Co., 1980.

Ford CW (ed): Clinical Education for the Allied Health Professionals. St. Louis, C.V. Mosby Co., 1978.

Ford CW, Morgan MK (eds): Teaching in the Health Professions. St. Louis, C.V. Mosby Co., 1976.

Gagné R: The Conditions of Learning, ed 4. New York, Holt, Rinehart & Winston, 1985.

Gagné R, Briggs L: Principles of Instructional Design, ed 2. New York, Holt, Rinehart & Winston, 1979.

Gerlach VS, Ely DP: Teaching and Media: A Systems Approach. Englewood Cliffs, NJ, Prentice-Hall, Inc., 1971.

Gilbert T: Human Competence. New York, McGraw-Hill Book Co., 1978.

Guinee K: The Aims and Methods of Nursing Education. New York, Macmillan, Inc. 1966.

Huckabay LMD: Conditions of Learning and Instruction in Nursing. St. Louis, C.V. Mosby Co., 1980.

Keller F, Gilmore S: The Keller Plan Book. Menlo Park, CA, W.A. Benjamin, Inc., 1974.

Kemp J: Instructional Design, ed 2. Belmont, CA: Fearon Publishers, Inc., 1977.

Kibler R, Barker L, Miles D: Behavioral Objectives and Instruction. Boston, MA, Allyn & Bacon, Inc., 1970.

Knopke HJ, Diekelmann NL: Approaches to Teaching in the Health Sciences. Reading, MA, Addison-Wesley Publishing Co., Inc., 1978.

Krathwohl DR, et al.: Affective Domain, Taxonomy of Educational Objectives, Handbook 2. New York, David McKay Co., Inc., 1964.

Mager R: Preparing Instructional Objectives, ed 2. Belmont, CA, Fearon Publishers, Inc., 1975.

Mager R, Pipe P: Analyzing Performance Problems: Or, You Really Oughta Wanna. Belmont, CA: Fearon Publishers, Inc., 1970.

Ortin J, Neuhaus O: Human Biochemistry. St. Louis, C.V. Mosby Co., 1982.

Ostmoe PM, et al.: Learning Style Preferences and Selection of Learning Strategies: Considerations and Implications for Nurse Educators. Journal of Nursing Education 23: 27–30, 1984.

Postlethwaite SN, Novak J, Murray H: The Audio-Tutorial Approach to Learning. Minneapolis, MN, Burgess Publishing Company, 1972.

Rankin M: Administering Intradermal Injections. Unpublished paper, The University of Iowa, 1984.

Segall AJ, Vanderschmidt H, et al.: Systematic Course Design for the Health Fields. New York, John Wiley & Sons, Inc., 1975.

Wales C, Stager R: The Guided Design Approach. Englewood, Cliffs, NJ, Educational Technology Publications, 1978.

3

Determining Strategies for Teaching

Helen L. Van Hoozer

OBJECTIVES

Upon completion of this chapter, you will be able to:

1. Identify twelve psychological conditions that can be manipulated and controlled by the teacher to promote achievement of specific learning outcomes.
2. Identify the primary advantages and limitations of fourteen types of teaching strategies to determine those best suited for particular learning experiences.
3. Identify physical and environmental factors related to sound, light, temperature, and design that can affect learning.
4. Consider learner characteristics, constraints of the teaching situation, and psychological, physical, and environmental conditions to determine teaching strategies that promote achievement of specific learning outcomes.
5. Given a learning outcome, select teaching strategies and plan a learning experience for a single learner or learner group, applying psychological, physical, and environmental conditions for learning and considering the primary advantages and limitations of teaching strategies and the constraints of the teaching situation.

INTRODUCTION

Ms. V., aged 46, is a college graduate and is a full-time professional employee responsible for a service agency. She is married and has three grown children. She is informed by her obstetrician that she will need a total hysterectomy because of prolonged recurring menstrual periods, heavy bleeding, and anemia. Other treatments have been tried, including dilation and curettage and hormonal drug therapy, but to no avail. Because of her age and the possibility of developing ovarian tumors later in life, a salpingo-oophorectomy is advised. Surgery is to be performed vaginally in three weeks. Surgery is carried out as planned. After surgery there are problems with fluctuating blood pressure and extreme nausea for several hours. These problems are eventually controlled. Prior to, during, and following surgery, several drugs were administered: diazepam, phenylephrine, fentanyl, thiopental, flurazepam, cefazolin sodium, cephradine, hydroxyzine, meperidine, prochlorperazine, and triazolam. Recuperation in the hospital is 5 to 7 days. She will then be discharged under the care of her husband. Are there pre- and postoperative implications for teaching?

You are a nurse-educator in a large university. After class one day you overhear a student saying he was bored just sitting and being "talked at." He complains that he had personal experiences, comments, and questions related to the topic but never had a chance to express them. You felt your presentation was well organized and the information was interesting and relevant to all nursing students in the class. The topic was one that reflected your professional expertise. What, then, is the problem? Are there ways to address the student's concerns or is it beyond your control?

Regardless of the setting, teaching is an important responsibility for the professional nurse. Determining the strategies that stimulate learners to achieve particular cognitive, affective, and psychomotor behaviors based on their needs, interests, and concerns is a major function of the nurse-teacher. This task can be a formidable one because of the large number of options available and lack of clear-cut guidelines on which to base decisions. This chapter presents several psychological, physical, and environmental conditions related to identification and selection of teaching strategies that should be considered when deciding on strategies to promote learning. Through examination and consideration of such factors, teaching and learning can be improved.

DIRECT AND INDIRECT TEACHING STRATEGIES

The actions taken by a teacher to promote change in cognitive, affective, and psychomotor behaviors have been labeled, categorized, and defined in various ways throughout the literature and in practice. Common terms include teaching methods, instructional strategies, media, materials, resources, and audiovisual aids. In this chapter, the terms *strategy* or *teaching strategy* are used to refer to all methods, techniques, and materials that embody and transmit particular conditions for learning. They are the tangible and intangible cues and treatments used by the teacher to facilitate achievement of learning outcomes. Strategies are the direct (natural) or indirect (contrived) methods, techniques, and materials that transmit information (sensory messages). They are the means of message delivery; a means to the end, the learning outcome.

Direct strategies, such as live lecture, live demonstration, role play, clinical practicum, and discussion are characterized by face-to-face teacher communication and interaction. They are the verbal and nonverbal signs and symbols—the actual movements, gestures, pauses, and oral communications of the teacher. On the other hand, indirect strategies, such as films, objects, books, and pamphlets contain the signs and symbols that stand for some object, event, relationship, or idea. Indirect strategies provide vicarious or substitute experiences through intermediary channels. The presence of the teacher may or may not be required. Like direct strategies, indirect strategies are "attending" stimuli (Table 3–1).

Both direct and indirect strategies transmit sensory messages. The sensory message impinges on one or more of the learner's senses, stimulating cue selection and translation. Thus the strategy is instrumental in focusing the learner's attention on objects, qualities, or relationships that are necessary for attainment of learning outcomes (Table 3–2).

Teaching strategies are the materials, persons, and events that embody and convey particular conditions that enable the learner to achieve knowledge, skills, and attitudes. They are employed by the teacher to direct attention, to prompt a response, to motivate, to evaluate, to stimulate thinking, or to test for transfer. Examples of such strategies include the teacher's voice, smile, or pat on the head, books, posters, objects, films, pictures, field trips, and laboratory experiences. Various learning outcomes require different types of learning. Different types of learning require different conditions. The conditions for learning are provided through the direct and indirect strategies that make up a total learning experience. Identifying, analyzing, evaluating, selecting, and using direct and indirect teaching strategies is a critical part of the teaching process.

Strategies motivate learners to use particular perceptual-cognitive processes.

TABLE 3–1. SELECTED INDIRECT TEACHING STRATEGIES

Still Projected Visuals

Slides or filmstrips
Overhead transparencies

Still Nonprojected Visuals

Books, articles
Pamphlets, brochures, flyers
Games
Objects, specimens
Models, mock-ups, simulators
Handouts: worksheets, outlines, case studies, drawings, diagrams, pictures
Photographs
Programed instruction
Computer-assisted instruction: tutorials, tests, simulations, games, drill and practice, problem solving
Posters, displays, exhibits, charts, dioramas
Tables, charts

Motion

Film: 16 mm, 8 mm
Games
Role play
Models, mock-ups, simulators
Video: simulations, role play, demonstrations, interview, conferencing

Auditory Only

Audio recordings
Phonograph records
Audioconferencing
Telephone
Radio

Combinations

Sound-slide, sound filmstrip
Modular instruction
Learning activity packages
Multimedia kits
Multi-image

TABLE 3-2. SELECTED STRATEGIES AND PRIMARY SENSORY INPUT

	Sensory Input				
Strategy	***Auditory***	***Visual***	***Tactile***	***Olefactory***	***Gustatory***
Direct					
Live lecture	X	X			
Discussion	X	X			
Role play	X	X	X		
Live demonstration with return practice	X	X	X		
Clinical practicum	X	X	X	X	X
Indirect					
Textbook, syllabus, print programed text		X			
Journal article		X			
Handout, worksheet		X			
Transparencies: slides, overheads		X			
Photographs, pictures, posters, charts, print case study		X			
Model, mock-up		X	X		
Specimen, object		X	X	X	X
Sound-slide or film, filmstrip, video demonstration, lecture, interview, conferencing	X	X			
Audiotapes, phonograph records, audioconferencing	X				
Computer-based		X	X		
Multimedia modular instruction	X	X	X	X	X
Games	X	X	X	X	X

The learner perceives the transmitted symbols and codes by means of the senses, processes and translates the message cognitively, and exhibits it as observable behavior. The teacher receives feedback from learner behavior, gives feedback to the learner on performance, and utilizes feedback to evaluate the effectiveness of strategies used (Fig. 3–1).

Teaching, then, is basically a sensory messaging process. It involves a two-way interactive flow of messages between the transmitter and the receiver through direct or indirect sensory strategies that convey conditions that influence learning. Through selection and use of appropriate strategies, many of the obstacles to effective learning can be overcome.

Traditionally, direct and indirect strategies have been identified, selected, and used according to type or circumstance. For instance, a teacher chooses to lecture because of class size or required hours of "seat" time; or to use a sound-slide pro-

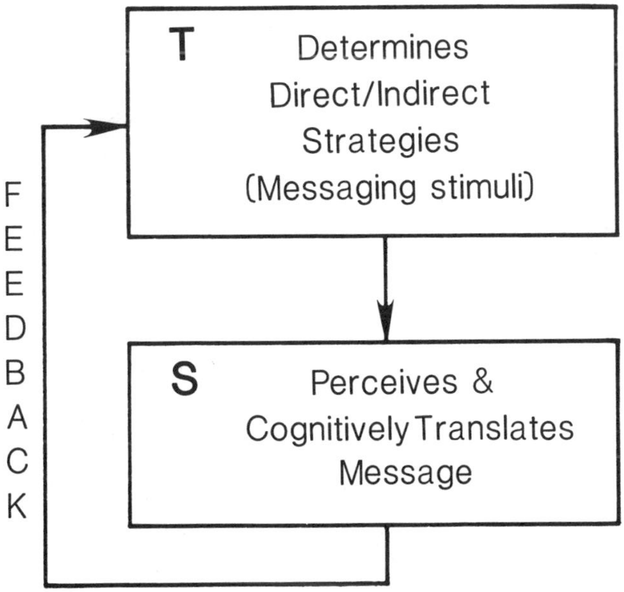

Figure 3-1. Sensory messaging process. T = teacher; S = student.

gram or film because it is "convenient" or "impressive" to do so, or because equipment is available. Research has been concerned with comparing one type of strategy to another to see if it makes a difference in learning. Such comparative research has, in most cases, been inconclusive. Under some circumstances and conditions, a particular strategy has made a difference in achievement and in others it hasn't. Researchers now contend that it is more valid to study particular attributes, qualities, or conditions embedded in or conveyed by a strategy (medium) rather than to compare one type with another. The contention is that it is not the medium that makes a difference in learning, but a specific attribute, quality, or condition that it entails.[1] These attributes or conditions have the potential to direct and hold attention and maintain an optimum level of stimulation to promote intrinsic motivation and translation of information into observable behaviors. Such conditions can be manipulated and controlled by the teacher.

The strategies that make up a total learning experience should be based on learner needs and characteristics, expected learning outcomes, conditions and principles necessary to achieve expectations, needs, and constraints relative to the situation (Fig. 3-2).

The process of determining teaching strategies involves analyzing learner characteristics, determining constraints in terms of time, setting, resources, and teacher preferences; stating specific learning objectives and subobjectives, considering principles of learning and forces that may influence learning, identifying psychological, physical, and environmental conditions that assist the learner(s) to attain expectations, and analyzing strengths and limitations of strategy options to determine those most practical and feasible for the learning experience. Data and decisions made at each point in the process lead to one or more strategies that make up a total learning experience. Table 3-3 presents an example of a planned learning experience.

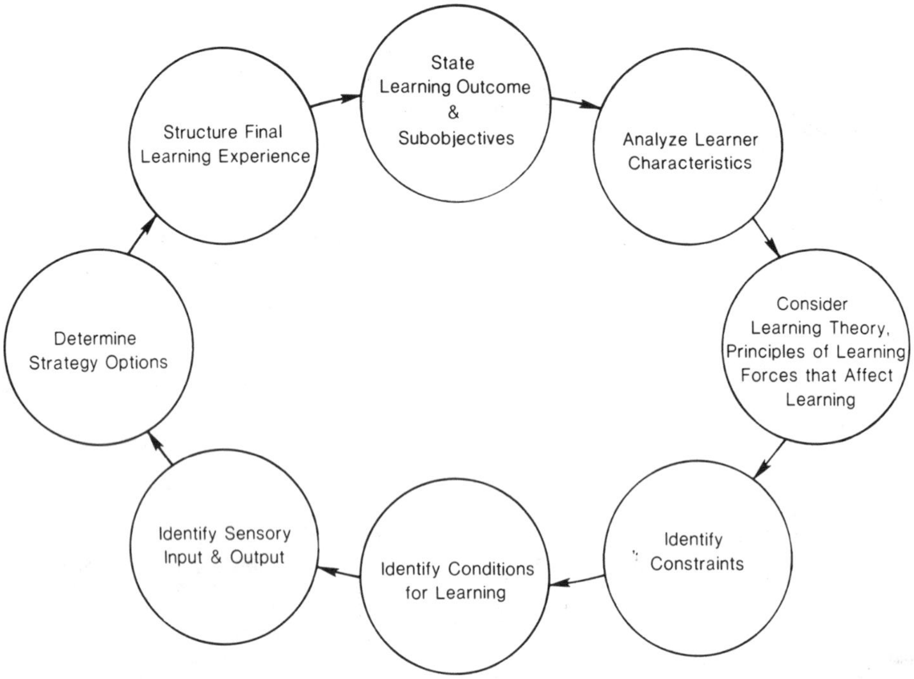

Figure 3-2. Determining teaching strategies: A process approach.

Perception and Cognition: The Basis for Determining Teaching Strategies

Understanding how to identify, select, and use direct and indirect strategies to promote achievement of learning outcomes is based on an understanding of the concepts of perception and cognition. Perception is the active sensory process through which individuals uniquely and selectively attend to, receive, and extract information from the environment and internally organize it for meaning. It is an early stage of the internal higher mental processes of cognition (concept formation, problem solving, imagination, and decision making). An individual's perception is influenced by culture, life experiences, developmental level, maturity, interests, motivation, selective attention, mind-set, perceptual style, and novelty. Thus, perception varies with the individual and depends on the psychological and physiological characteristics of the individual in addition to the stimulus event. The elementary process of sensation or receipt of information underlies the more complex perceptual process of translating sensory messages into meaningful information. The senses used to perceive a message depend on the object or event to be perceived, and perception immediately follows stimulation of the senses. How does the phenomenon of perception relate to the task of selecting teaching strategies?

The messages conveyed through direct and indirect teaching strategies are sensory events: they reach the learner through the senses. Information is not simply transferred intact from the environment or from humans to the perceiver's mind. It is transduced, translated, and transformed into meaning.[2] The learner must perceive before learning can occur. The learner sees, hears, touches, manipulates, smells, and tastes, transforming the message internally and exhibiting behaviors that can be observed and measured by the teacher. The internal and external status of the learner plays a major role in what message is received as well as how it is received. Therefore, it is important to avoid inaccurate perceptions. If the learner perceives the intent of a message incorrectly, inaccurate learning is the result.

The teacher should choose teaching strategies that embody and transmit conditions for learning based on what the learner is expected to do under particular circumstances and to what extent. For instance, if the objective is that the learner will correctly perform a breast self-exam, strategies and conditions—the constructs, codes, and treatments—should be designed to promote this primarily tactile outcome. The teacher considers the needs and characteristics of learners, including developmental level, age, abilities and disabilities, knowledge base, learning and cognitive style, modality strengths, preferences, interests, and level of motivation in relationship to the nature of the learning task to be achieved. The teacher's own teaching style, the resources available, constraints of the setting, and time factors will also influence decision making.

SUMMARY

It is the responsibility of the nurse-teacher to identify learning needs and to decide how to promote learning. This process involves identifying and selecting teaching strategies and designing learning experiences that activate the learner's perceptual-cognitive processes. The conditions for learning are critical because they will affect perception, cognition, and successful learning. The direct and indirect strategies that make up a total learning experience are considered in conjunction with the physical, psychological, cognitive, affective, and psychomotor idiosyncrasies of the learner who is to be taught. The strategies chosen and used by the teacher are relevant only to the extent that they influence in predictable ways the internal forms of representation and the mechanisms by which information is processed by the learner.

The nurse-teacher determines the signs, symbols, constructs, and treatments that call forth the desired verbal, nonverbal, auditory, visual, and tactile responses. The learner selectively attends to incoming messages, interprets them, and transforms them into meaning. The mechanisms used to communicate information are a part of the teaching-learning event. Use of different strategies based on expected learning outcomes and individual needs and characteristics can positively influence achievement of learning outcomes. The question is, what conditions or attributes will facilitate learning for what kinds of learners and what kinds of tasks? The focus is on internal perceptual and cognitive human processes that may be aroused by particular attributes of a direct or indirect teaching strategy rather than on the format of different teaching strategies.

TABLE 3–3. A PLANNED LEARNING EXPERIENCE

Learner Characteristics: A 40-year-old male with 2 years post-high school education; construction worker; lives alone in small apartment; job requires leaving home weeks at a time; works long hours; financial condition good when working; good outlook on life despite diabetic problem; complies with diet; knows etiology and treatment for diabetes and symptoms of insulin shock.

Constraints: One-on-one, 2 hour learning experience in home setting; limited resources available; have injection model and access to pamphlets and posters.

Learning Outcome/ Subobjectives	Psychological, Physical, and Environmental Conditons	Primary Sensory Input	Primary Output	Strategy Options	Learning Experience
The learner will self-administer insulin at home and in work environment with precision and accuracy	Teacher-learner (one-on-one) Cognitive, affective, and psychomotor learning Principle learning Chaining				Establish set reviewing objectives and relate content to past learning. Use poster to identify injection sites and point out sites; explain and discuss.
Identify injection sites	Association and discrimination, problem solving Mind-set and motivation Inductive, linear organization	Visual	Visual	Pictures with print, poster, pamphlet, live demonstration with model or client, discussion.	Point out injection sites on client's body. Prompt client to point out sites, giving positive reinforcement and feedback. Provide pamphlet showing injection sites. Explain and discuss site rotation plan.
Follow injection rotation schedule	Practice and repetition Positive reinforcement and feedback	Visual	Visual	Print instruction, print instructions with pictures, discussion.	Provide illustrated print handout. Prompt and prime client to orally repeat rotation schedule and give feedback and positive reinforcement.

					Demonstrate and discuss how to prepare injection site, first with model, then with client.
Prepare injection site	Active overt response Learner control over rate of presentation Eye-hand coordination Motion	Visual Tactile	Visual Tactile	Live demonstration with client or model, film, video, objects (supplies: alcohol, swabs, soap and water).	Prompt and prime client to prepare site, give feedback, and reinforce correct procedure. Demonstrate and discuss how to handle a syringe and needle, rotate insulin bottle to mix, and draw up correct dosage (water).
Draw up correct dosage and inject	Cognitive closure Informal home environment Time depends on client's work schedule and preference	Visual Tactile	Visual Tactile	Live demonstration with client or model, film, video, objects (insulin bottle, disposable syringe and needle, alcohol, cotton balls, swabs).	Demonstrate and discuss how to inject insulin using model. Prompt and prime client to practice, first with model, then self; give feedback and reinforcement.
Care for insulin, syringes, needles		Visual Tactile	Visual Tactile	Print, print with pictures, discussion, slide presentation, objects (bottle of insulin, syringe and needle, cotton balls, alcohol swabs).	Discuss and demonstrate how to dispose of syringe and needles and how to transport insulin and supplies. Prompt client to practice and give feedback and positive reinforcement. Follow-up discussion and performance testing.
Prepare insulin and supplies for transport		Visual Tactile	Visual Tactile	Discussion, live demonstration, print, print with pictures, poster, objects.	

PROVIDING CONDITIONS FOR LEARNING THROUGH DIRECT AND INDIRECT TEACHING STRATEGIES

Conditions or attributes with the potential for influencing the attainment of learning outcomes that the teacher can manipulate and control include: providing for positive reinforcement, feedback, practice and repetition, priming and prompting responses, considering perceptual capacity or information load, organizing, grouping, and patterning information in different ways, adapting rate of presentation and pacing, establishing mind-set and promoting cognitive closure, conveying color or movement, promoting participation in learning, and determining the appropriate physical and environmental conditions for the learning environment. It is the responsibility of a teacher to consider such conditions when determining teaching strategies for particular learning experiences. The teacher receives input from the learner, considers learning needs and learner characteristics, decides on the objectives and the conditions necessary to promote achievement, and determines the strategy or combination of strategies that can provide the necessary conditions for learning. The direct and indirect strategies selected convey the messages that evoke perceptual-cognitive processes. For instance, let's assume Mary Jones, aged 43, is under considerable stress because of family and job pressures. She needs to use progressive muscle relaxation and visualization techniques to relax. What conditions must be provided to promote achievement of this task? Is reinforcement and feedback necessary? Will Mary need to practice? If so, to what extent? Will the use of prompts, primes, movement, color, or repetition promote learning? If so, how can these conditions be provided? How should information be organized? What amount of information is appropriate? Should Mary be able to control the rate of presentation of information? How can mental set be established? How can cognitive closure be prompted and how will you know when Mary has achieved cognitive closure? Will Mary learn more efficiently and effectively if she participates actively in learning? Will she need to respond overtly as well as covertly? What type of physical environment is necessary for effective learning?

Reinforcement

The condition of reinforcement and its role in learning comes from associationism, classical and operant conditioning, and Gestalt-field learning theory. Reinforcement is a universal condition for learning. It is based on established principles of learning: (1) that personal satisfaction is necessary for learning to occur, (2) that a praised response will be remembered longer than one that is not, (3) that reinforced responses tend to be committed to memory, and (4) that the strength of a rewarded response increases with the number of positive reinforcements.

Reinforcers can be either positive or negative, tangible or intangible. A positive reinforcer is a reward that strengthens behavior and increases the probability that the behavior will be repeated, whereas a negative reinforcer is an undesirable event, such as withholding a positive reinforcer or punishing behavior in some other way. Negative reinforcers are administered to help eliminate unwanted behavior and to elicit desired responses; however, a negative reinforcer usually only slows down the rate at which a response is exhibited and does not totally eliminate the behavior. Both positive and negative reinforcers must be perceived as such by the individual receiving the reinforcement. When it comes to the matter of teaching desirable responses, whether in a school, home, hospital, or work setting, positive reinforcement, such as giving verbal praise, gold stars, awards, correct answers, or a gentle touch, should be used liberally and negative reinforcement used sparingly. The emotional accompaniments and untoward effects of negative reinforcement can seriously disrupt the learning process. Also, the more closely the positive reinforcer follows the desired response, the more effective the reinforcer will be in building a strong response.

When a teacher gives tokens or allows the learner to engage in a special activity after a desired response, positive, tangible reinforcement is being used. The activity and tokens are positive reinforcers. Also, if the teacher says or writes "Good idea!" "That's correct!" or smiles, nods, or puts a hand on the learner's shoulder following a response or to encourage a response, the teacher is using direct, positive reinforcement to strengthen the response. Programed and computer-assisted instruction are good examples of indirect strategies that usually incorporate mechanisms that provide positive reinforcement. Consider the following example:

> Large molecules and solid particles may be "eaten" by the plasma membrane. *Phago* means "eat" and *cyto* means "cell," so this process of "cellular eating" is called ——.
>
> Phagocytosis is correct. Keep going, you're doing great!

In this example, the learner is told the correct response and is rewarded for giving the correct response.

The condition of positive reinforcement can easily be incorporated and conveyed through all types of direct and indirect teaching strategies. The principle of positive reinforcement emphasizes that responding favorably to a person's actions will affect later behavior. In other words, success breeds success. Giving immediate, positive rewards may be more important during the early stages of learning tasks, whereas rewards can be delayed and reduced later on as the learner becomes more familiar and confident about learning.

Positive reinforcement is an important condition for learning no matter what the learner's age or developmental level. Yet, there should be a slow shift away from extrinsic, tangible rewards toward the more intrinsic, intangible rewards of self-satisfaction and mastery performance. The question is, how can a person's intrinsic motivation for learning be used and increased? If we are intrinsically motivated to learn something, we are likely to spend more time and effort learning, feel better about what is learned, and be more likely to apply what has been learned in the future. An activity is said to be intrinsically motivated if there is no obvious external reward associated with it.

To increase intrinsic motivation, the learning environment should be stimulating and challenging, and it should invoke curiosity and sometimes even fantasy. A challenging environment should provide for multiple-level goals. An environment will not be challenging either if the person is certain to reach a goal or is certain not to reach a goal. Attention-attracting events evoke sensory curiosity. For example, television stimulates the sensory curiosity of the viewer through technical events, such as camera angles, zooms, close-ups, and so on. These sensory events capture our attention, apart from the message. Most television commercials average 20 to 30 technical events per minute, whereas regular programming averages 8 to 10. Perhaps this is why even two- and three-year-olds find commercials attractive and are soon able to recite the message after listening and viewing only one or two times. Popular educational television programs like "Sesame Street" and "Electric Company" have capitalized on the attention-attracting value of changes in light, sound, movement, and other conditions to evoke curiosity. Another way to engage the curiosity of the learner is to present just enough information to promote a desire for cognitive completeness and consistency.

The value of fantasy for motivating learning has often been overlooked. A fantasy-inducing environment is one that evokes mental images of things not present to the senses or within the actual experiences of the person involved. These mental images can be either physical objects or social situations. For example, analogies can often help a person apply old knowledge to understand new things. Video games can provide an outlet for aggressive feelings. Many children's games and books include elements of fantasy, which maintain optimal levels of mental arousal. Maurice Sendak's book, *Where the Wild Things Are,* is one example. Through the use of fantasy, the author helps children deal with fears and emotions. Malone found that children and adults preferred games that actively involved them in a fantasy situation.[3]

Feedback. Feedback is a subset of reinforcement that refers to providing information about the quality or accuracy of a response immediately or shortly after it is given. Like reinforcement, feedback can be positive or negative. It can reinforce correct responses. Orally telling a learner that a response is correct or incorrect and *explaining why* is one example of direct feedback. Feedback can help to correct a response if the nature of the mistake is made clear, but simply telling the learner whether the response is right or wrong is not sufficient to promote understanding and change behavior.

Feedback generally increases motivation and usually improves subsequent performance. The more specific the knowledge of performance, the more rapidly performance will improve. Excessively detailed feedback on early trials or complex tasks may prove to be confusing and even detrimental to learning, however. If knowledge of results is not provided by the teacher, learners tend to develop substitutes. For example, they may watch peers to decide whether their performance is better or worse. This can result in misinformation and inaccurate learning.

Feedback on performance is important for all types of learning, whether cognitive, affective, or psychomotor; however, it is an especially important condition for psychomotor skills learning. When learning a skill, feedback should be given regularly, especially during the first practice sessions. It should be detailed enough to encourage systematic improvement in later sessions and include information on both correct and incorrect action. As performance improves, direct oral feedback from the teacher becomes less necessary and in most cases should be gradually reduced and withdrawn. As learners become more familiar with tasks, they can be encouraged to provide their own feedback. For example, teachers can structure conditions so that learners evaluate their own performance after practice. Self-evaluation can then be compared to objective feedback. The following example illustrates the use of direct and indirect feedback in both direct and indirect teaching strategies:

OBJECTIVE: Applying strict aseptic technique, the learner will scrub, using correct, full-hand-forearm technique two out of three times.

INDIRECT TEACHING STRATEGY: The student will:

1. View a five-minute video demonstration and explanation of full-hand-forearm scrub.
2. Practice and record, on videotape, performance of the full-hand-forearm scrub.
3. View the recorded performance and evaluate it, using a checklist that specifies steps in the full-hand-forearm scrub and compare performance with the model video demonstration (indirect videofeedback).
4. Repeat the strategy until mastery.

DIRECT TEACHING STRATEGY: The student will demonstrate performance of the full-hand-forearm scrub in the presence of the teacher, who will evaluate performance, using the checklist, and give verbal feedback on correct and incorrect action (direct feedback from the teacher).

When feedback is an integral component of teaching strategies, the learner receives information on how well a task is performed. This increases the likelihood that achievement and performance will improve. Feedback from learners also helps teachers to know what effect the learning experience has had on learner behavior and how to achieve better communication to facilitate change.

Practice and Repetition

In the full-hand-forearm-scrub example, it was assumed that practice and repetition were important conditions for learning. Research indicates that in most cases practice and repetition are essential conditions for learning. Many psychologists have shown that the more thoroughly something is learned at first, the better the chances are that it will be retained. Providing practice and repetition through a variety of strategies is one way of improving retention and promoting transfer of learning to new situations. For example, a study by Young and Morgan indicated that a treatment for enuresis that required children to maintain bladder control for 14 nights beyond the regular mastery period resulted in more permanent effects after treatment than did the clinic's less demanding treatment program.[4] It appears that practice and repetition, or overlearning, are beneficial for physical, social, and intellectual behaviors. The question is, how much practice or rehearsal is necessary to promote retention and how can practice and repetition be effectively used by the teacher to promote learning?

Researchers have repeatedly found evidence that distributed practice (short practice periods at spaced intervals) leads to better performance than massed practice (one long practice period), particularly when the task to be learned is complex.[5] It is suggested that distributed practice allows for and encourages more rehearsal than does massed practice and that people actually spend less time studying during massed practice. Also, information becomes more redundant in massed practice sessions, which leads to a decrease in interest and attention. Distributed practice, on the other hand, helps to connect new information with what is already known, and associations tend to grow stronger with later exposure. Going back to the full-hand-forearm-scrub example, it seems that relatively short practice periods with short rest periods would be best for the first exposure to the aseptic skill, followed by additional short practice sessions and rest periods until mastery, depending on the learner's strengths and weaknesses. Thereafter, strategies should be designed to provide periodic practice and application of the skill in varied contexts to increase retention and transfer.

The arrangement of practice time is critical because performance (particularly of skills) tends to drop off between practice sessions. The longer the period of time between trials or practice sessions, the greater the loss. Likewise, the longer a person practices, the more likely boredom and fatigue will result. The teacher will notice this circumstance if performance begins to decline after a series of repetitive trials. It is important that conditions for practice and repetition be correlated with the complexity of the task and be as similar to the real situation as possible.

Too frequently, concepts are taught and treated as discrete units that may never be used again. In fact, repeated use of concepts enhances learning. One way to ensure repeated use of concepts is to organize a curriculum around basic concepts. Important concepts are thus threaded throughout a program of study. This is the basis for the integrated nursing curriculum. Initially the learner is exposed to concepts like research and communication by using simple, familiar examples and non-examples (examples that do not represent the concept). Repetition and practice with the concept becomes progressively more complex throughout the curriculum, yet builds upon previous learning.

Similarly, repetition of a message directs attention. A repeated message has a better chance of catching the learner's attention, and the repetition increases perceptual sensitivity or alertness to the message. Therefore, it is good teaching to devise conditions so that learners have the opportunity to repeat information more than one time in a variety of ways. For example, articles, films, video, and computer programs, as well as other types of indirect strategies with the same message, can be placed in a learning resource center, allowing almost unlimited review of information. Some types of indirect strategies are particularly suited for providing repetition of information because of their portable nature and lack of the need for adjunct equipment. These include: books, handouts, pamphlets, pictures, programed texts, and some types of games, objects, and models.

Priming and Prompting as Conditions for Learning

Simply waiting indefinitely for a desired behavior to occur so that it can be reinforced is not efficient or effective teaching. It is necessary to prime and prompt desired responses. It is true that information may be available in the learner's cognitive structure, but it may not be immediately accessible without a prime or prompt to stimulate recall. As Susan Markle states in *Good Frames and Bad: A Grammar of Frame Writing,* priming is analogous to the old water pump. If you remember, we had to pour a little water in to get water to flow. Similarly, teachers "prime" students by giving them messages to help them give a particular response or one that bears close resemblance to the desired one. *Prompting* means providing only a clue or hint that assists the learner to make the response. In other words, primes usually show or tell the learner the exact response, whereas prompts only hint at the response. The teacher's role is providing primes and prompts and the learner's role is active participation in learning by responding.

The Prime. According to Susan Markle, there are three major types of primes: copying, echoing, and imitation, or modeling.[6] Copying and echoing are low-level primes. *Copying* involves telling the learner something and asking that it be repeated exactly. The following excerpt from a sound-slide program on female reproductive physiology illustrates the copying prime. In this case, the copying prime is both visual and auditory, and the response is the act of writing the correct response. The copying prime is narrated while it is pictured on a graphic slide. The student's response is written on a study guide during a pause.

> At three months gestation, the fully-functioning placenta takes over for the duration of pregnancy as the primary source of estrogens and progesterone. The placenta takes over as the primary source of ______ and ______ at three months gestation.

Markle writes that an *echoing* prime is similar to a copying prime, except that the stimulus is a sound pattern and the response is reproduction of the sound. The following example illustrates the echoing prime:

OBJECTIVE: The learner will be able to correctly pronounce ten medical terms.
STRATEGY: The student will listen to each word as it is pronounced on an audiorecording, echo the word while recording it, listen to the word repeated once more, and pronounce the word again.

The *imitation, or modeling,* prime involves directly showing the learner how to do something or indirectly giving the learner a set of written directions that is read and followed step by step. Let's suppose we need to teach a class how to set up and operate the audio recorder so they will be able to complete the medical terminology lesson previously described. We could either directly demonstrate the procedure while the class (or individual) watches and then have each student imitate our model demonstration, or we could give each learner a set of written and illustrated instructions, which the learner would read and follow to set up and operate the recorder. Either strategy would prime the response: operating the audio recorder.

When priming, the teacher's role is providing priming conditions and giving feedback on response. The learner's role is active, overt participation. It should be emphasized that priming is not a guarantee that the learner will be able to give the response without the priming condition. Telling a response and having the learner repeat it does not always lead to mastery or transfer of learning. Other conditions, like reinforcement, feedback, practice, and repetition will be needed as well.

The Prompt. A *prompt* is a hint or cue that helps the learner come up with a correct response. Unlike a prime, a prompt does not tell the learner the correct response. Either pictorial or verbal (oral or written) strategies can provide prompting conditions to elicit desired responses. Markle classifies prompts as two major types: formal and thematic. *Formal* prompts provide knowledge about the form of the expected response, such as providing a hint as to the number of letters in a word, supplying the initial letter for a word, or giving a multiple-choice item. Formal prompts do not necessarily insure that the learner will understand the meaning of the response. Formal prompts can be readily identified in programed and computer-assisted teaching strategies. Other types of indirect and direct strategies also include formal prompts or serve as formal prompts in and of themselves. The following excerpts illustrate each of the three types of formal prompts within a print-programed text.[7]

Initial Letter Supplied

> Charting is the concise, accurate, factual documentation and communication of events and situations pertaining to a particular client. Charting is required for each medication, treatment, and nursing intervention that you initiate or implement, be it within the hospital or in another health care setting, clinic, or the client's home.
>
> Charting is a means of c___________ pertinent aspects of health care relating to a particular person.

Communicating is correct. The health record that results from charting communicates information on the details of care for a particular client to all health care team members and to other health care agency personnel.

Number of Letters Supplied

> Avoid personal opinions or biased findings. Do not allow your observations to be clouded by someone else's opinion. Be objective.
>
> Charting entries should be free from ____ and should be stated ___________.

Bias and *objectively* are correct.

Multiple-choice Item

You can print or write in longhand, but writing must be legible. Complete statements are not necessary, but the meaning must be clear.

Bad example: Talking about committing suicide. Encouraged.
Better: Encouraged to express feelings about suicide.

Which of the following is the better example of a legibile, comprehensible chart entry?

(a) To BR with assist. Encouragement needed.
(b) Got up to go to BR

(a) is right! (a) reflects the event more completely and is therefore a better chart entry.

You will notice that feedback explaining the correct response is provided in two of these examples and positive reinforcement is given in all three. It should be remembered that formal prompts provide the learner with information about the structure of a response and may tend to reduce the learner's attention to important discriminations and meanings. On the other hand, *thematic* prompts promote understanding of the meaning of the response but do not cue the exact structure of the response. Thematic prompts depend upon the learner's ability to form meaningful associations and draw inferences. Questions to be answered and blanks to be completed in print materials are examples of thematic prompts.

When a teacher asks questions to stimulate discussion, thematic prompting is being used. The following excerpt from a lecture on life-style serves to illustrate thematic prompting as an embedded attribute of this strategy.

TEACHER: "Let's think about a theoretical model of life-style change composed of three steps. Let's start with the third step, which is actual change." (Thematic prompt)

QUESTION: "What do you think would have to happen before this third step, 'actual change,' could occur?"

In this instance, students are not actually told the response or the structure of the response but are prompted to recall information, form associations, and draw inferences in order to supply the first two steps of the life-style change model after being given the third step in the model. Additional prompts or primes may have to be given to elicit the desired response. Entire filmstrips, films, video programs, and so on can serve as prompts and primes to elicit responses.

Visual Prompting and Priming. Visual elements within illustrations and visual materials themselves, such as pictures, overhead transparencies, slides, and print text can serve as prompts and primes. Visual signs and symbols and elements, such as color and shading, underlining, boxing, capitalizing, italicizing, circling, varying style or size of print, directional arrows, and varying design or format, stimulate the visual sense and direct attention to important constructs to promote translation and transformation of the message.

A text design called "information mapping" developed by Robert Horn illustrates how text can be presented in a diagrammatic form to facilitate information scanning and retrieval.[8] The fundamental unit of information mapping is an information block. Each block has a functional label, and only one kind of information is included in a block. Information blocks are combined in various ways into larger units called information maps. The page labels, diagrams, tables, flow charts, and symbols within a map prompt and direct the learner's attention to key information (Fig. 3–3). Information mapping does not guarantee that a particular response will be made or motivated, but it does ensure that the material will be clear and consistent, which should enhance learning. The information mapping format has been the topic of research studies, and evidence indicates that it can have a positive effect on learning.

Research does indicate that varied methods of cuing can be used to heighten learner interest and enthusiasm; however, it appears that too many or too few cues

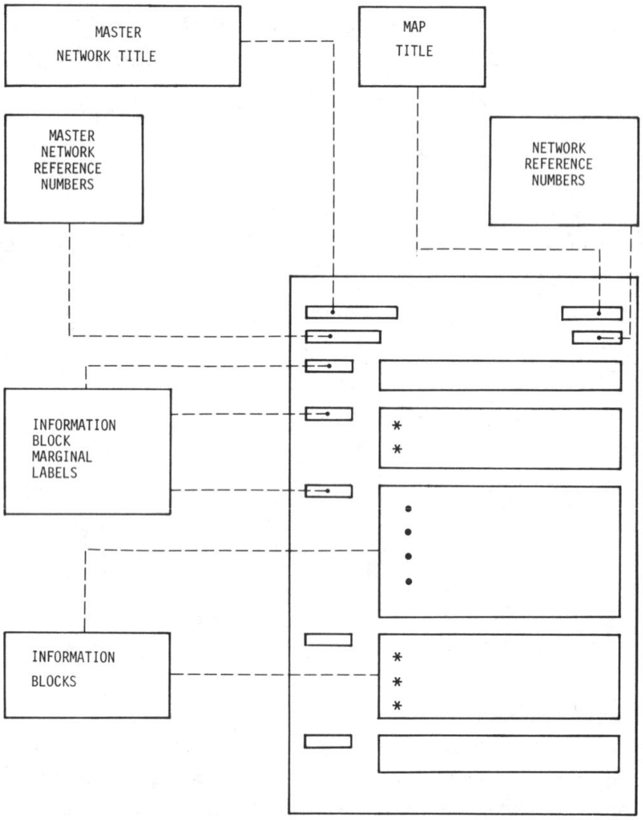

Figure 3–3. Information mapping: Basic format. *(Adapted from Horn RE: Information Mapping for Learning and Reference. Paper available from Information Resources Incorporated, Box 417, Lexington, MA, 02173.)*

may adversely affect learning. Constant repetition of a single type of cue may produce lack of interest and boredom. In addition, all types of attention-directing cuing mechanisms are not equally effective.[9] Cultural differences can influence perception. There is some evidence that when a visual strategy is used, a visual prime should be included in the testing situation. Requiring the learner to transfer completely verbal (aural) information to a visual testing situation or the opposite is clearly inappropriate. For instance, if the learning outcome reflects complex psychomotor behavior, lecture or discussion and readings are not appropriate teaching strategies. For the learner to exhibit the skill, the learner must *see* all the integrated steps performed in sequence.

Guidelines for the use of visuals as prompts for learning can be drawn from the extensive review of research done by Levie and Lentz.[10] In their report of the literature involving the effects of text illustrations on learning, they point out that when an illustration does not overlap text content, it will not have a motivating effect or facilitate learning, even though the illustration may be attention-getting. On the other hand, if illustrations complement the text or contain redundant information, learning will be enhanced for the particular content. In addition, illustrations can provide a context for organizing information in the text and prompt future recall of information. Photographs, drawings, diagrams, maps, and other pictorial forms can encourage visual thinking. They are often more effective than words. Learners must, however, be taught how to interpret complex diagrams and prompted to extract relevant detail from them. Some evidence suggests that poor readers may benefit more from visual prompts than good readers. Whether an individual is a "visual learner" or not will also influence learning from visual prompts and primes.

Perceptual Capacity or Information Load

Individuals differ as to the amount of information they can receive, code, store, and translate at any one time. Therefore, teachers must consider the perceptual capacity of learners in relation to the amount and type of information conveyed as well as how it is communicated. To a large degree, the amount of information that is appropriate will depend on the developmental and maturational level of the learner and how familiar the learner is with the information, its meaningfulness, and complexity. The question is, how do we determine the amount of information to prevent sensory overload?

Evidence indicates that some people can perceive at a glance and store in memory up to seven items at one time, although what constitutes an item is not clearly established.[11] The capacity to process information at any stage depends on the ability to attend. Attention is related to internal states of arousal and concentration; thus, there are implications for single and multisensory input strategies relative to attention and information-processing capabilities. Investigation has been made of both auditory and visual single and multisensory input strategies as they relate to perceptual capacity and effect on learning. It appears that the more difficult or complex and verbal the message, the greater the perceptual advantage of visual input (printed or pictorial) over auditory (spoken) input. Communicating information orally, either directly or indirectly, usually allows the learner only one opportunity to perceive. For example, when the teacher uses the pure live lecture as a means of communication, the learner may have difficulty stopping the speaker for clarification. Furthermore, extraneous noises (talkative neighbors, environmental sounds) and internal noises (decreased concentration because of worries, daydreaming, and so on) can influence perceptual capacity and interfere with information processing. When auditory information is recorded on tape or film, the learner may at least have the option of reversing the player or projector to review the information a second time, but there is no control over technically recorded noise.

Research to date indicates that perceptual capacity appears to increase when the message is received through two separate sensory channels, such as spoken words (auditory input) with related and relevant illustrations (visual input). On the other hand, if multisensory input contains *unrelated* verbal and pictorial cues, interference and decreased information gain will result. Also, if multisensory input is too rapid or too packed with information, the learner will be forced to make a choice between channels. For instance, if students are given a written handout and are expected to write responses as they view and listen to an audiovisual presentation, such as a film, video, or sound-slide program, and the message is presented too fast or there is too much information, they will usually give up looking at the pictorial information and concentrate on listening, reading, and writing responses. Learning problems result if the learner misses relevant information conveyed through the ignored visual input.

There is also evidence that interference will be more likely to occur when two tasks involve visual input, like slides and a print handout, rather than when one involves visual and the other involves auditory input, like slides and audiotape. When information is received simultaneously from several sources, one source can degrade, accentuate, or bias other sources. Most direct and indirect strategies are overloaded with information, and teachers need to be aware that sensory or information overload can interfere with the attainment of learning outcomes. Such strategies as multi-image and three-dimensional sound may be more appropriate for affective behaviors; however, cognitive and psychomotor learning outcomes may warrant input strategies that are organized and paced in relatively small steps or segments of information and involve only one or two senses. Johnson contends that three facts are the maximum for a one-hour live lecture, and that visuals such as slides or overhead transparencies should convey only one bit of information or a single idea.[12]

There is some evidence that we remember about 10 percent of what we hear, 75 percent of what we see, and 90 percent of what we see and hear.[13] Approximately 70 percent of the sensory perception reaching the brain comes by means of the visual sense. Therefore, the visual sense is by far the most effective channel for communication. The aural sense is secondary.[14] Of course, this circumstance varies from person to person.

Judgment is essential when identifying the sensory input needs and tasks of learners and assessing the amount of information in both direct and indirect teaching strategies as it relates to the characteristics of the learner and the learning outcomes to be achieved.

Organization, Grouping, and Patterning

Organization, grouping, and patterning of information are influential factors in the achievement of learning outcomes. Without organized perceptions—stability, order, pattern, predictability—we could scarcely cope with learning. Organization is in part determined by the event and in part by what the perceiver chooses to impose upon or construct from the situation because of past experiences and present interests and needs. It is the teacher's responsibility to select, arrange, and present information in a way that is most conducive to learning.

Information can be organized in various ways: from simple to complex, familiar to unfamiliar, specific to general, general to specific, certain to uncertain, and so on. The type or method of organization used depends on the outcome to be attained, the subject matter, and the characteristics of the learner. General-to-specific, or *deductive* organization starts with a general statement—a definition, concept, principle, or rule. This is followed by specific examples, illustrations, or applications. The learner is led to see the relationship between the generalization and specific examples that relate to it. The following example illustrates use of deductive organization of information. Frame 10 of a sound filmstrip visually and verbally presents the message: "Carbohydrates comprise the sugars and starches in the diet." This is the statement of principle. The example follows. Frame 11 presents examples visually and states: "Grains are starch-based carbohydrates. What are some examples of carbohydrates in these two groupings?" Students are asked to respond orally.

Specific-to-general, or *inductive,* organization reverses the process. Specific facts, examples, or situations are stated or observed first and from them the generalization is derived. Either the teacher or the learner might be the originator of the specific facts, examples, or situations. For instance, a teacher could show slides or photographs of various body types and verbally (orally or in print) explain the type of daily activity and dietary caloric intake related to each type. The relationship between energy input and output could then be generated as the gain, loss, or stability of body weight. The principle becomes the generalization drawn from the examples.

Both deductive and inductive organization and patterning of information can promote learning. Deductive organization allows the learner to test concepts, principles, or theories and their applications. Inductive organization helps the learner to generalize concepts, theories, and principles from examples. When rules or principles are presented first, care must be taken to provide sufficient and relevant concrete examples that illustrate the principle. The learner must be able to relate to the examples, incorporate the ideas in his or her cognitive structure, and form generalizations. The learner essentially organizes experiences so that they are meaningful and useful. The goal is that generalizations be retained and transferred to new situations.

Inductive organization prompts the learner with a set of specific, meaningful examples to stimulate generation of a principle to predict or explain the pattern of relationships. The following example further illustrates *inductive* organization of information during a seminar. To begin the seminar, the teacher presents two short vignettes:

> Jane is driving down the street and stops at a red light. As the light changes, she accelerates to proceed across the intersection. Just as she picks up speed, a boy on a bicycle appears in her peripheral vision. She slams on her brakes, and the boy whizzes by. Jane's heart is pounding, but she continues on her way to work. She relates her near-miss to friends at work and that evening relaxes in front of the television. Eventually she forgets all about the experience.
>
> Jill has been working overtime at the office to meet an important deadline. She is increasingly frustrated by interruptions and excess pressure placed on her by her supervisor. After hours of burning the midnight oil, the project is completed, and she and her husband leave for a two-week whirlwind tour of the western states. Jill arrives home exhausted. While preparing breakfast the next day, she slips on the stairs and sustains a serious back injury.

Following the vignettes, the teacher questions: Can you relate these two situations to the concepts of relaxation and stress? What stressors are there in each of the two situations? How did both Jane and Jill deal with stress? Did each of the two people deal appropriately with stress or was one method of relaxation more effective than the other?

Simple-to-Complex and Familiar-to-Unfamiliar Organization, Patterning, and Grouping. Relevant examples are extremely important for clarifying, verifying, and substantiating concepts, theories, and principles. It is important to begin with relatively simple, familiar examples and progress to more complex or unfamiliar ones. Helping learners generate examples from their own experience and knowledge reinforces learning and promotes transfer of learning.

Overhead transparencies, slides, drawings, and print text, such as handouts, as well as other strategies can be designed and used to visually convey simple, familiar information followed by more complex, unfamiliar information. Let's assume our objective is that students will be able to identify and explain components of the nursing process. One strategy would be to present a video simulation of a familiar nursing care situation as an example and then ask students to analyze the situation and identify and discuss the assessment, diagnosis, planning, intervention, and evaluation phases. This could be followed by a more complex, unfamiliar example. In this manner, higher-level problem solving is used to assist the learner to attend to and assimilate information. Contrast this strategy with the following one: Professor Jones places a complex model of the nursing process on the overhead projector and proceeds to explain each component of the process in detail. The students listen and take notes.

In your judgment, which of these two strategies would be more likely to effectively promote perceptual-cognitive processing and facilitate retention and transfer of the nursing process?

Linear and Branched Organization and Patterning of Information. Teachers need to consider whether information is best delivered sequentially in a hierarchical pattern, with one point leading to the next in a fixed, linear pattern, or whether it would be better to "branch" it so that learners who already have some knowledge can quickly move on to information with which they are unfamiliar or need to review.

When information is organized in a linear or fixed pattern, there is no variation in the sequence in which the information is delivered or received. The only way that linear sequencing can be adapted to individual learning differences is to vary the rate of time allowed for the learner to receive the message. Such linear organization and patterning of information is inherent in certain types of direct and indirect strategies. Sound filmstrips, 16mm film, video simulations, and formal, live lecture are examples. The information is predetermined, delivered and received by the learner in a fixed order. The message cannot be easily rearranged by the learner.

Unlike the linear format, branched organization and patterning allows the learner to control the sequence of information. For instance, the learner can read chapter 3 before chapter 1 in a textbook, redirect the flow and topic of conversation during a discussion, or select different options when receiving and responding to a computer program.

Robert Gagné offers a four-level framework that can be used to organize information sequentially and hierarchically.[15] The structure is composed of: (1) establishing a factual foundation, (2) developing conceptual understandings, (3) using principles and rules, and (4) engaging in problem solving and other applications. By attending to each of these four levels, the learner is guided to apply and use knowledge and/or skills gained. The structure can be applied to either direct or indirect teaching strategies.

At the first level, the factual foundation, the basic terminology, facts, and details establish the framework for the development of the second level—concept development. Concepts are formed from facts having common characteristics, from facts unrelated by class but that have a relationship that leads to the concept, or from a set of lower-level concepts that lead to a higher conceptual level. For example, the concept of blood is formed by perceiving the relationship among plasma, platelets, red and white blood cells, and other facts. The development of higher-level concepts resembles a chain in which each subsequent concept depends upon previous ones. The major outcome of any strategy is for learners to be able to generalize from the facts to form concepts on various levels.

The third level of organization, using principles and rules, involves assisting the learner to form relationships among two or more concepts. The learner must understand the facts and concepts contained in a principle before the principle can be understood. Application of the principle is the next essential stage. The learner may be required to apply the principle by solving problems, by explaining situations, by inferring causes, or by predicting consequences. Both direct and indirect teaching strategies can be organized to first establish a factual foundation; second, to develop concepts; third, to use principles and rules; and fourth, to promote application, critical thinking, and problem solving.

Advance Organizers as a Means of Organization. A teacher cannot assume that learners have formed concepts and principles and can recall them to understand new information. Ausubel suggests using advance organizers (expository, historical, or comparative) as general introductory information.[16] These organizers provide a framework for more detailed information that follows. A given advance organizer or a series of organizers are usually abstract, general, and inclusive in nature but not as detailed as the information the learner must acquire. They are designed to explain, integrate, and interrelate the information they precede. Advance organizers can take the form of an outline, a sentence or two, one or two paragraphs, or an entire chapter.

The advantage of using an advance organizer for each new unit of information is that it gives the learner a general overview of more detailed information to come and it provides an organizing framework for the information. Organizers are expressly designed to draw attention to and point out how previously learned related concepts are either basically similar to or essentially different from new ideas and information. Providing advance organizers should ensure that fewer ambiguities, fewer competing meanings, and fewer misconceptions result. All types of indirect and direct strategies can incorporate advance organizers or may serve as advance organizers themselves. For example, the information contained in a series of slides, overhead transparencies, or a modular learning package can be hierarchically ordered. Each organizer precedes its corresponding segment or unit of information and progressively differentiates between and integrates information. Chapter 1 of this text is an example of how an entire chapter serves as an advance organizer. The chapter is relatively abstract and general, yet it provides the conceptual framework for the chapters that follow. The headings in each chapter are also advance organizers, as well as the introduction sections.

Research indicates that when verbal advance organizers present relevant and appropriately inclusive concepts, better learning and retention of unfamiliar information will result. Advance organizers appear to be particularly helpful for individuals with relatively poor verbal ability and those who tend to structure information less efficiently and effectively.[17,18] Canelos, Taylor, and Altschuld investigated the effectiveness of a visual advance organizer.[19] The visual advance organizer was a series of slides showing the parts and names of a water-filter pump and another series showing the parts as a whole pump system. There was a direct analogous relationship to the parts of the heart in the heart presentation. The visual advance organizer was compared with a verbal advance organizer—listing the names of the components of the water-filter system orally only. The results of this study indicate that for spatial learning tasks in which the learner is required to remember locations of parts and their names, visual advance organizers are more productive than verbal (oral) organizers or no organizers at all.

Rate of Presentation

The rate at which a message is presented is another crucial variable for teachers to consider when determining strategies to promote learning. There is some evidence to suggest that even though information is well organized and of the appropriate amount, it can be presented too fast or too slow, thus interfering with learning. This condition for learning is especially important when the message is being delivered to a group of learners, because individuals vary as to the rate at which information can be received and processed. The rate depends on age, developmental level, maturity, abilities and disabilities, interests, motivation, and sensory strengths and weaknesses. The teacher should assess the characteristics of the learners, the learning outcomes expected, the nature of the learning situation, and the nature of the information to be transmitted to determine the rate of presentation. In general, the more familiar the learner is with the information and the more concrete and meaningful it is, the more rapidly it can be transmitted, perceived, and processed. When information is unfamiliar and abstract, it should be presented less rapidly, allowing the learner more control over the rate of presentation (Table 3–4).

TABLE 3-4. STRATEGIES AND DEGREE OF CONTROL OVER PRESENTATION BY LEARNER

	Degree of Learner Control		
Strategy	***High***	***Medium***	***Low***
Direct			
Discussion	X		
Role play	X		
Live demonstration with return practice		X	
Clinical practicum		X	
Live lecture			X
Indirect			
Textbook, syllabus	X		
Journal article	X		
Model, mock-up	X		
Specimen, object	X		
Handout, worksheet	X		
Slides	X		
Photographs, posters	X		
Pictures, charts	X		
Print case study	X		
Computer-based	X		
Print programed instruction, autotutorial	X		
Project	X		
Game	X		
Multimedia modular instruction		X	
Audioconferencing		X	
Videoconferencing		X	
Video demonstration, lecture, interview			X
Sound-slide, filmstrip			X
Film			X
Audiotape			X
Phonograph record			X

If a message is delivered through a mechanized device, the learner's control over the presentation rate may be reduced, depending on the nature of the equipment. For example, a film or sound filmstrip requires a projector, a sound-slide program requires a projector and tape-playing device, and a video program requires a video player and TV monitor or a video projector. In such instances, the rate of presentation of the message can be controlled only by forwarding or reversing the equipment. Computers are exceptions. Unless there is mechanical failure within the system, presentation rate can easily be controlled by the learner.

Travers has studied auditory-visual message delivery.[20] Evidence from his research indicates that multisensory input (more than two senses involved) is likely to be of value only when the rate of information delivery is relatively slow. On the other hand, at very high presentation rates (faster than 300 words per minute) the two-modality, auditory-visual condition appears to be superior. If an auditory-visual presentation is too rapid, the learner (perceiver) must choose between the two channels. Only at slower rates can both auditory and visual messages be interrelated efficiently and effectively.

Reiser examined the interaction effects of various pacing procedures and perception of locus of control on final examination performance in a personalized system of instruction.[21] The three pacing procedures employed were: (1) rewarding students if they mastered unit tests on or before deadlines, (2) penalizing them if they failed to pass unit tests on or before deadlines, and (3) informing students of deadlines but not rewarding or penalizing. Results indicate that the effects of various pacing procedures on final exam scores vary according to perception of locus of control of reinforcement. In this study, imposing a penalty on students with a high internal locus of control resulted in better performance than a reward. Among students with an external locus of control, a reward procedure and a neutral procedure seemed to work better than a penalty.

Set

Perception and cognition are strongly affected by what we expect to perceive. This expectation influences what we select from the environment and how we organize and interpret it. It is necessary for teachers to establish a mind-set that will help learners achieve cognitive closure—the act of making associations, drawing inferences, and organizing information for meaning so that transfer will result. In a theatrical production, the set creates mood, establishes tone, and facilitates transition from scene to scene. Similarly, in teaching, set predisposes the learner to perceive and approach information in a particular manner. It is an attitude of mind, the purposeful attention to sensory messages, a predisposer to cognitive organization. The actions taken to induce set by the teacher are, as a whole, called set induction. Such planned activities or conditions focus attention on expectations and help the learner to perceive the value of the learning task. Set arouses interest, focuses attention, provides a common frame of reference, establishes a link between past and present messages, and facilitates transition to future messages.

Inducing set is a teacher's way of controlling how the learner perceives the learning experience. For example, asking a particular question, posing a specific problem, reading a poem, or even providing a reading list or outline directs the learner's attention in a certain way.

Set can be restrictive. When the objective is to involve the learner in an open, creative way, it will be important to avoid establishing a predetermined set. In this case, open-ended questions could be posed, such as asking, "Why do you suppose this happened?"

All direct and indirect strategies, in part or whole, can establish mind-set. For example, textbooks contain a preface, introduction, and table of contents; a videorecording begins with a crisis or problem situation and poses questions for analysis; the teacher begins a lecture by displaying the objectives on an overhead transparency and then reads a short case study; the narration provides the set for the accompanying slide and the syllabus establishes set for the entire course.

Elements of set—arousal, incentive, and expectancy—provide cues to expectations and relieve anxiety. Set is an essential condition for learning—an adjunct to achieving cognitive closure. To arouse interest and establish expectancy, the objectives and key points to be covered can be identified in sequence as advance organizers. An explanation of why the content is important and how the content builds upon previous learning and applies to future learning (incentive) can then follow.

Either the inductive or deductive method of organization can be used when establishing set. For instance, a short role play depicting a specific familiar situation relating to psychological immobility can be presented to guide the learner to come up with the definition, concepts, and principles of psychological immobility. On the other hand, the deductive method would start with the definition, concepts, and principles of psychological immobility and be followed by the specific situation.

Johnson describes how he begins a lecture on child development.[22] First, a lively stereorecording is played to wake up the audience. This is followed by the wheeling in of a supposedly screaming newborn (a doll in a carriage with a concealed taped recording), whereby Dr. Johnson becomes progressively agitated and finally flings the doll into the audience. Can you imagine how effective this strategy would be for arousing attention and establishing incentive and expectancy for the lecture to follow?

Closure

Set is an essential condition for learning. It is an adjunct to achieving *closure*. Closure is derived from the Gestalt principle that behavior or mental processes tend toward a finished, stable, or completed state. Closure involves drawing together old and new information, establishing its relevance, and helping the learner to formulate meaningful associations, draw meaningful relationships, and organize information for transfer to new learning experiences. Both perceived set and cognitive closure affect learner achievement. The teacher is instrumental in helping the learner to achieve cognitive closure.[23]

Elements of closure include summarizing information, extending and applying information to new examples and circumstances, posing application experiences, and introducing new concepts and principles to facilitate transfer of learning to real-life situations.

Instructional closure helps the learner to attend, translate, and transform the message. The direct and indirect strategies used by the teacher should provide instructional closure to facilitate cognitive closure. Instructional closure is reached when the learning experience is completed and the teacher has linked past knowledge with new knowledge. Cognitive closure, however, is reached only when the learner has internally associated old and new learnings. Cognitive closure is the goal of instructional closure. The summary sections and the application activities in each chapter of this text illustrate how instructional closure can be provided within a book. Each of these components are designed to facilitate cognitive closure.

Motion and Color

In some cases, the qualities of motion (movement/action) and color may be crucial conditions for learning, in others they may not. For instance, if the learning outcomes are such that they require either the use of action or the identifying characteristic of color, then the strategies used by the teacher to facilitate achievement should include these attributes.

Motion. Human perception is extremely sensitive to movement. Motion attracts attention and influences feelings and emotions. Because of its realism, it is usually considered to be an effective motivator. According to a number of research studies, the value of motion as a necessary condition for learning is questionable unless the objective requires motion as a critical condition for learning. For example, it seems that when teaching a psychomotor skill, such as giving an injection, the learner needs to see the actual movements involved in technique; however, research indicates that when skills are relatively simple with few steps involved and the movements are separate rather than concurrent or interacting, they can be perceived without seeing movement. On the other hand, when skills are so complex that ambiguity or disorientation may result without the aspect of movement, then seeing the skill demonstrated in action may be beneficial to the learner.

Certain direct and indirect strategies convey movement and others do not. Motion strategies include models and mock-ups with moving parts, simulators, games, video and live demonstrations, and role plays. The illusion of motion or apparent movement can be conveyed through still pictures, film, drawings, and slides. Even computerized strategies can convey action and movement. The action-packed video or computer game is one example. There is also evidence that motion strategies may be instrumental in influencing attitudes, values, and emotions. The element of action appears to evoke emotional reactions and contributes to attitude change. Miller examined film motion and its relationship to emotional involvement and positive attitude response to a film.[24] Subjects who received the treatment with motion showed significantly higher attitude evaluation than those receiving nonmotion treatment.

Color. Attention is drawn to novelty and to anything that is perceived to be different. Color directs attention and conveys realism; therefore, it contributes to the perceptual-cognitive processes of sensory stimulation, cue selection, translation, and transformation of messages. When considering the use of color, the single most important question should be whether it will significantly contribute to achievement of the learning outcome. The use of color may be attractive and interesting, but it will not necessarily increase learning unless a color discrimination is involved or if the learner must perceive the dynamic features of a realistic event or object. If a learning outcome indicates that color differentiation is a mandatory condition for learning, then the strategies used to facilitate the outcome should convey color. For instance, if the learner is expected to perform a surface appraisal of the newborn or assess the condition of the skin, then the attribute of color is a critical condition for learning. Most direct and indirect strategies have the potential for conveying color. Exceptions are those that provide purely auditory input, such as audiorecordings and audioconferencing.

Researchers have for a long time been interested in the role of color in learning; however, most studies have resulted in inconclusive findings and consequently provide few guidelines for teachers. Depending on the individual, color cues may add to or inhibit information processing. It is assumed that the importance of color as a condition for learning rests primarily on the degree to which color cues facilitate structuring and organizing the information presented—the ability of color to delineate figure-ground relationships, to provide directional signs, to show interrelatedness, to make discriminations, and to organize a simplified whole into a complex whole.[25] Like motion, color may be instrumental for influencing attitudes and emotions. Donahue found that politicians and political advertisements were perceived more favorably after viewing a color film, as opposed to a black-and-white version, of a political commercial.[26] Color may also be a motivating force.

Active Involvement

Active involvement or active participation in learning refers to the learner's ability to actually react to or interact with the learning experience. This construct comes from stimulus-response theory, which proposes that the learner should be an active learner rather than a passive one who simply receives information from a direct or indirect source. Experimental evidence indicates that active, experiential sensory learning appears to maximize application and transfer of learning and suggests that direct active involvement in learning does change cognitive, affective, and psychomotor behaviors. For instance, assuming the role of another person through role play appears to change attitudes about the person portrayed.

Active participation in learning involves perceiving through the senses, carrying out physical actions, and using mental processes. Therefore, active involvement can be either covert or overt. Covert activity refers to internal responding, such as forming a mental image. A covert response is not observable. On the other hand, overt responding is observable—the learner writes a paper, takes notes, manipulates pieces to complete a puzzle, plays a game, or sets up an IV system.

Research indicates that we do not always have to exhibit an overt response to learn. For example, we can view and listen to a television program without taking notes and still attend to and translate the message. Yet, there is evidence that as the degree of activity increases (from covert to overt) the amount of learning also increases. Whether this is true or not depends to some extent upon the individual characteristics of the learner, including age, developmental level, learning style, modality strengths, cognitive style, and learning preferences. The teacher can influence achievement to some extent by providing appropriate organization, prompts and primes, type and amount of information, rate of presentation, and so on.

Active experiential learning through direct, hands-on manipulative experiences with objects and through varied positive and negative examples is particularly important for young children. If we want a child to learn to brush teeth daily in a particular way, we must provide conditions that enable the child to perceive how to brush, and structure conditions so that the child can actually brush each day. Just telling the child how to brush and when will probably not help the child to achieve the outcome. The child must see it done and do it properly.

Active involvement in learning is preferred by most adults and adolescents, as well as children. For instance, by actively participating in discussion following a film, we have the opportunity to discuss relevant content, relate it to previous learning, clear up misconceptions, engage in problem solving, and air personal attitudes and feelings. Active overt participation is particularly important for learning psychomotor skills. While knowledge of form and sequence can be acquired by observing a model, proficiency in action requires actual hands-on, overt practice and performance. Observation alone is not sufficient for learning complex psychomotor skills that are new to the learner. Yet, if the skill has been acquired previously but has not been used for a time, covert participation through observation may be sufficient to revitalize the skill. It should be evident that one advantage of providing conditions of active overt participation is that the teacher can observe performance and determine whether learning has occurred and to what degree. Changes in strategies and conditions can then be made on a more objective basis.

If the objective is such that active, overt participation is necessary for learning, we can use particular strategies that have this condition as an embedded quality. Examples are discussion, role play, live demonstration with return practice, clinical or laboratory practicum, models and mock-ups, specimens and objects, worksheets, programed instruction, modular instruction, videoconferencing, projects, and games. Other strategies can be adapted or combined to incorporate active overt involvement in learning (Table 3–5).

The live lecture frequently is only one-way communication without active, overt involvement. This may result in relatively passive covert learner response if, for instance, notes are not taken or learners do not even speak. Thus, learners are at the receiving level of the learning process and usually are not encouraged to go on

TABLE 3-5. PROVIDING FOR ACTIVE OVERT INVOLVEMENT

Strategy	Mechanisms for Providing Active Overt Involvement
Direct	
Live lecture	Present for 15 minutes. Pose 5-minute problem situation. Discuss. Repeat.
Indirect	
Textbook Journal article Print case study	Provide questions to answer in writing or outlines for notetaking. Incorporate discussion. Use adjunct models, objects, or projects.
Slides Video lecture Video interview	Incorporate print study guide with questions or problems to solve and space for notetaking. Incorporate videodisk and computer. Use programing techniques. Incorporate discussion.
Poster Photograph Picture Chart	Ask questions and promote discussion. Incorporate manipulative objects. Pose problems to solve. Provide worksheet. Use in conjunction with computer game.
Audioconferencing Audiotape Phonograph record Sound slide Film Filmstrip	Promote discussion and questioning. Incorporate role play. Provide manipulative models, mock-ups, objects, specimens, worksheets. Give pre- and posttests.
Video demonstration	Pretest. Require return practice. Provide help sessions. Use proficiency testing. Pause for practice. Incorporate videodisk and computer.
Overhead transparencies	Reproduce masters on a plain paper copier and assemble in a notebook. Record narrative on audio recorder and prepare study questions. Give pre- and posttest. Use programed transparencies at the end of a lecture to prime and prompt responses and then give feedback.

to a higher level of generating ideas and internalizing concepts and principles. They do not assume responsibility for their own learning. There are, however, things that the teacher can do to help the learner participate in the lecture. The "feedback lecture" is one way to adapt the one-way lecture to a two-way strategy with active, overt participation.[27] The feedback lecture is guided by a lecture study guide. The guide prepares the student for learning in advance of the actual presentation by suggesting specific methods and procedures for study. Components of the study guide include a pretest, a suggested procedure for studying, objectives, terminology, visuals, advance readings, and an introduction to the content to be presented. Lecture notes in outline form are handed out at the beginning of the lecture. They can also be incorporated in the study guide. After 15 to 20 minutes of lecturing, the instructor guides learners to discuss a question, problem, or situation relative to the content for 5 minutes in groups of two. The learners discuss and write their response and hand it in. During the learner activity session, the teacher circulates to the various teams (if the room allows), responds to individual questions, and gives feedback. After the written responses are collected, the teacher guides discussion or provides the answer to the question, problem, or situation. One point toward a final grade can be awarded for an appropriate response. This same format can be repeated for the duration of the lecture.

Other strategies that help to make the one-way lecture two-way, with active involvement in learning, include the following: (1) having learners identify questions they would like answered or problems they have experienced related to the topic, writing these on a chalkboard, flip chart, or overhead transparency and referring to them during and at the end of the session; (2) having students respond to a series of yes/no questions related to the topic throughout the session; (3) at the beginning of the session, giving a self-assessment quiz composed of true/false, multiple-choice, or short-answer items and addressing the information during the presentation; (4) giving students a handout to read at an appropriate point during the presentation, displaying questions for students to answer from the reading, and discussing their answers before the end of the session; (5) identifying a group of three to five students at the beginning of the session and asking them to stop you at any point during the session to explain confusing information; (6) asking three to five students to come to the front of the class and at appropriate points in the lecture, having this group discuss or analyze information presented (other students can interject information or ask questions of the student group); and (7) providing time for small group brainstorming on a problem situation. Students can be asked to generate all possible ideas and solutions. Students' ideas can be written on a chalkboard, flip chart, or overhead transparency, and the feasibility of each can be discussed.

Physical and Environmental Factors

Physical and environmental factors such as room temperature, lighting, noise, the individual's need for mobility, time of day, and seating arrangements are among the factors that can affect learning. According to Rita and Kenneth Dunn, these factors can be classified as sound, light, temperature, and design.[28] As well-known researchers on learning styles, they contend that some persons are comfortable learning in the presence of noise, whereas others need absolute silence. For instance, some people can read and concentrate without difficulty while watching television or listening to the radio, others cannot. Poor technical quality of film and tape recordings and outside environmental sounds have been known to inhibit attention and concentration, thus interfering with learning.

Some people prefer low light levels when learning, whereas others prefer a well-lighted environment. Fluorescent lights may bother some people. It should be remembered that certain types of audiovisual strategies require a low light level or even total darkness. Sixteen-millimeter film, slide, filmstrip, and opaque projection are examples. A suitable light level should be maintained for note-taking and other activities that require light. Sufficient light must be reflected from the chalkboard

to insure the contrast necessary for reading. Also, high light level at the front of a classroom tends to direct and hold attention; however, glare or unusual bright spots caused by the sun or other outside light source that reflects from surfaces should be avoided. Unwanted light can be controlled with shades, blinds, or dimmer switches. When images are projected on a screen, the light level should be controlled so that little or no light falls on the screen to distort projected images.

Temperature requirements also vary with the individual. Some learners prefer a cool place in order to be intellectually productive while others do not. Inadequate ventilation, high humidity, lack of fresh air, and stifling heat can decrease attention and concentration.

Many times, a formal environment with straight rows of chairs is the typical seating arrangement. Yet, some people prefer an informal setting with comfortable chairs, while others prefer to work alone in isolation. The seating arrangement should be an integral part of the teaching strategy. For example, if the strategy is group discussion, chairs should be arranged in a circular or semicircular pattern so that the environment promotes open interaction, feedback, and reinforcement. On the other hand, independent learning warrants a relatively closed, yet comfortable environment. Seating for a large group lecture should be flexible and arranged so that each learner can easily see the presenter and projected or displayed visuals. The room should allow for flexibility in message delivery so that the necessary conditions for learning can be provided and a multiplicity of strategies used. Traditional lecture halls should be replaced with multipurpose rooms to allow for different seating arrangements and to take advantage of the latest technology.

Strategies for teaching should include options to accommodate individual differences in peak performance time and mobility. Some people learn best early in the morning while others prefer late morning or afternoon hours. Lack of physical mobility may inhibit learning for those who prefer to be active while learning. Even eating or drinking may be an important condition for learning for some. An attempt should be made to match learning preferences and styles such as these with teaching strategies and learning events.

SUMMARY

Reinforcement and feedback can be incorporated in either direct or indirect teaching strategies. Specific praise, augmented with informative feedback emphasizing the positive, can improve performance and be a motivating force in learning. The information received by the learner through feedback focuses the learner's attention on critical aspects necessary for accurate learning. Video, computer- and print-programed strategies are some of the indirect strategies that, because of their inherent properties and potential capabilities, can be used by the teacher to convey positive reinforcement and feedback conditions for learning.

Practice and repetition are necessary prerequisites to and reinforcers for learning. The learner must, however, be aware of the goal to be attained and must desire to improve; otherwise repetition and practice may result in no improvement or even in inferior learning. Consideration should be given to the length of the practice and repetitive sessions in relationship to the complexity and nature of the task to be learned. When information is new to the learner, frequent, short practice periods interspersed with periods of rest are preferable to extended, continuous practice periods. Novice learners are more prone to lose interest and become inattentive when faced with something new and difficult to learn. Up to a certain point, it seems that practice continued beyond the stage of one perfect recital might help retention and transfer. The conditions of practice and repetition can be incorporated in both direct and indirect teaching strategies and they are embedded attributes in several types of indirect teaching strategies.

A teacher can elicit correct responses by using copying, echoing, or imitation primes and formal or thematic prompts. Such conditions help the learner to attend to key elements, recall information from memory, and assimilate new information. When a response is primed, the learner will be able to perceive the exact structure or nature of the desired response, whereas a prompted response only hints at the correct response. Thematic prompts are more likely to promote high-level association, discrimination, and comprehension behaviors than formal prompts. Visual prompting and priming techniques include using signs and symbols and varying embellishments and format to direct attention to important aspects, thus activating perceptual-cognitive processes. For example, adding a drawing to a verbal definition, underlining key words, and using line drawings instead of realistic pictures may be just what is needed to facilitate learning.

Priming conditions are provided through strategies that show how to do something or give information. Examples are actual demonstration, lecture with visuals, such as overhead transparencies, slides, chalkboard, and film. Just using visuals does not constitute a prime; rather, the message and how it is visually presented is the prime. Questioning and discussion or computer and programed instruction exemplify strategies that are particularly suited for establishing prompting conditions that magnify critical features of the message to elicit desired responses. Learning may be maximized when initial instruction is cued and when cues are added or removed gradually.

One of the most easily controlled conditions for learning, but one that is abused to a large extent, concerns the amount of information conveyed at one time. For example, it is common practice to lecture for two hours or to show a 50-minute film. In the majority of cases, too much information is covered in too little time. There are apparently outside limits to human ability to receive, perceive, and process information. It appears that the more mature and motivated the learner, the greater the perceptual capacity; however, attention is easily lost during one-way, one-modality, information-packed presentations. It is, therefore, important to limit the number of items per unit of time, to vary the sensory input, and to provide practice and overt response conditions with frequent periods of rest. More complex material should be conveyed through print or pictorial strategies rather than through the auditory mode.

Clear, logical organization of information is a basic condition for efficient and effective perception, cognition, and learning. The teacher is instrumental in influencing perceptual-cognitive processes and achievement of learning outcomes by the way messages are organized. Well-organized patterning of information into parts and wholes can improve the learner's ability to make associations, retain information, and transfer learning, no matter what type of teaching strategy is used. On the other hand, a disorganized teaching strategy can inhibit learning.

Messages can be organized deductively (moving from generalizations to concrete examples), inductively (beginning with specifics and progressing to generalizations), progressing from simple to complex, and from familiar to unfamiliar. Linear patterning and fixed sequencing of information is less flexible than branched patterning in that the learner must receive the information as it is presented in a predetermined order. On the other hand, branched organization allows the learner to rearrange information according to individual needs, strengths, and weaknesses.

The sequential, hierarchical organization of information combined with the use of advance organizers can positively affect learning because each new increment of information serves as an anchoring post for subsequent learning. Sequential organization presupposes that the preceding step is always clear, stable, and well-organized. If it is not, learning of subsequent steps is jeopardized. New information should not be introduced until all previous steps are thoroughly mastered. The visual (pictorial) advance organizer tends to provide the learner with an effective cognitive framework for relating new information and stimulating recall. Visual organizers can be imbedded in all types of teaching strategies.

The rate of presentation of a message is a crucial condition for learning that correlates closely with the amount of information presented. Depending on the learning outcome to be achieved, the characteristics of the learner or learner group and the content, it may be desirable to use strategies that allow the learner to have maximum control over the rate at which information is received and the pace at which the learner proceeds through the learning experience. Such is the case with mastery learning and learning that involves unfamiliar or abstract content. Without imposed deadlines, some strategies readily lend themselves to learner control over the rate of presentation, and hence, the pace of learning. Examples are discussion, role play, textbooks, sets of individual slides that can be advanced, stopped, and reversed manually, with accompanying print outlines or worksheets, some games, and computer-based strategies. On the other hand, the teacher, equipment, or a device may control the rate of presentation. Such controlled situations include live or recorded lecture, video demonstration, sound-slide or filmstrip programs, and film. Strategies such as clinical practicum, live demonstration with return practice, video- or audioconferencing, and multimedia modular instruction fall somewhere in between depending on the circumstances of the learning experience and the design of the strategy. In addition, placing external constraints on the learner, such as imposing deadlines for completing learning experiences or rewarding early completion, may influence individual achievement by controlling the pace of learning. The nature of the content, type of learning, and learning objectives influence selection of teaching strategies, which in turn influence the time required to achieve learning outcomes.

Of the factors that determine attention, mind-set is probably the most important. Set involves a readiness to think or respond in a certain way when confronted with a problem or situation. Set plays a major role in both what we select from the environment and how we organize and interpret it. For example, a parent may sleep through a ringing telephone, but the slightest sound from a sick child will bring immediate arousal. Set largely directs and orders perceptual experiences. Without it, perceiving would be largely at random, fluctuating with environmental stimuli. Human thought is governed by mind-set. The teacher is instrumental in establishing events that impose a particular set or expectancy for learning. The strategies and conditions selected and used by the teacher, including posing questions and problems, providing introductory information in the form of outlines, readings, and advance organizers, and establishing objectives and learning outcomes, help the learner to focus on key points and maintain attention throughout a learning experience. The presence and strength of a particular mind-set can influence alternative interpretations of a learning event and encourage or discourage convergent or divergent thinking. Inadequate set induction can lead to inaccurate perceptions and inhibit learning.

Set will also influence cognitive closure; that is, how and the extent to which the learner is able to link old and new learning, form meaningful associations and relationships, and process and organize information for transfer to new learning experiences. The conditions necessary for inducing cognitive closure can be embedded in both direct and indirect teaching strategies. For example, the teacher can provide a print or oral summary of information and structure application activities, such as requiring the learner to design a game or computer program that applies the facts, concepts, and principles just presented. In this manner, the learner will be able to achieve cognitive closure through high-level analysis, synthesis, and decision making processes.

Motion and color are considered to be effective attention-focusing and affect-inducing conditions for learning. Both attributes are capable of influencing and contributing to attitude change.

Indirect motion strategies, such as video programs and motion pictures, have been experimentally investigated for their worth in promoting psychomotor learning. Their value appears to be related to their capability of allowing the learner to view the task and analyze critically the body movements involved in the skill. Both film and video strategies are commonly used for modeling or demonstration purposes. Videorecording is particularly useful for providing instant visual feedback on action performance. The individual can immediately see how the skill was performed after a recorded session.

It would seem that motion strategies should facilitate achievement of all learning outcomes involving motor skill; however, some studies give only a slightly favorable indication of the value of motion strategies, while others indicate no difference in final skill proficiency. Similarly, color is a critical condition for learning when the learning outcome requires color for discrimination purposes.

The use of motion and color to focus attention, instill interest, promote the formation of associations, and differentiate between constructs depends upon what conditions are necessary for achievement of learning outcomes. Because of the lack of hard research data about the value of these two conditions for learning, common sense must rule decision making. It appears, however, that the judicious use of color and motion may influence improved learner achievement of particular objectives, if for no other reason than that their use provides realism and motivation.

Active, overt experiential participation in learning means "learning by doing." It is a condition for learning that cuts across age and developmental levels. Most of us can attest to the fact that we do learn through active "hands-on" involvement. Why is it, then, that most learning experiences, especially in a formalized classroom setting, are composed of strategies that require little or no active, overt response? Lectures, films, readings, videorecordings, and other auditory and visual strategies in which we become passive watchers and listeners are the rule, while role play, games, debating, brainstorming, computer-assisted instruction, and perhaps even discussion are seen as supplementary teaching strategies.

Active, overt involvement can be provided even when there are a large number of students in a class and when learning involves abstract concept and principle learning. Knowing the strategies that are particularly conducive to providing for active, overt response and creative teaching is the key.

There are a number of psychological conditions that may make a difference in learning. These include reinforcement, feedback, practice, and repetition, priming and prompting, perceptual capacity, organization, grouping and patterning of information, rate of presentation and pacing, set and closure, motion, color, and active participation in learning.

In addition, physical and environmental factors, such as lighting, noise, mobility, time of day, and seating arrangements can affect the extent to which learners achieve learning outcomes and program goals. Learner preferences for sound, light, temperature, and design should be considered in conjunction with constraints imposed by the teaching situation when determining the teaching strategies appropriate for learning experiences.

The inherent nature of teaching strategies themselves will affect environmental factors. They may dictate specific needs relative to lighting, sound, and design. They may inject noise, affect mobility, and even control the time and place for learning. Psychological, physical, and environmental conditions for learning and teaching strategies are intricately interrelated.

ADVANTAGES AND LIMITATIONS OF SELECTED DIRECT AND INDIRECT TEACHING STRATEGIES

Some teaching strategies have a geater potential for providing certain conditions for learning than others. For instance, video, film, real objects, models, simulators, clinical practicum, and lab experiences prime and prompt psychomotor skills. Film or video may be effective for priming and prompting psychomotor skills and attitudinal behaviors because realistic action is an inherent quality of these strategies. Such auditory, visual, motion strategies will enable the learner to see every action in a skill while hearing how the action should and should not be performed. Active, overt hands-on participation in learning is provided through live demonstration with return practice, computer simulations, real objects, models or simulators, games, programed or modular instruction, role play, laboratory experiences, and clinical practicum. Two-way feedback and reinforcement is apparent in live discussion, live demonstration with return practice, audio- and videoconferencing, clinical practicum, programed and computer-based learning strategies and role play. The learner can easily repeat information delivered through such strategies as textbooks, games, handouts, pamphlets, and computer programs. Color can be conveyed through use of overhead transparencies and slides during a live lecture, and it is usually an embedded quality in sound-slide or filmstrip programs, color video demonstrations or interviews, pamphlets, motion films, and books.

Live, formal lecture incorporating overhead transparencies or individual slides and other visuals, video lecture, textbooks and readings, audioconferencing, sound-slide or filmstrip, 16-millimeter film, and some types of simulations and games are appropriate for large groups, whereas discussion, computer-based strategies, objects and models, live demonstration with return practice, field trips, and clinical practicum are more effective for small-group, team, or individual learning experiences. Modular, programed, computer-based strategies, learning activity packages, or contract learning lend themselves well to individualized, independent, self-paced learning. Audio- and videoconferencing, radio, broadcast television, and computer-based networking strategies are particularly appropriate for long-distance learning. Other types of indirect strategies can be combined and incorporated for use at distant sites. Textbooks, computer-assisted strategies, programed instruction, discussions, and videodisks facilitate branched organization of information. Computer games and simulations are particularly useful for providing high-level active, overt response, corrective feedback, positive reinforcement, and repetition.

Live, formal lecture tends to be limited to one-way communication as do film, sound-slide, filmstrip, radio, and video presentations unless mechanisms for interaction are built in. Modular instruction and other learner-directed strategies may lead to learner procrastination (Table 3–6).

Each strategy, then, because of its inherent properties, has particular attributes that make it more suitable for particular learning events and learners. For example, consider computer-assisted strategies, which are being recognized as effective and efficient ways of delivering nursing and client education. Ball and Hannah state the major advantages of computer-assisted learning as: (1) being applicable to independent study, (2) capable of facilitating development of creative and flexible approaches to problem solving, (3) lending continuity to situations in which there is a shortage or turnover of nursing educators, (4) providing more effective use of teaching and learning time, (5) promoting effective learning, (6) facilitating lesson updating, (7) providing motivation through immediate feedback, (8) being compatible with multimedia, multisensory approaches to learning, and (9) being consistent, patient, fair, tolerant, and approving of each and every learner.[29] In addition, Ball and Hannah point out limitations related to cost, content control, altered professional roles, the technology itself (standardization), deficits relating to learning theory and computer-assisted instruction (CAI), and lack of formal communication among users. Table 3–7 presents several strategies, their advantages, and limitations.

When a teacher chooses to use a particular teaching strategy, certain demands are imposed upon the learner. For example, a one-hour live, formal lecture may require the learner to adapt to relatively abstract, aural symbol decoding, linear organization of information, and lack of immediate reinforcement, feedback, and overt participation in learning. Studies dealing with learning and cognitive style indicate, however, that individuals do have unique strengths and preferences that determine to some extent how successfully they will learn when confronted with strategies that may or may not be in accord with modality strengths. It appears that many individuals can change their learning styles in response to demands of the teaching-learning experience and content. People can learn to cope with demands placed upon them by a particular strategy.[30] Therefore, it seems that one of the major responsibilities of the teacher is to teach students how to learn from particular teaching strategies before they are used.

TOOLS FOR SELECTING TEACHING STRATEGIES

Teachers also have unique teaching styles and preferences for teaching. Teachers tend to teach the way they learn best and to model the behaviors of their own teachers. It is also true that conditions relative to the setting, time limitations, societal influences, equipment and facility needs, and budget place constraints on what is taught as well as how it is taught. There is an extraordinary relationship among the teacher, the learner, and the psychological, physical, and environmental conditions that influence how successful an individual will be in learning. The knowledge, skill, and judgment of the teacher in regard to selecting teaching strategies are critical to effective teaching and learning.

Determining teaching strategies for learning experiences requires careful, critical analysis and evaluation. The selection process takes into consideration knowledge of the learner(s), the purpose of the learning experience, and the learning objectives to be achieved. The particular advantages and limitations of strategies, their potential for conveying the necessary conditions for learning, and their relative value for particular learning experiences should be thoroughly assessed before use. A multitude of forms have been developed just for this purpose. Such forms are valuable tools that help a teacher systematically decide which strategies to use for a particular learning event. Although most forms have been designed for appraisal of audiovisual strategies, they can be used for other types of strategies as well. Typically, they include provision for assessing conditions for learning inherent in the strategy relative to a predetermined purpose and to specific learning objectives for a particular learner or learner group. Descriptors usually reflect content, psychological factors, and technical and environmental variables. (*See* the Appendix for sample forms.)

TABLE 3-6. PRIMARY ADVANTAGES AND LIMITATIONS OF SELECTED STRATEGIES

Conditions for Learning / Strategy	Formal, live lecture with still visuals	Live discussion	Textbook, journal article	Live demonstration with return practice	Computer simulation	Video lecture, demonstration, interview	Audioconferencing with slides and handouts on site	Sound-filmstrip or sound-slide	Real object	Model, mock-up	Film	Board or card game	Clinical practicum	Modular instruction or learning activity package with multisensory components and return practice	Programed instruction: Print or audiovisual	Role play	Audiotape	Radio	Videoconferencing
Auditory and visual stimuli	X	X		X	X	X	X	X	X	X	X	X	X	X	X	X			X
Auditory stimuli only																	X	X	
Visual stimuli only			X									X			X				
Tactile and visual stimuli		X		X	X				X	X		X	X	X	X	X			
Olefactory or gustatory stimuli									X				X						
Color stimuli	X	X	X	X	X	X	X	X	X	X	X	X	X	X	X	X			X
Active, two-way interaction		X		X	X		X					X	X	X	X	X			X
Immediate feedback and reinforcement		X		X	X		X		X	X		X	X	X	X	X			X
Active, overt hands-on participation and practice				X	X				X	X		X	X	X	X	X			

Learner control over rate of presentation		X	X	X	X		X		X	X		X		X	X	X			
Information load easily adapted to learner needs		X	X	X	X		X			X		X	X	X	X	X			X
Branched information to accommodate individual needs		X	X	X	X		X			X		X	X	X	X	X			X
Information easily repeated by learner			X		X	X		X	X	X	X	X		X	X		X		
"Real" motion stimuli				X	X	X			X	X	X	X	X	X	X	X			X
Alteration of time, place, space, size, or distance			X		X	X	X	X		X	X	X		X	X	X	X	X	X
Immediate recognition of consequences of actions		X		X	X		X		X	X		X	X	X	X	X			X
Independent, self-directed learning			X		X	X		X	X	X	X	X		X	X		X	X	
Same information to large group of learners at same time (50–100+)	X		X			X	X	X			X					X	X	X	X

TABLE 3-7. MAJOR ADVANTAGES AND LIMITATIONS OF SELECTED TEACHING STRATEGIES

Strategy	Advantages	Limitations
Live, formal lecture with overhead transparencies or slides	Auditory, visual sensory input Same information delivered to large group of learners at one time Linear message delivery	Primarily one-way communication Immediate feedback and reinforcement limited or nonexistent
Discussion	Highly interactive Immediate feedback and reinforcement Flexible sequencing of information Branched organization of information	Lack of participation by some learners Message delivered to limited number of learners at one time Message not the same from one group or individual to another from time to time Primarily auditory input
Textbooks, readings	Same information conveyed to large group of learners at one time Flexible or fixed sequencing of information Highly portable Easy to repeat information	Visual input only Reading level may not be appropriate for all learners May lack immediate feedback and reinforcement
Live demonstration with return practice	Personalized role modeling Fixed or flexible sequencing of information Immediate feedback and reinforcement Step-by-step disclosure of information Active, overt, hands-on participation in learning	Not appropriate for large numbers of learners at same time Relatively expensive in terms of teaching time, equipment, and facility needs Scheduling problems
Computer-assisted	Saves teaching and learning time Branched sequencing of information Immediate feedback and reinforcement Message easily repeated and manipulated Highly interactive Random access to information	Learner dependent on hardware System "down time" Inadequate programing Scheduling problems Limited to 1 to 3 learners at one time Equipment expensive
Video: lecture, demonstration, interview 16-mm film	Auditory, visual sensory input Fixed sequencing of information Saves teaching time	Learner dependent on hardware Rate and pace controlled by hardware

TABLE 3-7. ***(continued)***

Strategy	Advantages	Limitations
	Overcomes barriers of time, size, space, distance Conveys real action (motion) Message can be repeated Adaptable to group or individual	Fixed sequencing of information Difficult to update and revise Equipment expensive Scheduling problems Usually lacks immediate feedback and reinforcement
Audioconferencing	Overcomes barriers of distance Flexible message delivery Highly interactive Immediate feedback and reinforcement Personalized Same information delivered to large group of learners at one time	Primarily auditory input Equipment malfunction Equipment and line time expensive Scheduling problems Message not easily repeated
2 × 2 slides	Easy to rearrange Fixed or flexible sequencing of information Adaptable to group or individual learning Multiple images can be displayed at one time Conveys realism Step-by-step disclosure of information	Still, visual input May lack immediate feedback and reinforcement Learner dependent on hardware May be lost or damaged by learners
Filmstrip	Fixed sequencing of information Step-by-step disclosure of information Adaptable to group or individual learning Message can be repeated Conveys realism	Still, visual input Difficult and expensive to revise Learner dependent on hardware Easily damaged
Objects, models, mock-ups, simulators	Multisensory input Conveys realism Concrete, hands-on, overt participation in learning Immediate feedback and reinforcement	May oversimplify reality Damage, loss of parts Not suitable for large numbers of learners at same time
Teacher-directed clinical practicum	Real experiential learning Multisensory input Hands-on, overt participation in learning	Limited to one-on-one or small groups of learners Facilities, scheduling problems

(cont.)

TABLE 3-7. *(continued)*

Strategy	Advantages	Limitations
	Immediate feedback and reinforcement Personalized	Great amount of direct teaching time required
Games, simulations, role play	Can be highly interactive or provide for independent participation in learning Consequences of actions realized Hands-on, overt participation in learning Immediate feedback and reinforcement Flexible sequencing of information Makes learning fun, rewarding Can simulate lifelike experiences	May distort reality May be limited in scope May foster anger or frustration Props may be needed
Modular instruction, learning activity packages	Multisensory input Can accommodate individual learning styles and preferences Facilitates mastery learning Step-by-step disclosure of information Highly organized Linear or branched organization of information Active, overt response Guided practice Easy to repeat information Learner can proceed at own rate and pace Objectives and procedures stated Immediate feedback and reinforcement	Allows learner procrastination
Independent projects, contracts	Personalized Individualized Active, overt participation in learning	Instructor's management, record-keeping time great
Print programed instruction	Individualized Small, step-by-step disclosure of information Linear or branched organization of information Saves teaching and learning time	Visual input only Readability may be a problem May foster boredom Allows learner procrastination

TABLE 3-7. (continued)

Strategy	Advantages	Limitations
	Active, overt participation in learning Portable Easy to repeat Learner can proceed at own rate and pace Immediate feedback and reinforcement	

In addition to using selection forms, the following questions should also help to guide decisions as to teaching strategies appropriate for learner needs and content:

1. Prelearning preparation. Does the learner have the background needed for understanding?
2. Motivation. Is the learner interested in this particular mode of learning?
3. Individual differences. Does the content meet the learner's needs? Is it appropriate to the learner's ability level, handicap, attention span, etc.?
4. Active participation. What response activity is required?
5. Knowledge of results. Does the material provide feedback for self-evaluation?
6. Successful achievement. Is the content structured so the learner is challenged, yet is reinforced successfully enough to continue?
7. Practice. Does the material provide ample opportunity for the learner to use newly acquired knowledge and skills?
8. Rate of presentation of information. Does the rate and amount of information to be learned at any one time relate to the complexity and difficulty of the information in terms of learner ability?
9. Graduated sequencing of content. Are the steps and sequence of the content too large or too small? Out of task order?
10. Instructor attitude. Do I as the teacher have a positive attitude about the strategy and content?

Selection of the "best" teaching strategy or combination of strategies for a particular learning episode presupposes knowledge of how to identify different types of strategies as well as of resources for obtaining them. Auditory, visual, and tactile materials can be purchased or rented from associations, societies, foundations, commercial publishers and distributors, universities, colleges, libraries, and drug companies. They can be adapted or created to meet specific needs. Free or inexpensive materials can also be obtained with a little ingenuity. (*See* the Appendix for a limited listing of sources.)

When selected strategies promote the understandings, skills, and attitudes sought, then proper selection has taken place. Effectiveness can be checked through observation of student behavior, various types of tests and measurements, and student application and extension of learning experiences.

Traditionally, the teacher has looked upon auditory and visual strategies as simply aids to instruction. The teacher was viewed as information provider. The film, filmstrip, or whatever was only a means of supplementing the oral message. Today, there is a growing awareness that indirect strategies are not simply adjunct or supplementary materials. Instructional television was one of the first technological advancements to foster this broader view. Today's modular, computer-based learning packages and systems, audio- and videoconferencing technologies, interactive videodisk programing, and other self-contained and combined strategies allow the teacher to become a facilitator and manager of humanistic learning experiences based on individual needs. A new paradigm is being created, one that has far-reaching implications for nurse-teachers and learners.

SUMMARY

The conditions necessary for promoting achievement of cognitive, affective, and psychomotor learning outcomes may be conveyed through either direct or indirect teaching strategies. These strategies are the means for conveying messages that stimulate the learner's perceptual-cognitive processes, activating attention, cue selection, translation, and transformation of information into observable behaviors. Each strategy has potential advantages as well as limitations that may help a teacher determine which to choose when devising learning experiences for particular learners, tasks, content, and settings. The learner's age, developmental level, physical and psychological maturity, abilities and disabilities, interests, motivation, and health status, along with your preferences for teaching must be considered when selecting teaching strategies. Resources such as assessment tools are available to help make decisions more objective.

We have moved into a more sophisticated era of thinking about learning as an internal process controlled by the learner and engaging the whole being in interaction with the environment. In this context, teaching is viewed as a decision-making process. The nurse-teacher, with input from the learner, determines and provides certain psychological, physical, and environmental conditions that stimulate learning and make it observable so that it can be evaluated. In the past, it has been functional to think about improving learning in terms of discovering and developing new devices for making it more interesting, but we can no longer afford this luxury. We have moved beyond talking about gimmicks to innovative theories, processes, and conditions for learning.

Specific conditions for learning that guide selection decisions can be derived from stimulus-response, cognitive, and humanistic theories of learning. From stimulus-response theory, we learn that a person should be active rather than a passive listener or viewer, that frequency of repetition and practice is important for acquiring knowledge and skill and for retention and transfer, that correct responses should be positively rewarded, that novelty enhances learning, and that priming and prompting can facilitate learning. From cognitive and humanistic theory, we see that perception is an important condition for learning and that clear, logical organization of information should be a primary concern of the teacher. Feedback confirms correct knowledge and corrects faulty learning. Collaborative goal setting by the teacher and the learner is important to motivation. The learner's culture, abilities, developmental level, maturity, interests, preferences, and attitudes are as important as hereditary and congenital determiners. Hence, learning will be affected by variables such as rate of presentation, amount of information, and physical and environmental factors within the learning climate.

The nurse-teacher is instrumental in providing the external conditions that, when combined with internal learner capabilities, bring about desired behavioral change. There are numerous ways to establish these conditions in the learning environment, and many combinations of direct and indirect strategies may be employed to do so. The important point is that the conditions for learning should guide decision making, and various teaching strategies need to be carefully considered as components of a holistic learning experience. The professional nurse-teacher as a facilitator of learning is instrumental in diagnosing learning needs and creating a climate conducive to effective cognitive, affective, and psychomotor learning for all students in his or her charge.

SELECTED RESEARCH ON TEACHING STRATEGIES

Since the early 1950s, there has been a multitude of studies comparing one type of strategy (medium) to another; however, contemporary researchers agree that such studies have not been significant and are inconclusive. The experimental studies that have been done conclude only that a particular strategy under certain conditions can affect learning. No broader generalization can be made. Therefore, teachers cannot glean much from such gross comparative studies to guide selection and utilization decisions. It appears, however, that the research exploring particular attributes, qualities, conditions, or elements conveyed or embedded in a specific strategy and the role that such attributes play in learning can guide decision making. Following is a summary of selected research findings involving particular attributes, qualities, or conditions for learning according to type of strategy. More experimental research is needed.

Sixteen-millimeter Film

Studies by Briggs, Hoban, MacLennan, Wendt, Dayton, and others appear to indicate that: (1) increased learning will result from film if viewers are told what they will be expected to do as a result of viewing, (2) increased learning will result with repeated viewing, pretesting, posttesting, and feedback, (3) more learning will occur if printed study guides are used before and after viewing, and (4) stopping films periodically for questions and note-taking has been found to contribute to learning.[31-35] In addition, one viewing of a film dealing with a complex skill may not be sufficient. Films can provide a model for guided mental practice. A skill can be partially learned by viewing it on film and imagining performance. Viewing a series of films for a half hour daily for many months can lead to unfavorable attitudes by both students and teachers. Learning will increase when films have built-in participative activities and planned redundancy or repetition, or when teachers provide these conditions for learning apart from the film. There appears to be no doubt that the insertion of questions into motion pictures can increase learning under proper conditions. Furnishing knowledge of results of the learner's overt response during a film also has a positive effect upon learning from film.

Knirk's review of the literature on film and its effect on learning reveals that when a film incorporates cues to guide the audience in making correct responses, superior learning results.[36] Slow motion has a slight tendency to produce better learning of a simple perceptual motor task. Inserting attention-gaining devices (not attention-directing devices) does not improve performance and may actually detract from the effectiveness of a demonstration. There is some evidence that when color is an essential cue, more learning may result. Written practice with feedback and correction produces significantly better results than practice alone. Guidance by means of prompting produces better results than unguided practice with feedback. Nearness of an item to a reward sequence in a film may have a significant effect on learning.

Chute found that color helped students of all ability levels in a fourth and fifth grade class to learn information from a color film, but that it affected learning of task-relevant information differently, depending on ability level.[37]

Print Text

Schramm analyzed the research and concluded that: (1) more learning is achieved when the print medium is used to reinforce another medium, but the added channel must provide added interpretation; (2) the human eye can adapt to different type styles and sizes and lengths of lines, but conditioning of readers with respect to these variables is important; (3) readers may resist less-expensive book production practices, such as nonjustified right margins; (4) color illustrations gain attention and interest, but there is no evidence that they produce greater learning unless color itself is a necessary and integral component of the concept to be learned; (5) some evidence exists to support the fact that a writing style in which examples and special cases are subordinated to general explanatory principles elaborated in the text conveys more meaning than a style in which example and principle have the same emphasis; and (6) overlap and repetition appear to benefit comprehension in print materials.[38]

Dayton found that the insertion of factual postquestions in written instructional materials can result in increased learning of both intentional and incidental information.[39] An analysis of intervening variables suggests that post-questions are beneficial for mature readers only, result in an increase in study time, and are more effective for learners who are not highly motivated. Additional evidence suggests that intentional learning will increase when higher order questions requiring comprehension, application or analysis, and knowledge of correct response are provided.

Autotutorial, Programed Instruction (PI), Self-instruction

Fisher found that students valued the self-paced independent study, group study, and mastery learning components of autotutorial strategies. The audiovisual components may be significant in providing motivation. Autotutorial instruction may differentially benefit low-ability students. No consistent differences between sexes were observed in Fisher's review. The tendency to be serious-minded and responsible appears to give significant trait/treatment interaction, so that high achievers with low verbal aptitude and low restraint may learn more from autotutorial instruction. Initial cost investment is moderately high, and savings are purportedly realized over a period of years.[40]

Research on PI confirms that students can effectively learn, often more effectively, from all types of PI, whether linear or branching, and from programs on machines such as computers, or in texts. Equal amounts of information are learned in far less time. Several studies have shown that significantly superior learning results from programed strategies.[41]

Anderson states that organization is a plus of self-instructional strategies. Such teaching strategies usually specify objectives, include advance organizers, and are organized inductively or deductively in a clear and purposeful manner.[42]

Computer

The literature regarding the effectiveness of computer use in learning has been concerned with achievement gains. Reviews of the literature support the notion that supplementary instruction with CAI leads to higher achievement and that the amount of time needed to learn is significantly reduced. Time is saved in terms of completion of a course of study and achievement is increased per unit of time. The capability of the computer to present a stimulus, and review and evaluate a response has generally been successful. Efforts to use the computer to simulate complex models and phenomena have been very successful. Students with higher ability appear to profit more from computer strategies[43]; however, more research is needed. Teachers also save time in actual content delivery when computer-assisted strategies are used. The number of hours spent in lecturing has been reduced as much as 66 percent according to studies done by Joseph Lagowski, at the University of Texas, Austin.[44] Okey and Majer found that as many as four students could use a computer terminal simultaneously and learn as much as students who worked alone.[45]

Murphy's review of the nursing and education literature related to the effectiveness of CAI reveals that: (1) there appears to be equal learning by students using computer tutorials, (2) CAI requires less time to complete when compared to more traditional types of strategies, (3) CAI may lead to greater transfer of learning than more traditional strategies, such as lecture-discussion, (4) CAI can teach psychomotor skills like intravenous rate calculations and regulation, as well as a skills laboratory, (5) despite student preferences for paper-and-pencil simulations, students admit that CAI simulations offer more immediate feedback and are more efficient than paper-and-pencil simulations, and (6) some students prefer CAI to more conventional teaching strategies.[46]

Filmstrip

When concepts or skills involve motion, filmstrips are likely to be less effective than motion strategies. If deficient in detail, definition, or clarity they fail to contribute to learning and may even inhibit learning.[47] Vandermeer found that captions make a difference in learning from a given filmstrip frame.[48] The caption should be at the bottom of the frame in words rather than numbers and should be exact and succinct. Captions can be improved by redundancy and by capitalizing or underlining key names. Labels and directional arrows improve filmstrips, and hence, improve learning. Pictorial or graphic elements in filmstrips should closely resemble their referrants.

Kendler, Kendler, Desiderato and Cook in 1953 found that there was no discernible effect on either learning or performance on an examination when they showed a full-color, sound-filmstrip of the gory results of automobile accidents as an external motivator in conjunction with a sound-filmstrip demonstration of safety measures. They did find, however, that the filmstrip motivator did produce some anxiety in the viewers.[49]

Slides

A review of the literature by Briggs indicates that slides are especially suited for learning when conditions warrant individual pacing and learner participation.[50] In addition, slides with declarative or imperative captions appear to facilitate learning significantly better than slides with questions as captions. Three-dimensional projections of objects on slides are most advantageous where spatial concepts are important, such as size and form in space.

Reiser and Andrews investigated the use of slides instead of drawings as stimuli in an individual testing situation and found that when the same medium (slides) was used for testing as was for teaching, student performance and attitude improved, as did instructor attitude.[51] Both internal and external test validity also increased. Interchangeability of slides resulted in improved test security.

Dayton concluded that inserting postquestions in slide-tape presentations can result in increased incidental learning if the auditory mode is the active ingredient in the teaching strategy.[52]

Overhead Transparencies

Research on teaching with transparencies has been limited, but there is evidence that the investment of time in their preparation and use can improve instruction and save teaching time. It appears that overhead transparencies increase interest on the part of both learners and teachers. Maddox and Loughran explored the use of previously prepared and of built-up transparency diagrams of moderate complexity by testing the recall ability of 54 senior undergraduate students in geography at the end of lecture.[53] Responses to an accompanying questionnaire showed that students preferred that diagrams be built-up during lecture rather than shown already completed. The reasoning was that they could see the sequence in which a fairly complex diagram was constructed and had time to copy it. The researchers concluded that extremely complex materials should be duplicated and handed out to students.

Illustrations

Winn examined the different effects of presenting items as words, black-and-white pictures, or color pictures on the structure of multiple free associations in response to stimulus items.[54] He found no differences in responses to color as opposed to black-and-white pictures, but words elicited more common associations than did pictures. Color, when it was a critical attribute of the concept, emerged as a part of the associative structure.

Jahoda, Cheyne, et al. concluded from their research that in general, pictures with words were more effective than either alone and that the pattern of learning as well as recall was similar across different cultures.[55] The sample was composed of secondary school students in India, Scotland, and Africa.

Dwyer studied the effectiveness of using black-and-white and color versions of four types of illustrations of the heart to complement oral instruction to determine which type of visualization would be most effective in facilitating the achievement of students of different IQ levels and found that there was a significant interaction between IQ and instructional treatment.[56] The line and detailed line drawings in color were most effective in facilitating student achievement. The factor of realism was not a reliable predictor of learning efficiency. Apparently excessive detail in the more realistic illustrations interfered with the transmission of the intended message and reduced effectiveness.

Holliday found that diagrams alone were more effective than either text alone or a combination of text and diagram.[57]

Games

Malone investigated children's and adult's preferences for particular computer games and found that the most important feature determining game popularity was whether the game had an obvious goal and whether players were active participants in a fantasy situation. In addition, children in the sample disliked games that were too hard or too simple.[58]

Posters

Camer found that nurses who viewed posters on cardiopulmonary resuscitation (CPR) techniques for 12 weeks prior to taking a written and practical test scored higher than nurses who had not seen the posters.[59] But the researcher concluded that posters are not useful for initial CPR training and that they have limitations for reinforcing already learned techniques, since even nurses with CPR certification who saw the posters averaged lower-than-passing grades on practical CPR tests.

Video

Weiss found that television was chosen by the general public over magazines, newspapers, and radio as the source of general information because of its "visual" and "live" qualities.[60]

Henderson and Swanson found that linearly sequenced television instruction was most effective when used with active, directed learner participation and corrective feedback, but this, as well as amount of knowledge and skills learned, varied with the age of Head Start preschoolers on an isolated Papago reservation in Arizona.[61]

Coldevin found that spaced treatment of review material (information repeated after each subunit, preceded by a five-second pause) was superior to summary treatment (information repeated at the end of conceptual units) or massed treatment that repeats information after each subunit within a conceptual unit without a preceding five-second pause.[62]

Dwyer investigated the relative effectiveness of three methods of cuing (prompting) in televised instruction and found that when subjects received televised presentations containing motion as a cue, they received significantly higher scores on criterion measures than students who received arrows as cuing devices.[63] Knowledge of the objectives to be achieved, however, almost completely eliminated the effect of different types of cuing used to focus attention on essential information.

A review of the literature by Briggs provides evidence that: (1) learning will increase when methods are built into the televised instruction to ensure that students will make correct responses, and (2) active response groups perform significantly better than no response groups.[64] Programed TV lessons requiring active response may also yield significantly greater achievement.

Yarlow and Bruhn report that a series of sixteen 20-minute role plays were designed to help nursing service personnel care for client needs.[65] Each of the programs presented an actual nursing situation that could portray good, mediocre, or inappropriate nurse behavior. The role plays showed the nurse assessing client needs in a variety of care situations. They illustrated the attitudes and behaviors of the nurse and coping mechanisms. Topics included anxiety, impending death, uncertainty, mental confusion, fear, and dependency. Nurses viewed a presentation and then discussed the subject with the help of a discussion leader. When the ratings of all groups were considered, it was found that the groups achieved higher scores on discussing attitudes and behavior of the nurse and patient in the role plays than they did on recommending solutions to problems. Those who had the ability to empathize with the situation within the role play were more successful in reaching solutions to the nursing care problems.

Griffin, Kinsinger, and Pitman tested the hypothesis that the use of closed circuit television (CCTV) in the hospital would enable an existing number of nursing instructors to teach an increased number of students effectively while using the same clinical facilities.[66] The study demonstrated that: (1) one clinical instructor using CCTV and audio equipment could teach 15 nursing students just as effectively as a teacher who had only 10 students and who used more conventional methods of instruction; (2) the increased frequency of observation of students by CCTV increased the possibility for individualized instruction and the opportunity to control safety factors in patient care; (3) clients did accept having care televised to a monitor room, and hospital personnel did not seem to resist this teaching strategy because normal hospital routine was not disrupted; (4) nursing instructors could adapt their clinical teaching skills to use CCTV; and (5) clinical teaching was facilitated by having students learn and practice technical skills or tasks in the classroom laboratory before actual practice in the clinical area.

Valentine and Saito report that core lectures, guest lectures, and segments of lectures that outline specific techniques can be taped and used either in lieu of live presentations or for reinforcement purposes.[67] This strategy makes possible repeated viewing by students. The researchers do not recommend regular taping of full-length lectures because the speaker appears to students as a talking head, which does not stimulate learning. Videotape can be a valuable evaluation-feedback tool for psychomotor or interpersonal skills. Students receive feedback permitting correction of errors before performing in the clinical setting.

Harvard faculty have their teaching techniques videotaped for criticism and evaluation. Faculty are able to "see" what works, and it promotes discussion of what turns students off. Staff reaction is reported as positive.[68] This feedback attribute of video has been investigated by a number of researchers. Ellett and Smith found that the teaching effectiveness of 20 teachers improved after watching their performance on videotape and answering a specifically designed self-evaluation questionnaire, as compared to 20 teachers who did not view the taped performances or answer the questionnaire.[69] Copeland explored possible relationships between the direct and indirect intervention behaviors of cooperating teachers and the classroom exhibition of skills acquired in microteaching training sessions by student teachers.[70] The findings provide evidence that for the student teachers in this study who were taught the skill of "asking probing questions," the intervention provided by the cooperating teachers interacted significantly with the microteaching training received by the student teachers. Only when microteaching training was complemented by appropriate intervention behaviors and reinforcement of the cooperating teacher in the field did any significant behavioral differences result.

Nadelson and Bassuk cite numerous instances in the literature where videofeedback has been used successfully in psychotherapy to realistically assess behaviors for self improvement.[71] Moore, Chernell, and West found that self-viewing improved client behaviors, even though oral feedback was not provided by therapists during viewing.[72]

Videoconferencing

Galdi found that videoconferencing seemed to be as effective for studio audiences at remote locations as it was for live audiences—at least where information dissemination was the goal.[73]

Audioconferencing

A review of research on audioconferencing indicates that there is no difference between indirect telephone-based instruction and direct face-to-face instruction in terms of learning cognitive outcomes. In addition, attitude surveys indicate a high level of user satisfaction.[74]

Williams and Chapanis found that information transmission, problem solving, decision making, generating ideas, and interviewing tasks could be effectively facilitated through audioconferencing.[75]

Wilson reports that the biggest advantage to Oklahoma nurses enrolled in a year-long continuing education workshop seemed to be the opportunity for professional peer interaction through audioconferencing.[76]

POSTTEST

MULTIPLE CHOICE

DIRECTIONS: Circle the *best* answer. More than one response may be correct.

1. Teaching a client how to deep-breathe and cough in preparation for the postoperative period is a common teaching event. The teaching strategy selected should provide which of the following conditions for learning to ensure that the client will be able to breathe deeply and cough effectively after surgery?
   a. Visual priming and prompting
   b. Positive reinforcement and corrective feedback
   c. Covert involvement in the learning experience
   d. Massed practice and repetition
2. You are preparing a class on the physiology of menstruation for six prepubertal girls. As you determine the teaching strategies for this learning experience, which of the following conditions for learning are important?
   a. Guiding each girl to establish a positive mental set toward pubescence and menstruation by beginning with a familiar example
   b. Providing the greatest amount of information in the least amount of time through a direct, auditory, sequentially organized teaching strategy
   c. Organizing information from simple to complex, familiar to unfamiliar, incorporating real, familiar examples early in instruction
   d. Stimulating the girls to generate examples and express feelings and questions using visual primes and prompts
3. Given normal circumstances and assuming that students are college-level, which of the following teaching strategies would be best to use for this objective:

"From a given list, correctly choose the word to complete the definitions for anxiety and fear, conscious and unconscious, observable and unobservable behavior, repression, and defense mechanism."

a. An audiocassette
b. A video interview
c. A handout or worksheet
d. A sound-slide presentation

4. Given normal circumstances and college-level students, which of the following teaching strategies would be best to use for this objective: "The learner will be able to discriminate among abnormal and normal chest sounds with 90 percent accuracy."

a. A live lecture with visuals
b. Discussion
c. A textbook or readings
d. An audiotape recording

5. You are to teach a seminar on oral medications. The class will be composed of 15 nursing students at the undergraduate level. The content is new. One of your objectives is that nine out of ten times the student will be able to identify the physical properties of the following pharmaceutical preparations: aqueous solution, syrup, emulsion, spirit, elixir, tablet, troche, capsule, and enteric-coated tablet. Which of the following teaching strategies would best facilitate achievement of the learning outcome?

a. Real objects
b. Sound filmstrip
c. A computer program
d. A 16-millimeter film

6. During a clinical experience, you observe that students need further instruction on principles of therapeutic communication. You are planning a learning experience for the seven senior nursing students on the topic. The purpose of one session is to explore how a nurse feels when confronted with a stressful client situation, how to be aware of feelings, accept them, and deal with them so that therapeutic communication is not inhibited. Your objectives are that the student will be able to: (1) identify specific actions or reactions of the client that may cause negative feelings; (2) express feelings invoked by these negative encounters; (3) identify effective ways to handle negative feelings; and (4) act in an appropriate manner when dealing with negative client encounters.
The learning experience and the teaching strategies of which it is composed should provide which of the following conditions for learning to promote achievement of the objectives?

a. Immediate verbal or nonverbal praise and positive feedback when students exhibit behaviors that reflect appropriate ways of dealing with negative feelings

b. Immediate and regular corrective feedback when early behaviors reflect inappropriate ways of dealing with negative feelings
c. Active, overt repetitive practice involving handling negative client encounters in the clinical setting as a real-life application experience
d. Priming by telling students all possible specific actions or reactions of clients that may cause negative feelings and ways they can handle such feelings, and asking students to orally repeat information conveyed
e. Control of rate of presentation by the direct or indirect strategy with deductive organization of information in a fixed linear pattern, establishing facts, developing concepts, using principles and advance organizers
f. Establishment of a positive set in regard to therapeutic communication, with reassurance that it's all right to have negative feelings if they are handled appropriately

7. Which of the following strategies would be most suitable for providing the conditions necessary for learning in the preceding teaching-learning situation?
   a. Print modular instruction incorporating a video and computer program and game
   b. Formal live lecture with sound-slide program
   c. Discussion with short video vignettes or trigger films
   d. Clinical practicum
   e. Role play
   f. Posters and audiotapes
   g. Audio- or videoconferencing
   h. Live demonstration
   i. Print programed instruction with pictures
   j. Computer simulation

8. As a part of the staff development program, you are to teach a refresher course on the recognition and interpretation of specific heart rhythm disturbances as shown by ECG wave patterns. All nurses have a basic understanding of cardiac electrophysiology and the ECG. Nurses are on flexible schedules and must fit the course into their schedules as well as they can. By the end of the first part of the course, all nurses are expected to correctly identify sinus node and atrial arrhythmias. Which of the following is the primary sensory input modality required to facilitate learning?
   a. Visual
   b. Auditory
   c. Tactile
   d. Olefactory
   e. Gustatory

9. Consider the nature of the preceding situation, principles of learning, conditions necessary for achievement of the learning outcome and determine which of the following teaching strategies would be most likely to facilitate achievement.

a. Live demonstration with a model and return practice
b. Textbook and journal articles
c. Overhead transparencies
d. Modular instruction incorporating real objects and examples

10. Travis, aged three and one half, is going to have a tonsillectomy. This is his first hospital experience. To alleviate some of his fear about the surgery, which of the following strategies would be most appropriate?
    a. A 5-to-10 minute animated video program
    b. Role play using puppets
    c. A 30-minute realistic film
    d. Poster with words and print worksheet

POSTTEST ANSWER KEY

1. b
2. a, c, d
3. c
4. d
5. a
6. a, b, c, f
7. c, d, e, j
8. a
9. d
10. a, b

SUGGESTED APPLICATION ACTIVITIES

1. You are to give a presentation on infant care. The topic is "Bathing Your Baby." Your audience will be composed of 15 expectant mothers and fathers. This child will be their first. Education and socioeconomic background varies from person to person. The average age of the group is 25 years. The class is to be held in a room in the community recreation building where other activities are going on at the same time, including active sports events.
   a. State the learning outcome(s) and the subobjectives that you would want the participants to achieve.
   b. Describe learning theory, principles of learning, and forces that could affect learning, as well as the constraints within the teaching-learning situation.

   c. Consider sensory input and output modality, list and describe all strategies that might be appropriate for the teaching-learning experience.
2. You are to teach a class of junior nursing students how to assist persons with chronic low back pain to develop skills to care for and protect the back and how to assist them to learn ways to think and act to minimize discomfort and increase mobility.
   a. State the learning outcome(s) and subobjectives for this learning experience.
   b. List learner characteristics that you would consider and explain how you would analyze learner characteristics. Include prerequisite knowledge and skill required.
   c. Describe constraints relative to the situation.
   d. Describe principles of learning and forces that may affect learning and list conditions necessary for learning required by the learning outcome(s).
   e. Determine the primary sensory input and response mode(s) needed.
   f. List the most feasible teaching strategies for each subobjective.
   g. Outline the total learning experience.
3. Through a needs assessment, you have found that a large number of full- and part-time employed nurses throughout the state are interested in learning how to conduct an adult physical assessment. Educational background and prerequisite learning varies with potential learners. You don't know the specifics. Some are new graduates and need limited review, while others have been out of school for a number of years. A grant has been awarded to cover all costs related to the course, and time is not a concern.
   a. Consider factors relative to the teaching-learning need, including conditions for learning and advantages and limitations of teaching strategies. Decide on the best teaching strategy and justify your choice.
4. State one behavioral objective for each of the three domains of learning for a particular learner or learner group. Analyze conditions for learning and factors that may affect learning and determine the teaching strategy that would be most likely to help the learner achieve each of the learning outcomes. State factors that guided decision making.
5. State, in behavioral terms, a learning outcome that would require auditory, visual, and tactile sensory input (including motion and color) as critical conditions for learning. Determine the most appropriate teaching strategy to promote achievement of the outcome. Analyze at least two available strategies to determine whether they meet the requirements of the teaching-learning need.
6. Observe a teaching-learning experience and analyze how the teacher provides conditions for learning through direct or indirect teaching strategies. Pay particular attention to how the teacher uses and controls or manipulates reinforcement and feedback, prompting and priming, practice and repetition, establishes set, and facilitates closure, provides for active learner involvement, controls the rate of presentation, and organizes information.
7. Observe a teaching-learning environment and analyze physical and environmental conditions for learning prior to a teaching-learning experience. Then observe and analyze how the teacher manipulates and controls these conditions to promote learning.

8. Describe a learning need or problem, including information relating to learner characteristics and number to be involved, the setting for learning and constraints relative to the situation. State the learning outcome to be achieved and enabling objectives. List necessary conditions for learning and determine appropriate teaching strategies for each objective. Then outline the total learning experience in detail.
9. Design and carry out a research study to explore the effects of a particular condition for learning embedded in a specific teaching strategy, such as feedback, motion, rate of presentation, reinforcement, or method of information organization.
10. Select one contrived teaching strategy and list particular attributes of the strategy. Design a research study to explore the effect that one of these attributes has on the achievement of a specific learning outcome for a sample population.

REFERENCES

1. Salomon G: Interaction of Media, Cognition and Learning. San Francisco, Jossey-Bass Inc., Publishers, 1979, p. 6.
2. Fleming M, Levie H: Instructional Message Design: Principles from the Behavioral Sciences. Englewood Cliffs, NJ, Educational Technology Publications, 1978, p. 27.
3. Malone TW: What Makes Things Fun to Learn? A Study of Intrinsically Motivating Computer Games. Palo Alto, CA, Xerox, August 1980, pp. 1-9, 49-64.
4. Young GC, Morgan RT: Overlearning in the Conditioning Treatment of Enuresis: A Long-term Follow-up Study. Behavior Research and Therapy 10:409-410, 1972.
5. Ciccone DL: Massed and Distributed Item Repetition in Verbal Discrimination Learning. Journal of Experimental Psychology 101:396-397, 1973.
6. Markle SM: Good Frames and Bad: A Grammar of Frame Writing, ed 2. New York, John Wiley & Sons, Inc., 1969, p. 60.
7. Van Hoozer H, Ruther L, Craft M: Introduction to Charting. Philadelpia, J.B. Lippincott Co., 1982, pp. 13, 47, 48.
8. Hartley J: Designing Instructional Text. New York, Nichols Publishing Co., 1978, p. 62.
9. Dwyer FM: Behavioral Approach to Visual Communications. Washington, D.C., Association for Educational Communications and Technology: Instructional Communications and Technology Research Report 11:21-25, 1980.
10. Levie WH, Lentz R: Effects of Text Illustrations: A Review of Research. Educational Communications and Technology Journal 30:195-232, 1982.
11. Miller GA: The Magical Number of Seven, Plus or Minus Two: Some Limits on our Capacity for Processing Information. In RN Haber (ed), Contemporary Theory and Research in Visual Perception. New York, Holt, Rinehart & Winston, 1968.
12. Johnson CF: Avoiding Soporific Soliloquies. Medical Opinion 4:33, 35, 37, 41, 1975.
13. Stecker EH: Visual Speechmaking. Audiovisual Product News 2:78, 1980.
14. Braselman HP: Instructional Films: Asset or Liability? Audiovisual Instruction 23:14, 1978.
15. Gagné R: The Conditions of Learning. New York, Holt, Rinehart & Winston, 1970.
16. Ausubel DP: Cognitive Structure and the Facilitation of Meaningful Verbal Learning. In HF Clarizio, RC Craig, WA Mehrens (eds): Contemporary Issues in Educational Psychology. Boston, Allyn & Bacon, Inc., 1970, pp. 206-209.

17. Ausubel DP: The Use of Advance Organizers in the Learning and Retention of Meaningful Verbal Material. Journal of Educational Psychology 51:267–272, 1966.
18. Ausubel DP, Fitzgerald D: Organizer, General Background and Antecedent Learning Variables in Sequential Verbal Learning. Journal of Educational Psychology 53:243–249, 1962.
19. Canelos J, Taylor W, Altschuld J: Effectiveness of a Visual Advance Organizer and a Verbal Advance Organizer When Learning From Visual Instruction for Later Performance on Two Types of Learning Tasks. Paper presented at the National Convention of the Association for Educational Communications and Technology, New Orleans, LA, 1983.
20. Fleming M, Levie H: Instructional Message Design: Principles from the Behavioral Sciences. Englewood Cliffs, NJ, Educational Technology Publications, 1978, p. 60.
21. Reiser RA: Interaction Between Locus of Control and Three Pacing Procedures in a Personalized System of Instruction Course. Educational Communications and Technology Journal 28:194–202, 1980.
22. Johnson CF: Avoiding Soporific Soliloquies. Medical Opinion 4:33, 35, 37, 41, 1975.
23. de Tornyay R, Thompson MA: Strategies for Teaching Nursing, ed 2. New York, John Wiley & Sons, Inc., 1982, pp. 81–85.
24. Miller WC: An Experimental Study of the Relationship of Film Movement and Emotional Involvement Response and Its Effect on Learning and Attitude Formation. Los Angeles: University of Southern California, 1967. (ERIC Document Reproduction Service No. ED07172)
25. Chute AG: Effect of Color and Monochrome Versions of a Film on Incidental and Task-Relevant Learning. Educational Communications and Technology Journal 28:10–18, 1980.
26. Donahue TR: Viewer Perceptions of Color and Black-and-White Paid Political Advertising. Journalism Quarterly 50:660–665, 1973.
27. Osterman DN: Feedback Lecture: Increasing Individual Involvement and Learning in the Lecture Style. Paper presented at the National Convention of the Association for Educational Communication and Technology, Dallas, TX, 1982.
28. Della-Dora D, Blanchard LJ (eds): Moving Toward Self-Directed Learning: Highlights of Relevant Research and of Promising Practices. Alexandria, VA, Association for Supervision and Curriculum Development, 1979, pp. 23–24.
29. Ball MJ, Hannah KJ: Using Computers in Nursing. Reston, VA, Reston Publishing Co. Inc., 1984, pp. 78–79.
30. Gregorc AF: Learning/Teaching Styles: Potent Forces Behind Them. Educational Leadership 36:234–236, 1979.
31. Briggs LJ, Campeau PL, Gagné RM, May MA: Instructional Media: A Procedure for the Design of Multi-media Instruction, A Critical Review of Research and Suggestions for Future Research. Pittsburg, PA, American Institute for Research, 1967, pp. 109–116.
32. Hoban CF: The Usable Residue of Educational Film Research. In W. Schramm (ed): New Teaching Aids for American Classrooms. Stanford, CA, Institute for Communication Research, 1960, pp. 95–115.
33. MacLennan W: Research in Instructional Television and Film. Washington, DC, U.S. Office of Education, Bureau of Research, 1967.
34. Wendt PR, Butts GK: Audi-visual Materials, Instructional Materials: Educational Media and Technology. Review of Educational Research 32:141–155, 1962.
35. Dayton DK: Inserted Post-questions and Learning from Slide-tape Presentations. Audiovisual Communications Review 25:140, 1977.

36. Knirk FG: Instructional Technology: A Book of Readings. New York, Holt, Rinehart & Winston, 1968.
37. Chute AG: Effect of Color and Monochrome Versions of a Film on Incidental and Task-Relevant Learning. Educational Communications and Technology Journal 28:10–18, 1980.
38. Schramm W: The Publishing Process. In LJ Cronback (ed): Text Materials in Modern Education. Urbana, IL, University of Illinois, 1955, pp. 145–155.
39. Dayton DK: Inserted Post-questions and Learning from Slide-tape Presentations. Audiovisual Communications Review 25:136, 1977.
40. Fisher KM, MacWhinney B: AV Autotutorial Instruction: A Review of Evaluative Research. AV Communications Review 24:229–261, 1976.
41. Moldstad JA: Selective Review of Research Studies Showing Media Effectiveness. AV Communications Review 22:396–399, 1974.
42. Anderson J: Nutrition Programs Improve Classroom Instruction. Carrboro, NC, Health Sciences Consortium, Inc. 64:3, 1979.
43. Billings K: Research on School Computing. In MT Grady, JD Gawronski (eds): Computers in Curriculum and Instruction. Alexandria, VA, Association for Supervision and Curriculum Development, 1981, pp. 12–18.
44. Magarrel J: Self-paced Instruction Seen Benefiting Students. The Chronicle of Higher Education 13:6, 1976.
45. Okey JR, Majer K: Individual and Small Group Learning with Computer-Assisted Instruction. AV Communications Review 24:79–86, 1976.
46. Murphy MA: Computer-based Education in Nursing: Factors Influencing its Utilization. Computers in Nursing 2:219–220, 1984.
47. Briggs LJ, et al.: Instructional Media: A Procedure for the Design of Multi-media Instruction, A Critical Review of Research and Suggestions for Future Research. Pittsburgh, PA, American Institute for Research, 1967, pp. 161–240.
48. Vandermeer AW: Three Investigations of the Improvement of Informational Filmstrips and the Derivation of Principles Relating to the Improvement of This Media. AV Communications Review 12:494–497, 1964.
49. Cook JO: Research in Audio-visual Communication. In Knirk FG: Instructional Technology: A Book of Readings. New York: Holt, Rinehart, and Winston, 1968, p. 261.
50. Briggs LJ, Campeau PL, Gagné RM, May MA: Instructional Media: A Procedure for the Design of Multi-media Instruction, A Critical Review of Research and Suggestions for Future Research. Pittsburgh, PA, American Institute for Research, 1967, pp. 128–132.
51. Reiser RA, Andrews DH: Using Non-print Media for Assessment Purposes. Paper presented at the National Convention of the Association for Educational Communications and Technology, New Orleans, LA, 1979.
52. Dayton DK: Inserted Post-questions and Learning from Slide-tape Presentations. Audiovisual Communications Review 25:139, 1977.
53. Maddox H, Loughran RJ: Illustrating the Lecture: Prepared Diagrams vs. Built-up Diagrams. AV Communications Review 25:87–90, 1977.
54. Winn W: The Structure of Multiple Free Association to Words, Black and White Pictures and Color Pictures. AV Communications Review 24:273–293, 1976.
55. Jahoda G, Cheyne WB, et al.: Utilization of Pictorial Information in Classroom Learning: A Cross Cultural Study. AV Communications Review 24:295–315, 1976.
56. Dwyer FM: The Effect of IQ Level on the Instructional Effectiveness of Black and White and Color Illustrations. AV Communications Review 24:49–62, 1976.

57. Holliday WG: Teaching Verbal Chains Using Flow Diagrams and Texts. AV Communications Review 24:63–78, 1976.
58. Malone TW: What Makes Things Fun to Learn? A Study of Intrinsically Motivating Computer Games. Englewood Cliffs, NJ, Educational Technology Publications, 1978, pp. 11–48.
59. Camer R: Toilet Training. Psychology Today 16:82, 1982.
60. Weiss W: Mass Communication. Annual Review of Psychology 22:309–366, 1971.
61. Henderson RW, Swanson RA: Age and Directed-participation Variables Influencing the Effectiveness of Televised Instruction in Concrete Operational Behaviors. Educational Communications and Technology Journal 26:301–312, 1978.
62. Coldevin G: Spaced, Massed and Summary Treatments as Review Strategies for ITV Production. AV Communications Review 23:289–303, 1975.
63. Dwyer FM: The Effect of Varied Cueing Strategies in Facilitating Student Achievement of Different Educational Objectives. Philadelphia, Pennsylvania State University, 1981, pp. 19–22.
64. Briggs LJ, Campeau PL, Gagné RM, May MA: Instructional Media: A Procedure for the Design of Multi-media Instruction, A Critical Review of Research and Suggestions for Future Research. Pittsburg, PA, American Institute for Research, 1967, pp. 104–109.
65. Yarlow DJ, Bruhn JG: Role Plays on Television. Nursing Outlook 21:242–244, 1973.
66. Griffin, GJ, Kinsinger RE, Pitman AJ: Clinical Nursing Instruction by Television: A Report on a Two-year Experiment Using Closed Circuit Television to Teach Clinical Nursing. New York, Columbia University Teachers College, Bureau of Publications, 1965.
67. Valentine NM, Saito Y: Videotaping: A Viable Teaching Strategy in Nursing Education. Nurse Educator:8–17, 1980.
68. Video Helps Harvard's Faculty Sharpen Its Teaching Skills. Video User 3:10, 1980.
69. Ellett LE, Smith EP: Improving Performance of Classroom Teachers Through Videotaping and Self-Evaluation. AV Communication Review 23:277–287, 1975.
70. Copeland WD: Some Factors Related to Student-Teacher Classroom Performance Following Microteaching Training. American Educational Research Journal 14:147–157, 1977.
71. Nadelson CC, Bassuk EL: The Use of Videotape in Couples Therapy. International Journal of Group Psychotherapy 27:241–253, 1973.
72. Moore RJ, Chernell E, West MJ: Television as a Therapeutic Tool. Archives of General Psychiatry 12:217–220, 1965.
73. Galdi V: Teleconferencing Scores High Grades on Effectiveness. Video User:18, 1982.
74. Monson M: Bridging the Distance: An Instructional Guide to Teleconferencing. Madison, WI, University of Wisconsin Extension, Instructional Communications Systems, 1978, p. 59.
75. Williams E, Chapanis A: A Review of Psychological Research Comparing Communications Media. In L Parker, B Riccomini (eds): The Status of the Telephone in Education. Madison, WI, University of Wisconsin Extension, Instructional Communications Systems, 1976, pp. 164–168.
76. Wilson JS: Bridging the Gap in Communication Among Nurses: Use of Teleconference. Journal of Nursing Education 18:14, 1979.

BIBLIOGRAPHY

Ball MJ, Hannah KJ: Using Computers in Nursing. Reston, VA, Reston Publishing Co., 1984.

Briggs, LJ: Handbook of Procedures for the Design of Instruction. Pittsburg, PA, American Institutes for Research, 1970.

Brown JW, Lewis RB, Harcleroad FF: AV Instruction: Technology, Media and Methods, ed 2. New York, McGraw-Hill, Book Co., 1977.

Chance P: Fred Keller: The Revolutionary Gentleman. Psychology Today, 18:43–48, 1984.

de Tornyay R, Thompson MA: Strategies for Teaching Nursing, ed 2. New York, John Wiley & Sons, Inc., 1982.

Fleming M, Levie WH: Instructional Message Design: Principles from the Behavioral Sciences. Englewood Cliffs, NJ, Educational Technology Publications, 1978.

Grobe SJ: Computer Primer and Resource Guide for Nurses. Philadelphia, J.B. Lippincott Co., 1984.

Guinee KK: Teaching and Learning in Nursing. New York, Macmillan Inc., 1978.

Haney JB, Ullmer EJ: Educational Media and the Teacher. Dubuque, IA, Wm. C. Brown Co. Publishers, 1970.

Huckabay LM: Conditions of Learning and Instruction in Nursing: Modularized. St. Louis, C.V. Mosby Co., 1980.

Kemp JE: Instructional Design: A Plan for Unit and Course Development, ed 2. Belmont, CA, Fearon Publishers, Inc., 1977.

Knopke HJ, Diekelmann NL: Approaches to Teaching in the Health Sciences. Reading, MA, Addison-Wesley Publishing Co., Inc., 1978.

Knowles M: The Adult Learner: A Neglected Species, ed 2. Houston, TX, Gulf Publishing Co. Book Division, 1978.

McKeachie, WJ: Teaching Tips: A Guidebook for the Beginning College Teacher, ed 7. Lexington, MA, D.C. Heath & Co., 1978.

Ostmoe P, Van Hoozer H, et al.: Learning Style Preferences and Selection of Learning Strategies: Considerations and Implications for Nurse Educators. Journal of Nursing Education 23:27–30, 1984.

Pohl ML: The Teaching Function of the Nursing Practitioner, ed 2. Dubuque, IA, Wm.C. Brown Co., Publishers, 1968.

Roberts K, Turston H: Teaching Methodologies: Knowledge Acquisition and Retention. Journal of Nursing Education 23:21–26, 1984.

Salomon G: Interaction of Media, Cognition and Learning. San Francisco, Jossey-Bass Inc., Publishers, 1979.

Smith L, Hudson M: Physical Assessment Rounds as a Teaching Strategy. Journal of Nursing Education 23:30–32, 1984.

Verduin JR, Jr, Miller HG, Greer CE: Adults Teaching Adults: Principles and Strategies. Austin, TX, Learning Concepts, Inc. 1977.

4

Selecting Clinical Teaching Strategies

Donn Weinholtz and Patricia M. Ostmoe

OBJECTIVES

Upon completion of this chapter, you will be able to:

1. Cite seven factors and three general dimensions suitable for differentiating effective from ineffective clinical teachers.
2. State a rationale for the clinical instructor's use of a clinical education guide and develop an outline for such a guide.
3. Design a set of instructional strategies to promote student development and provide a rationale for the strategies according to situational leadership theory.
4. Explain the importance of feedback within the clinical evaluation process and suggest an overall strategy for providing feedback regarding students' affective behavior.
5. Evaluate a lecture using ten criteria for organization and clarity.
6. Develop a rudimentary skill analysis checklist.
7. Explain the rationale for active listening and experiment with the skill.
8. Explain the rationale for using "I-messages" and experiment with the skill.
9. Explain the rationale for "no-lose negotiation" and experiment with the skill.
10. Evaluate self-performance as a discussion group leader, conducting a problem-solving discussion.
11. Self-assess level of proficiency in three professional skills areas: knowledge, clinical competence, and modeling of professional characteristics.

INTRODUCTION

Clinical education involves experiential learning. Although experiential learning is an elusive concept, Carl Rogers attempted to describe its essence as follows: "It has a quality of personal involvement—the whole person in both his feeling and cognitive aspects being in the learning event."[1] Experiential learning occurs in the clinical setting in response to a rich and steady stream of educational opportunities flowing from daily client health care demands. Learning results, both in a potentially positive or negative sense, as events force students to act or observe others act, and then to experience or observe the consequences of the action.[2]

Clinical instructors need to anticipate potential learning opportunities, recognize unanticipated learning situations when they arise, and design instruction that amplifies the positive learning events critically important to students' professional development.

The responsibilities of clinical instructors are highly diverse. They include identifying client populations for learning experiences, finding space for clinical conferences, determining objectives for clinical experiences, diagnosing individual students' learning needs, planning clinical rotations and schedules, providing for student orientation, selecting learning experiences, demonstrating professional skills, communicating with agency staff, evaluating learning experiences, and providing and facilitating student learning. While these tasks sound relatively easy, in practice they are extremely challenging. Teaching is hard enough in a classroom setting where the teacher has a high degree of control over the nature and sequence of events, but the difficulty of teaching in the clinical setting is compounded by the fact that many events are far beyond the instructor's control. Indeed, this difficulty led Reichsman, Browning, and Hinshaw to conclude that the clinical teacher's task is unique in the entire realm of teaching. In no other field does the nature of the material demand of the teacher this degree of preparedness without preparation.[3] We suggest that the problem of learning how to teach as a clinician deserves much thoughtful study.

In spite of difficulties inherent in the process, clinical nursing instruction can be very rewarding. For example, because of the nature of the student-teacher relationships that develop in an experiential learning environment, nurse-faculty frequently report that their greatest rewards come from observing a dramatic growth in individual student's professional abilities. The progress clients make toward achieving health as a result of students' interventions and interactions also brings satisfaction to the clinical nursing instructor. For the clinical instructor who is interested in improving client care through nursing research, the opportunities for problem identification associated with clinical instruction can be very satisfying. Frequent client contact, routine communication with agency personnel, and the penetrating creative questions of students all facilitate the exchange of ideas for clinical nursing research.

The challenges and rewards of clinical instruction all indicate the richness of the clinical setting as a teaching and learning environment. Experiential learning rarely occurs to an optimal extent, but it is most likely to occur when clinical instructors cultivate effective teaching practices.

Clinical Instruction

Clinical instruction or clinical teaching can be defined as acting and interacting with students, clients, and other health professionals in settings where people are in need of health care to promote both the maximum learning of students and the maximum health of clients. When applied to clinical instruction in nursing, this definition acknowledges dual responsibility for clinical instructors—that is, a responsibility both to students and to clients. While this notion of dual responsibility deviates from the beliefs and practices of some current nurse-educators, this concept must be acccepted by academic nursing if nurse-educators are to legitimize their credibility and visibility as health care providers. This definition also recognizes the diversity of health care settings in which contemporary nursing education occurs—the ambulatory clinic, health support group, school, and doctor's office among others, all of which are ideal sites for clinical instruction in nursing. The acute-care hospital, which has traditionally been almost the exclusive clinical setting for learning nursing practice, is no longer sufficient to provide essential learning experiences for nursing students. The term *client*, therefore, is used to emphasize the importance of identifying a wide variety of potential clinical learning settings.

Schweer's and Gebbie's overview of the history of nursing education between the years of 1890 and 1915 uncovers a number of problems addressed and questions raised by clinical nursing instructors in that era.[4] More recently, a group of faculty and graduate students in nursing identified another set of questions and problems related to current clinical instruction.[5] Table 4–1 compares these two sets of questions and concerns. As Table 4–1 shows, the paucity of nursing research in the area of clinical instruction has resulted in over 75 years of unanswered questions and unresolved problems. While these concerns do not all relate directly to clinical teaching strategies, they point out the complexities surrounding clinical teaching. Also, the limited amount of actual research in the area of clinical instruction causes some controversy as to what are optimal clinical teaching behaviors.[6] Nevertheless, there

TABLE 4-1. HISTORICAL COMPARISON OF CLINICAL INSTRUCTION CONCERNS

1890/1915	1980s
How can we provide more time for skill development?	Is effective use being made of the supervised clinical hours available?
How do we increase students' interest in learning in a skills laboratory?	What is the purpose of the skills laboratory?
How do you make staff nurses aware of what students are taught?	How do you correct staff misconceptions of the student role?
How do you decrease the discrepancy between how procedures are taught in the classroom and how they are performed in the hospital?	"Students learn one thing but don't see staff nurses carry it out in the way it was learned."
"Students are meeting staffing needs, not their own learning needs."	"Students are counted on as 'staff' in terms of planning clinical coverage for patients."

have emerged a few research findings in this area that provide direction to clinical instructors committed to excellence. Some of the most useful clinical teaching research has been conducted by Irby. His review of the clinical teaching literature and his own research have indicated seven factors that differentiate the best from the worst clinical teachers.[7] The factors are: the instructor's approach to clinical supervision, enthusiasm, organization and clarity, group instructional skills, knowledge, clinical competence, and modeling of professional characteristics.

These seven factors provide the framework used in the remaining part of this chapter to examine clinical teaching in nursing. The first factor is discussed under a dimension called Supervisory Skills. The second, third and fourth factors are combined into a dimension labeled Instructional Process Skills. The last three factors are combined into a dimension called Professional Skills. Within each of the three categories, specific suggestions are made for clinical nursing instructors to consider when designing and providing clinical nursing instruction.

SUPERVISORY SKILLS

An effective clinical teacher should develop supervisory skills that augment instructional efforts. A competent clinical instructor must be a manager who possesses a high degree of skill in planning, directing, and controlling (evaluating).

Planning

An effective supervisor's plan must demonstrate understanding of organizational complexities and show how efforts fit into the organizational plan.[8] When this principle is applied to clinical instruction, it dictates that clinical instructors be responsible for recognizing how their contributions articulate with other aspects of the nursing curriculum.

Nursing curriculums are more than a collection of courses or an outgrowth of individual faculty members' expertise. They are, instead, well-organized and logical entities. Cognitive, affective, and psychomotor learning experiences are designed in some rational sequence. An instructor who is unaware of the overall curriculum design is unlikely to contribute in an effective way to students' clinical learning experiences. For example, if the curriculum design dictates that the clinical instructor select early learning experiences that facilitate the development of students' abilities to teach individual clients, but instead the instructor chooses experiences designed to enhance students' psychomotor competencies, these students will be disadvantaged in subsequent courses when the curriculum design emphasizes client-teaching competencies. Curriculums are designed to build on students' prior learning and to reinforce learning. Clinical instructors must provide the learning experiences required in a particular course if their students are to be successful in subsequent courses.

Going one step further, clinical instructors are responsible for helping students to see how their clinical experiences integrate with other aspects of the nursing curriculum. In the example just cited, the clinical instructor should not only provide learning experiences that develop the student's individual client teaching skills but should also relate why it is important to master this skill before attempting to teach groups of clients. Obviously, instructors must understand the rationale and design of the entire curriculum if they are going to be able to interpret it to their students effectively.

The classic recommendation among educators for assuring this kind of curricular coherence is for instructors to specify, understand, and communicate both their own and their program's educational objectives.[9] This recommendation has been repeatedly emphasized in the nursing education literature.[10-13] Nevertheless, research indicates that clinical instructors are often uncertain of objectives and are unlikely to make objectives explicit to their students.[14,15] One way to alleviate this problem is for each clinical instructor to design a clinical education guide for distribution to students and to set aside time to thoroughly explain the guide to students.

Ford described the clinical education guide as "consisting of written information that is used to help the various constituencies of the clinical experience understand the process of the procedures."[16] Ford's recommendations for using the clinical education guide are geared to the program level, that is, one guide to explain an entire program; thoughtful, creative clinical instructors can, however, develop their own guides focusing on their particular instructional areas. Such guides can emphasize the importance of a specific clinical experience in the overall curriculum.

The components of this sort of clinical education guide can parallel the components suggested by Ford for a program guide.[17] These include sections containing: (1) an overview explaining the role of the particular clinical experience in the students' overall professional education and other general orientation information (for example, major responsibilities, key dates, and so on); (2) assumptions about the entry-level competencies of students; (3) the objectives of the particular clinical learning experience; (4) an explanation of how the instructor will evaluate the students; (5) a description of policies and regulations; and (6) an appendix with any supplementary information that the instructor wishes to include. By adopting this one procedure alone, any clinical instructor can elevate the quality of his or her clinical instruction above the standard norm. Stritter and Flair emphasize that communicating goals and expectations are among the most important behaviors a clinical instructor can perform.[18] The very act of compiling a clinical education guide can augment an instructor's effectiveness while providing an instructional strategy of substantial merit.

The development of the clinical education guide provides students with ready access to necessary information and efficiently communicates expectations of faculty, curriculum, and agency. Students are free, then, to concentrate their learning efforts on meeting the clinical objectives of the course. Information that orients the student to the idiosyncratic procedures or routines of a particular clinical area are especially useful and should be included in the guide. The guide is also beneficial in helping to orient clinical personnel to the purposes of the clinical learning experience. Too often, agency nursing and medical staff who have the opportunity to facilitate students' clinical learning experiences lack understanding of students' previous educational and clinical experiences and, therefore, expect too much or too little of students. If, however, the staff, faculty and students all have similar expectations and goals, the experiential learning that occurs is more likely to be appropriate to the course objectives and therefore most effective in facilitating the students' professional education.

Directing

An effective supervisor's style of directing should encourage the professional development of supervisees. A clinical instructor's approach to supervision should be compatible with and augment students' professional development. Although professional development should be lifelong,[19] the process of professional development of nursing students can be inaugurated during their initial clinical learning experiences. Hersey and Blanchard address the responsibility of promoting professional development as a general leadership responsibility in their "situational leadership theory." [20] Drawing on the findings of the Ohio State Leadership Studies and the work of Blake and Mouton,[21] Hersey and Blanchard propose that individuals' leadership styles tend to fall into one of four major categories depending on the amount of emphasis the leader places on task or relationship behaviors. "Task" behaviors are leadership behaviors that focus directly on the type of work that is to be accomplished. "Relationship" behaviors are leadership behaviors that focus on group process and followers' interpersonal needs. Hersey and Blanchard's four major categories are: (1) high task-low relationship (telling), (2) high task-high relationship (selling), (3) low task-high relationship (participating), and (4) low task-low relationship (delegating). The four styles are adapted and are illustrated in Table 4-2.

Hersey and Blanchard also propose that each of these leadership styles may be more appropriate in certain situations and that a leader's effectiveness is determined

TABLE 4-2. FOUR LEADERSHIP STYLES AVAILABLE TO CLINICAL INSTRUCTORS

Style	Instructor Behavior
Telling (High task-low relationship)	Instructor dominates communication, providing learners with information and/or directions concerning responsibilities expected of them in the future.
Selling (High task-high relationship)	Instructor closely controls the flow of communication, but fosters two-way communication with learners and reinforces them for their contributions.
Participating (Low task-high relationship)	Instructor stimulates free communication among learners, offering occasional information and reinforcement as needed.
Delegating (Low task-low relationship)	Instructor allows the learners to control the learning situation and serves primarily as an observer or low-profile participant.

by whether or not he or she can offer the appropriate leadership style when the situation demands it. They agree that a leader can grow beyond dependence on a single dominant leadership style to develop a repertoire of styles. Thus, if trained to diagnose the leadership needs of the situation, the leader can adjust behavior in order to enhance leadership effectiveness.

Within Hersey's and Blanchard's scheme, the primary variables that a leader must diagnose are individual and group maturity. *Maturity* is defined as "the capacity to set high, but obtainable goals (achievement-motivation); willingness and ability to take responsibility; and education and/or experience."[22] While recognizing that individuals or groups are never mature or immature in any total sense, Hersey and Blanchard argue that all individuals and groups "tend to be more or less mature in relation to a specific task, function or objective that a leader is attempting to accomplish through their efforts."[23] Thus, maturity is situational in nature.

Situational leadership theory recognizes four general maturity levels: (1) the individual or group is neither willing nor able to take responsibility, (2) the individual or group is willing but not able to take responsibility, (3) the individual or group is able but not willing to take responsibility, and (4) the individual or group is willing and able to take responsibility. Given followers with low maturity, leaders should emphasize task behaviors at the expense of relationship behaviors, but as the level of maturity of their followers continues to increase in terms of accomplishing a specific task, leaders should begin to reduce their task behavior and increase the relationship behavior until a group or individual reaches a moderate level of maturity. As the individual or group begins to move into an above-average maturity level, it becomes appropriate for leaders to decrease not only task behavior but also relationship behavior.[24]

Hersey and Blanchard assume that when individuals are mature enough to receive delegated responsibility, they are quite capable of providing their own socioemotional support without reverting to dependence on the leader. The movement away from dependence (both task and socioemotional) on the leader is at the heart of the theory. Hersey and Blanchard assert that leaders should meet their followers' dependent needs at the appropriate times, but they also emphasize that leaders should develop their followers by giving them increasing responsibility. Table 4–3 relates the changes in leadership style recommended to promote growth in maturity level.

TABLE 4–3. PROGRESSION OF INDIVIDUAL OR GROUP MATURITY AND LEADERSHIP STYLES

Individual or Group Maturity Level	Leadership Style
Low	Telling
Low-moderate	Selling
Moderate-high	Participating
High	Delegating

Adapted from Hersey P, Blanchard K: Management of Organizational Behavior, ed 3. Englewood Cliffs, NJ, Prentice-Hall, Inc., 1977, pp. 164–168. Courtesy of Prentice-Hall, Inc.

Based on situational leadership theory, it is possible to derive leadership scenarios for clinical teaching in a variety of settings. The following example indicates how professional development might be promoted among nursing students. The example illustrates how a clinical instructor might exert leadership using the "telling-selling-participating-delegating" continuum that is central to the situational leadership perspective. The assumption is that a major goal of the clinical instructor is to promote individual and group maturity among nursing students.

PHASE

1. During the first few meetings between the clinical instructor and designated clinical student group (orientation phase), the instructor clearly explains (tells) the expectations for individual and group behavior during the students' length of time for clinical experience and assigns students appropriate learning experiences that enable the instructor to assess students' capabilities.
2. Based on assessments, the clinical instructor selects (sells) learning experiences aimed at developing the knowledge and skills of individual students in those areas congruent with course clinical objectives. The clinical instructor plays a major role in identifying learner needs and maintains a high level of relationship behavior by providing *positive feedback* to students.
3. As the students' experiences in the course and on a specific clinical area increase, the clinical instructor gradually tries to limit the students' dependence. In this phase quite frequently the instructor will give students the option of selecting their own learning experiences, although the instructor is available as resource adviser and source of emotional support (participating). Student group members begin to rely on each other for assistance and feedback rather than looking strictly to the instructor for guidance and evaluation.
4. Near the end of the clinical experience, students assume responsibility for their own learning and initiate client care activities with little reliance on the clinical instructor, who now assumes the role of an observer (delegating). The instructor assesses individual student performance in preparation for completing clinical evaluations on each student.

A critical assumption underlying this pattern is that the students will not continually be confronted by new demands for which their task maturity (that is, capability of completing a task) is low. Under such circumstances, situational leadership theory indicates that to ensure proper client care, the clinical instructor must maintain a high level of direction and control. It is also assumed that the degree to which students move from Phase 1 to Phase 4 is in part dictated by their level in the curriculum. For example, one would expect senior students about to graduate to move more rapidly from Phase 1 to Phase 4, while beginning students would not achieve the magnitude of independence normally seen in Phase 4.

Situational leadership theory is not a panacea for understanding all the complexities of clinical teaching or for correcting all counterproductive teaching behaviors. It provides a useful heuristic that can be used by concerned clinical teachers to guide experiments with their own teaching behavior. Only through such experimentation can teaching be improved.

Evaluating

Not only must the effective supervisor be an expert planner and leader, but he or she must also be a competent evaluator. Lawrence and Lawrence suggest that clinical evaluation is ultimately a means for promoting quality client care and, as such, is a critical parameter that must be addressed by the nurse-educator.[25] Because clinical evaluation occurs in complex situations in which students are required to demonstrate multiple behaviors in the cognitive, psychomotor, and affective domains, Wood asserts that clinical evaluation presents the nurse-educator with unique problems not inherent in classroom evaluation.[26] Classroom teachers have more control over the learning environment and can therefore systematically plan evaluation activities. Clinical instructors, however, must often contend with several variables that affect evaluation opportunities and over which they have no control. Examples of such variables include: a sudden change in a client's health status, an unanticipated change in the client's daily routine, a change in the client's setting (for example, hospital to home), and variations in students' opportunities for learning. In spite of these obstacles, a clinical instructor can develop effective clinical evaluation strategies if there is a clear understanding of the purpose for clinical evaluations. Such an understanding should be relatively simple to develop, but often in reality it is not. A helpful approach to understanding the purpose of clinical evaluation is to identify the dichotomies associated with the terms *purpose*, *clinical*, and *evaluation*. Once a clinical instructor clearly comprehends the complexities associated with these terms, he or she will be better equipped to identify and develop valid and reliable clinical evaluation strategies.

Purpose. *The American Heritage Dictionary* defines *purpose* as "the object toward which one strives or for which something exists; goal; aim." It should be easy, then, to decide on the purpose of clinical evaluation. All one needs to know is: What is the main reason for doing the clinical evaluation? In answering this question, the first dichotomy becomes apparent. In the real world of nursing education, we have at least two purposes. One of these is related to determining a grade, or in some way assessing a student's terminal performance (summative evaluation). The other purpose is associated with an ongoing evaluation process which exists to assist the student in learning (formative evaluation). These two purposes are mutually exclusive and cannot be achieved by using the same data collection tools or methods. Learning most often occurs in an atmosphere of free and open communication about standards, values, and expectations. Learning most often takes place when one can question, experiment, or try new approaches. A student cannot learn in an atmosphere where every act, judgment, or decision made at every moment is evaluated and taken into consideration to determine a grade. Failure to recognize the dichotomy between formative and summative evaluation often causes the greatest difficulty for clinical instructors. Both forms of evaluation are necessary, but clinical instructors must develop strategies that clearly differentiate the promotion of learning from the assessment of terminal behavior.

Feedback is an important aspect of evaluation. Providing constructive feedback to promote achievement demands substantial effort on the part of the instructor. Instruments in the form of checklists or structured anecdotal notes should be carefully designed to collect data on all aspects of student clinical performance, including knowledge and attitudes as well as psychomotor skills. The techniques necessary to ensure reliable and valid evaluation data require a highly detailed explanation transcending the scope of this chapter. Consequently, a very good source on the topic edited by Morgan and Irby is recommended.[27]

When some sort of scheme for collecting student performance data is implemented, it is the clinical instructor's responsibility to interpret that data and feed back the interpretation, along with necessary recommendations, to the student. For a number of reasons about which we can only speculate, many clinical teachers perform this task poorly.[28] One explanation for this poor performance might be that providing feedback is a delicate communication problem that easily leads either to overkill or avoidance by the instructor.

Overkill occurs when the instructor uses evaluation to bludgeon a student into repentence for previous errors. Overkill is probably rarer than avoidance, which occurs when the clinical instructor shies away from confronting the student. Both overkill and avoidance probably occur because providing feedback is an anxiety-producing experience. A few individuals may respond to this anxiety by overcompensating with hyperconfrontative behavior, while a larger group copes by means of denial and of paying greater attention to the ever-present distractions (i.e., other job responsibilities) in the clinical setting. Of course, the only consistently sound mechanism for providing feedback involves a steady, tempered, and helpful approach. Feedback should facilitate growth and to do so it must be organized and clear.

Michael Gordon offers suggestions on how feedback can be organized and delivered to promote student growth.[29] His clinical model of affective assessment is designed to deal with one of the more complicated instructional problems, that of changing student attitudes. But it can easily be adapted to providing feedback on cognitive and psychomotor skills. Gordon's model involves eight different steps. The first five are ordinary steps often used in the routine monitoring and feedback of student performance. The final three are extraordinary steps that may have to be taken as a part of the summative evaluation process.

Ordinary Steps (Formative Evaluation)

1. Stating objectives: Prior to any significant clinical experience, students are oriented to the objectives of the experience. Of course, such objectives must be congruent with the overall objectives of the nursing program.
2. Screening for potential problems: During the course of the clinical experience, data is collected on all major aspects of student performance. Ex-

emplary performance is noted and reinforced, while problem performance is noted for corrective action. Such action may be handled through immediate feedback or through a conference when chronic problems arise. Clinical instructors must constantly keep the course objectives and level of student in mind when collecting data. Failure to do so may result in expecting either too much or too little of students.

3. Clarifying problems: If a chronic problem is detected, the instructor confronts the student in a private conference, interprets the problem and opens the door for joint exploration of the root cause.
4. Assessing specific behaviors: To the extent that there is any disagreement between the instructor and the student over the nature of the problem, the student's specific performance record is analyzed. This step involves further clarification and will most likely be necessary only in situations where clear value differences exist.
5. Providing assistance: The instructor and student develop a plan to overcome whatever deficiency the student is experiencing. Such a plan may involve additional study (reading and so on), increased practice of certain skills, or attempts to interact with clients in a different manner.

Extraordinary Steps (Summative Evaluation)

6. Determining potential seriousness of problems: If the student's deficiency persists in spite of previous attempts to resolve it, the instructor must determine if the problem is serious enough to warrant unilateral action by the faculty. Responsibility for resolving less serious problems may be left to the student's discretion. In the case of more serious problems, the instructor may require departmental help.
7. Inspecting performance: A panel of faculty reviews the student's past behavior and monitors future performance.
8. Taking administrative action: Based on the results of the comprehensive performance review, the student is given a choice of quitting the program or taking one last opportunity at demonstrating competence.

Obviously, the extraordinary steps recommended by Gordon are rarely needed and, if they are, they require the support of clear departmental guidelines to be effectively implemented. The first five steps, however, should be consistently applied to promote student development. Toward the end of the clinical experience, all students should be provided opportunities for summative evaluation. While clinical instructors frequently focus their summative evaluation attention on students who have demonstrated performance problems throughout the course, such an opportunity is equally important for students who have consistently received positive feedback.

A number of techniques for summative evaluation are suggested in the nursing literature. Simulated clinical experiences and observations by an evaluator who is not the student's clinical instructor have been used successfully by Morgan, Luke, and Hebert.[30] In addition, video testing programs have been developed and used by a group of psychiatric clinical instructors at Harris College of Nursing in Texas. These faculty members concluded that the videotaped examination offered a more consistently objective and accurate method of summative student evaluation.[31]

Regardless of the specific evaluation technique used, a systematic attempt to provide summative evaluation will enable the clinical instructor to accurately assess the extent to which all students have met course clinical objectives.

Clinical. *The American Heritage Dictionary* defines *clinical* as "of or pertaining to direct observation and treatment of patients." The term *clinical* in nursing education usually refers to those activities that students engage in while providing nursing care to or for clients. The dichotomy that needs to be recognized in evaluating the clinical performance of nursing students is the difference between nursing knowledge and the application of knowledge. Dunn's 1970 research study found no relationship between nursing performance and theoretical test scores.[32] Those nurses who scored high on the test *did not* necessarily demonstrate this knowledge in the observed performance of nursing procedures. Although knowledge and application of knowledge cannot be separated for learning purposes, clinical instructors need to determine the extent to which their evaluation methods evaluate knowledge versus performance. Clinical instructors who weigh heavily students' written papers and oral reports when determining clinical grades may in fact be evaluating knowledge, not application of knowledge. Clinical instructors must, however, keep the goals of the educational program in mind when determining the amount of emphasis they place on knowledge as opposed to the application of knowledge. No doubt the weight given these two components will be and should be different in different nursing education programs.

Evaluation. The final term to be discussed in relation to developing valid and reliable clinical evaluation strategies is *evaluation*. Two definitions are included in most dictionaries: first, to determine or set the value or worth of; appraise, estimate, judge; and second, to ascertain the numerical value of some attribute. These two definitions are the source of many of the difficulties in clinical evaluation. Many behaviors of nursing students are valuable but can they be assigned a numerical value? Especially if the numerical value must be chosen from a five-point scale? The advent of behavioral objectives and level objectives has helped instructors assign numerical values, but perhaps clinical evaluation could be simplified if educators accepted that certain skills in nursing can't be differentiated by a number while others can. Behaviors that deal with attitudes and psychomotor skills are among the most difficult to differentiate numerically. No one will deny, however, that these skills are relevant and valuable in nursing practice. Clinical instructors who easily assign a numerical value to performance likely are evaluating the rate at which a student learned or the consistency of the behavior rather than the quality of performance itself. This problem is not easily resolved, but clinical instructors who clearly understand the difference between measurement and evaluation are well on their way to improving their clinical evaluation skills.

SUMMARY

Effective clinical teachers must be expert planners, directors, and evaluators. Clinical teachers deal with experiential learning in diverse settings populated by people of all ages in need of health care, health promotion, and health maintenance. Thus, clinical teachers must deal with issues and responsibilities involving both students and clients. To be effective, a clinical teacher should possess certain supervisory, instructional process, and professional skills. Supervisory skills are designed to augment instructional efforts. These skills include those associated with planning, directing (leading), and evaluating.

Planning skills include recognizing the articulation between the curriculum and clinical learning experiences and the ability to communicate this relationship to students through teaching strategies, such as a clinical education guide.

Directing abilities address the responsibility of the clinical teacher to foster the professional development of students through application of appropriate leadership styles according to the situation and the maturity level of students.

Evaluation abilities of the clinical teacher revolve around developing and using valid and reliable strategies whereby students' cognitive, affective, and psychomotor clinical competencies are measured, interpreted, and communicated to promote student growth with the ultimate goal of quality client care.

INSTRUCTIONAL PROCESS SKILLS

Specific teaching behaviors used to transmit knowledge, shape attitudes, or develop psychomotor abilities can be called instructional process skills. The broad criteria recommended by Irby to distinguish effective from ineffective instructional process skills are: organization and clarity, group instructional skills, and enthusiasm. Providing organization and clarity is always important when teaching, especially while lecturing and teaching specific clinical skills. Certain communication skills and behaviors are desirable when a clinical instructor conducts discussions or attempts to promote clinical problem solving. Communicating enthusiasm is an important baseline teaching requirement.

Communicating Enthusiasm

Whether in the classroom or the clinical setting, enthusiasm is an important teaching attribute. Although enthusiasm itself cannot be learned, most teachers experience a certain level of enthusiasm at some time or other, and ability to *express* enthusiasm can be learned. Nursing instructors who do not regularly feel enthusiastic when teaching should probably look for another way of practicing their profession. Instructors who feel enthusiastic but do not communicate enthusiasm to students should make a conscious effort to do so.

McKeachie discusses the role of "ego ideal" that the teacher can play for the student and argues that the "key attribute of the teacher as ego ideal is commitment, or as it is sometimes referred to, enthusiasm."[33] The goal of the teacher as ego ideal is "to convey the excitement and value of intellectual inquiry in a given field of study." Again, if we do not regularly feel this sort of excitement, we will not be able to stimulate our students. If we do feel it, we should work at sharing it with our students. Some people naturally communicate enthusiasm, whereas others must work at it.

A constant danger the clinical teacher faces is that high work demands will interfere with time for informal discussion with students. Yet it is within such periods of interaction that a clinical teacher may most readily communicate enthusiasm and the deep satisfaction derived from being a nurse. A conscious effort should be made to set aside time for informal discussion, either at lunch or coffee breaks. The less "vibrant" one is in other teaching tasks, the more important this teaching strategy becomes. Just because we are not dynamic performers does not mean we cannot communicate enthusiasm to students. We must simply take the time to find the proper approach.

It is possible, for example, to convey enthusiasm in one's written comments on students' papers (for example, nursing process, interaction, or health assessment assignments). The midterm and final evaluation conference also provide opportunities to convey one's zeal for nursing and teaching. An appropriate sharing of one's most rewarding personal client-care experiences or research can be a highly effective teaching strategy, especially if it is relevant to a student's present clinical situation. No strategy, however, is probably more effective than demonstrating to students warmth and effectiveness as a nurse in a client-care setting. By serving as a role model, the clinical instructor can in fact dispute the old adage "do as I say, not as I do."

Providing Organization and Clarity

As indicated earlier, organization and clarity are important teaching attributes that can affect learning. Clinical teachers can enhance organization and clarity while demonstrating clinical skills and lecturing.

Providing Organization and Clarity While Lecturing. The lecture is usually thought of as a classroom rather than a clinical teaching method, but clinical instructors may often have the opportunity to use this strategy for topics of clinical interest. Since such on-the-spot lectures may have to be brief because of competing clinical care demands or may be delivered to students distracted and tired after a full day of client-care responsibilities, organization and clarity of presentation is critical.

Whereas discussion and discovery techniques are more appropriate for shaping attitudes and promoting problem solving, lecture is best suited for straightforward delivery of information. Lecture is especially appropriate when teaching time is limited and when other suitable materials are not available. For example, a clinical nursing instructor might choose to draw on years of experience to synthesize the clinical implications of findings from several recent research studies.

When lecturing, the clinical instructor is advised to adhere to certain guidelines described by Holcomb and Garner.[34] These include: (1) knowing the subject thoroughly, (2) explaining the purposes, objectives, and relevance of the subject to students, (3) following an organized and logical sequence, (4) maintaining eye contact with students, (5) speaking clearly with an appropriate vocabulary, (6) illustrating main points with appropriate examples, (7) allowing opportunity for student questions and opinions, (8) using appropriate auditory, visual and/or tactile materials, (9) reiterating main points during the lecture, and (10) summarizing the main points while closing.

The first point addresses the commonsense notion that we should not try to tell others about something we do not know about. This is especially true in the case of clinical instructors holding appointments in educational institutions, who may sometimes be viewed as outsiders in a health care agency. Lectures provide an opportunity to build or destroy a clinical teacher's credibility. Consequently, the decision to lecture should not be made haphazardly or be abused through overuse. As a rule, lecture when you know a topic very well and have something unique to offer.

The remaining points listed deal with the process of lecturing. In combination, they illustrate the importance of moving forward in a logical fashion and ensuring that listeners are with you as you proceed. The recent explosion of knowledge in biomedical and clinical sciences lends itself to the abuse of lecturing as a teaching strategy. There is a tendency for lecturers to try to cram as much relevant information as possible into the available time. Unfortunately, verbal communication is not well suited for such overloading. Consequently, the effective lecturer must carefully choose and limit the main points to be covered. A good rule of thumb is that listeners will probably only be able to remember four or five key points the day following a lecture. Therefore, it is important to select the four or five points that you most want students to remember, alert your audience at the beginning of the lecture to what these main points will be, illustrate and summarize each main point with several common examples, vary sensory stimuli, provide opportunities for questions, and remind the audience of the main points as you finish speaking. By following these simple steps, lecture organization and clarity can be substantially enhanced.

Providing Organization and Clarity When Teaching Skills. Much clinical instruction involves teaching psychomotor skills. Foley and Smilansky have provided several helpful suggestions for ensuring the organization and clarity of skill lessons.[35] The steps they suggest include:

1. Performing a skill analysis. This step involves developing a written checklist describing in detail the component behaviors required to perform the skill.
2. Modeling the skill. The step involves accurately demonstrating the skill so that students can witness all of the necessary details, observing the checklist as the instructor proceeds.

3. Facilitating students' practice. When necessary, simulated practice on peers and models should be provided prior to performance on clients.
4. Providing supervision and evaluation. The instructor should arrange to provide feedback at practice sessions and to provide a summative evaluation based on the students' performance either in a simulated laboratory or in a client-care situation.

The planning necessary to organize and facilitate such skill classes may be discomforting to some, but, as with any teaching responsibility, planning is always more time-consuming the first time around. The major obstacles in the process described are the performance of the skill analysis and determining appropriate practice opportunities for students. The former is a straightforward analytic problem, the latter is a complicated managerial dilemma. The solution is dependent on the complexity of the skill, the risk to the client, and the practice resources available. It should be noted that under no circumstances should the distribution of skill checklists be viewed as a wholistic learning experience and substitute for other teaching strategies, such as direct or contrived skill demonstrations. The primary value of the skills checklist is to assist the instructor to analyze the skill in order to teach it most effectively, to assist the student to learn the steps in the skill procedure, and to guide evaluation of student performance of the skill. A skill analysis checklist is illustrated in Table 4–4.

Group Instructional Skills

The clinical instructor must be able to teach groups of students. Such teaching requires certain competencies. The behaviors that Irby clusters under the heading "group instructional skills" are: (1) establishes rapport with the class, (2) creates a climate of mutual respect, (3) shows sensitivity to student responses, and (4) stimulates active participation in discussion.[36] How can a clinical teacher implement these rather general behaviors? First, we will examine how the instructor might establish rapport, create a climate of mutual respect, and show sensitivity to student responses, all of which involve common communication strategies. Then we will examine multiple ways that the instructor might stimulate problem-solving discussions on particular client-care topics.

Communication in Groups. As with all teaching, the cornerstone of effective instruction is effective communication; however, communication during small-group instruction, as occurs in clinical settings, differs substantially from communication during large-group instruction. The former is far more interactive than the latter. Small group size invites free exchange. To teach effectively, the clinical instructor must take full advantage of this potential for interactive communication.

Of course, it is possible to spend years studying the communication process or a lifetime refining one's skills. Busy clinical teachers may not have the time to devote to such an enterprise. Consequently, it is best to focus on certain base-line communication skills likely to yield maximum benefit with minimum investment. The

TABLE 4-4. FULL-HAND-FOREARM HANDWASHING PERFORMANCE CHECKLIST

Action	Performance +	Performance −
The student:		
1. Identifies "clean" and "contaminated" objects in the immediate environment.		
2. Checks availability and condition of equipment and supplies.		
3. Cuts fingernails if needed.		
4. Removes all jewelry and rolls up sleeves.		
5. Adjusts water flow and temperature.		
6. Wets hands, applies sufficient soap to work up a good lather.		
7. Scrubs hands using friction movements including interlacing fingers, backs of hands, palms, and around fingernails for at least 15 seconds.		
8. Rinses hands under running water from tips to wrists, keeping hands level or pointing upward (clean to dirty) so water will not go from contaminated area to clean.		
9. Cleans fingernails.		
10. Wets one forearm and with a sufficient amount of soap, works up a good lather in both hands. With the opposite hand, beginning at wrist, works upward in a circular motion around the forearm. When the elbow is reached, stops, does *not* go backwards. This would contaminate the "clean" forearm.		
11. Rinses hands and forearm going from fingertips toward elbow.		
12. Repeats steps 10 and 11 for opposite forearm. Then washes hands again.		
13. Dries both hands first with paper towel, discards paper towel, then dries one forearm with a patting motion working upward around forearm without going backwards or lowering forearms. This would comtaminate the "clean" forearms. Uses as many towels as necessary. Repeats procedure for opposite forearm.		
14. Discards towel without transferring it to other hand *or* lowering hand so water will run down and contaminate clean areas.		
15. Uses last towel to turn off faucet.		
16. Discards towel without contaminating hands.		
17. If any contaminated article is touched by hands or arms, repeats procedure.		
Satisfactory _____ Unsatisfactory _____		

Used with permission of Nursing I faculty, The University of Iowa College of Nursing, Iowa City, IA, 1982.

skills—active listening, "I-messages," and "no-lose negotiation"—have been described in detail by Thomas Gordon.[37]

Active Listening. Active listening is a skill designed to increase empathy and acceptance among individuals engaged in conversation. In doing so, it fosters mutual problem solving rather than antagonism and conflict. A rather simple technique to describe, active listening merely requires that a listener restate in the listener's own language the impression of the message expressed by the person to whom he or she is listening. By doing so, the listener confirms that the message was accurately heard and interpreted.

Although useful in a wide variety of situations, active listening is particularly helpful when talking with somebody who is frustrated or angry. Such situations often arise in dealing with clients experiencing emotional problems or staff conflicts. The following few hypothetical conversations illustrate how a clinical nursing instructor might take the opportunity to use active listening.

Student: "I can't believe how nasty Mr. Johnson treats me. Sure he's very sick, but I'm trying to help him. You'd think he'd show some appreciation."

Instructor: "You're really upset over the way he is behaving."

Student: "That doctor infuriates me. She always insists that we drop everything we are doing to help her and then she has the nerve to constantly criticize us."

Instructor: "It sounds as if you're very angry at Dr. Johnson."

Student: "I know that I should be doing a better job giving these injections, but I can't seem to get over my nervousness."

Instructor: "So, giving injections really makes you anxious."

While active listening appears simple, it actually takes a great deal of practice to implement effectively. Probably, the main reason it is a difficult skill to master is that most of us are inclined to try to solve people's problems for them. Consequently, we immediately resort to providing solutions rather than being sounding boards. Gordon refers to such solution responses as "roadblocks," and he provides the following twelve classic examples: (1) ordering, directing, commanding, (2) warning, admonishing, threatening, (3) moralizing, preaching, imploring, (4) advising, giving suggestions or solutions, (5) persuading with logic, lecturing, arguing, (6) judging, criticizing, disagreeing, blaming, (7) praising, agreeing, evaluating positively, buttering up, (8) name-calling, ridiculing, shaming, (9) interpreting, analyzing, diagnosing, (10) reassuring, sympathizing, consoling, supporting, (11) probing, questioning, interrogating, and (12) distracting, diverting, kidding.[38]

Another reason that active listening is difficult to master is that people may overuse the skill. The great irony of active listening is that if it becomes a reflex response in virtually all communication situations, it too, can become a roadblock. Therefore, active listening should be used regularly, but judiciously. Virtually every day, several opportunities for effectively using active listening occur. These opportunities should be seized, but forced opportunities should be bypassed.

I-Messages. The I-message is a skill designed to ensure that communication remains a two-way process. While active listening is a very effective tool for understanding a student's problem, the I-message enables the instructor to communicate a problem to the student. In many cases, the instructor's problem is caused by the student's behavior. If the instructor wants the student to alter behavior, the needed change in behavior must be clearly explained. The I-message can be used in this instance. It contains three basic components: (1) a brief description of the behavior found to be unacceptable, (2) the instructor's feelings, and (3) a precise explanation of the effect of the behavior. Gordon provides the following simple formula to help us remember the I-message: Behavior + Feeling + Effect = I-message.[39]

While all the three components should be present, they do not necessarily have to be expressed in this order. The following hypothetical statements illustrate how a clinical instructor might effectively use I-messages:

> "Harry, your repeated unwillingness to prepare a thorough nursing process paper distresses me. Based on your performance to date, I'm afraid that I am going to have to submit a failing grade."
>
> "I'm dissatisfied with the way that you are dispensing medications. I believe that you must demonstrate much more care when checking the medication kardex."
>
> "Chris, your failure to acknowledge the contributions of the other members of the team upsets me. I get the impression that you don't value their efforts."

From these examples, it is readily apparent that I-messages may often evoke a strong reaction in the student. Nevertheless, while they may make a student cower or want to argue, I-messages are less likely to cause communication breakdowns than mere statements of instructor feelings or exclamations of dissastisfaction with student behavior. By providing a concise but accurate account of the cause and effect of the problem, the I-message maximizes the opportunity for resolution of the problem through negotiation. Immediately after delivering an I-message, an instructor will probably have to resort to active listening in order to assess the impact of the message on the student. Ultimately, the instructor should try to resolve the problem through "no-lose negotiation."

No-lose Negotiation. Whether in a supervisory or teaching capacity, the clinical instructor can benefit substantially from knowing the conflict resolution technique called no-lose negotiation. The no-lose method is designed to provide for the mutual need satisfaction of the participants through a joint problem-solving process. As such, it requires some restraint by the party holding the greater amount of power. In any case, the clinical teacher must abstain from reflex responses that exert power over students every time a conflict arises. Of course, this recommendation must be tempered by common sense. Inevitably, situations arise where a clinical instructor must simply pull rank. A client's health may depend on it. Furthermore, many conflicts are simply not important enough to warrant a time-consuming negotiation process. The no-lose method should be adopted in situations where it is clearly in everyone's interest to pursue a solution systematically. Also, clinical instructors should model the no-lose process so their students might emulate it when needed. Negotiation skills will be invaluable to them in their nursing careers.

No-lose negotiation requires the use of active listening and I-messages to ensure communication throughout the problem-solving process. This process involves six steps: (1) identifying and defining the problem, (2) generating alternative solutions, (3) evaluating the alternative solutions, (4) decision making (choosing preferred solution), (5) implementing the decision, and (6) following up to evaluate the solution.[40] The time required to proceed through these steps may vary greatly depending upon the number of people involved. In a case where the clinical instructor is dealing with a single student, the first four steps may be carried out in a single meeting and steps five and six implemented soon afterward. When the instructor must deal with a group of several people, a number of meetings might be necessary to reach step four.

The following case study illustrates how a clinical instructor might use the no-lose process to negotiate a change in a single student's behavior.

Instructor: "Sally, I'm very upset that you aren't better organized. It is already 1:00 and you should have completed the care of your client two hours ago. No matter which client you care for, you never finish on time."

Sally: "Well, if I didn't have to wait for *you* all the time, I could finish earlier. You are never available when I need help."

Instructor: "You are frustrated because I make you late?"

Sally: "Well, you always seem free to help other students, but I can't ever find you when I need help."

Instructor: "Sally, let's try to figure out why I don't seem to be free when you need me. What could account for this situation?"

Sally: "Well, maybe you like the other students better or maybe you don't think I'll need help, or maybe you are trying to see how I can do by myself."

Instructor: "Do you need my help every morning?"

Sally: "Well, no—but sometimes I just need to check to make sure I'm doing things right—I'm afraid to go ahead with some aspects of care without checking with someone."

Instructor: "You are insecure without checking with me?"

Sally: "Yes and no. I could ask the staff or other students, but *you* are my instructor, and I feel better checking with you."

Instructor: "Sally, you've never appeared to want my help and I didn't know you felt this way. It sounds as if we need to devise a plan that will help you to provide care with more confidence."

The essence of the no-lose negotiation process is achieved at this point. If the instructor and student can arrive at a plan that involves an identification of each of their mutual responsibilities, the approach can be tried and evaluated in the following weeks.

Promoting Learning Through Group Discussion. Clinical experiences provide many opportunities for group discussion. These discussions may occur spontaneously or may be carefully planned by the clinical instructor. In either case, the instructor's responsibility is to promote the best possible discussion eliciting full student participation. When students freely participate in discussion, the clinical instructor can assess understanding of critical content, thereby identifying students' strengths as well as needs for further instruction. McKeachie points out that discussion also provides students with the opportunity to formulate applications of principles, to practice thinking using subject matter, evaluate the logic of, and evidence for, their own and others' positions, to formulate problems using information gained from readings, lectures, or experience, and to develop motivation for further learning.[41]

A variety of skills are required by anyone attempting to lead an effective discussion. Hyman provides a thorough, excellent description of the skills briefly summarized here: introducing, questioning, contributing, crystalizing, focusing, supporting, and closing.[42]

Introducing. It is important to keep the introduction component of discussion sessions brief and succinct in order to clarify the topic at hand and to establish a climate of group participation rather than leader domination. One of the best ways of opening a discussion is with a question. Foley and Smilansky point out that open-ended questions can be used to promote student reasoning through clinical problem-solving discussions.[43] Comments and questions such as those that follow might be used to open a discussion focusing on application of the nursing process.

Instructor: "We decided yesterday we would use this clinical conference to develop a plan of nursing care for Mr. Hall, the patient with a medical diagnosis of acute pulmonary failure. At our last meeting we agreed all students would review Mr. Hall's chart and spend some time observing and talking with him."

Or

Instructor: "I'd like to begin this morning's clinical conference by asking Ms. Solberg, who is caring for Mr. Hall, the patient with acute pulmonary failure, what her assessment data indicate as this patient's priority nursing diagnosis."

An additional aspect of the introduction is a clear indication of how the discussion should proceed. Foley and Smilansky present a set of problem-solving steps that can be used to structure clinical problem-solving discussions in a wide variety of health fields.[44] These steps include: (1) explaining what is known and formulating tentative hypotheses, (2) gathering further data, (3) interpreting data by organizing it, selecting groups of data related to the problem, identifying various relationships that may exist, stating hypotheses to explain the data; and (4) testing the hypotheses by gathering further data, planning experimentation, or initiating a treatment. These steps are not new to the professional nurse or nurse-educator. Though the terms are different, they are in fact the essence of the approach used in the nursing process. The nursing process, therefore, provides a logical framework for organizing a clinical nursing problem-solving discussion. If the time for the clinical conference is limited, the instructor may want to limit discussion to one or two steps of the nursing process. For example, an alternative but reasonable approach might be to focus on assessment and diagnosis or intervention and evaluation. Whatever the circumstances, the learning needs of the students should always be considered when planning the specific procedural elements to be employed.

Questioning. While a well-formulated question is an important component of a discussion's introduction, a discussion leader must demonstrate questioning skill throughout the entire discussion. Questions are generally used to seek new information and to probe for responses. The first purpose is rather straightforward and is quite appropriate when gathering data in a clinical problem-solving discussion. The following example illustrates use of a data-gathering question:

Instructor: "Do the results of Mr. Hall's PO_2 and PCO_2 laboratory tests indicate any change in his condition?"

Probing is a more subtle questioning skill that can be used for a variety of reasons. Hyman points out that there are probes that ask for specifics, clarification of an idea, consequences of a suggested course of action, elaboration of a point, parallel cases, implementation of a proposed idea, relationships to other issues, comments from the perspective of another person, explanation of how one arrived at a position, or explanations of causes or purposes of a suggested idea.[45] Any of these probes might be used at different times by a clinical instructor, but a particular challenge is choosing the appropriate probes to facilitate clinical problem-solving. The following exchange illustrates how an instructor might proceed:

Instructor: "Can you elaborate on why you think Mr. Hall gets frustrated and angers easily?"

Student: "Well, he has a tracheostomy and receives intermittent ventilation by a respirator and, therefore, it is very difficult for him to communicate his needs."

Instructor: "Is there anything else that you think contributes to Mr. Hall's communication difficulty?"

Student: "Yes, I guess so. Writing on paper is hard for him because of his weakened condition."

Instructor: "Would your approach to thinking about Mr. Hall's frustration and anger be any different if he could communicate more easily?"

Contributing. Although the clinical instructor should guard against becoming the sole source of information in a group discussion, she or he should not hesitate to make contributions at appropriate times. Contributions by a discussion leader typically fall into three categories: substantive, socioemotional, and procedural.[46] Substantive contributions address the content issues of the discussion. Socioemotional contributions focus on the interpersonal realm, and procedural contributions provide direction for the flow of discussion. Here are examples of each type of contribution in our clinical problem-solving discussion:

Substantive

Instructor: "Ms. Solberg's concern about the effect of frequent suctioning on Mr. Hall's hypoxemia level is worth pursuing. I recently read in a research study in

Heart and Lung that hypoxemia resulted when endotracheal suctioning was performed without preoxygenation."[47]

Socioemotional

Instructor: "You're right, Jean, it is difficult to take the brunt of a patient's anger. Perhaps if we can focus on the reasons for anger, it will be easier for all of us to accept it."

Procedural

Instructor: "At this point, we can continue to discuss our feelings about working with angry patients or we can move to planning specific nursing interventions. I think we have all developed an understanding of Mr. Hall's anger and I suggest we move ahead to his plan of care."

Crystalizing. The crystalizing skill requires the instructor to concisely state the essence of a student's remarks. By rephrasing student comments through brief summaries, the instructor can clarify the discussion as it proceeds. Either the tone or content of a discussion can be crystalized. Typical techniques involve using analogies, declarative statements, or questions.[48] The following example illustrates how a clinical instructor might crystalize the content of a clinical problem-solving discussion using an analogy:

Instructor: "Jim and Diane both seem to be saying that this patient's condition seems so hopeless that it is hard for them to think realistically about a restorative plan of care. Am I interpreting your comments correctly?"

Focusing. Since discussions often go astray, it is important that the discussion leader be able to focus the discussion through remarks that keep participants addressing pertinent issues. This is particularly important during problem-solving discussions in situations where there is limited time available. Comments such as those that follow can be used to focus such a discussion:

Ms. Solberg: "Mr. Hall requires a lot of attention and care. It takes me all morning just to complete his bath and routine procedures."

Student B: "Does it seem impossible to think of doing anything more or of spending more time with him?"

Ms. Solberg: "Yes, and what am I going to do after graduation when I have more than one patient to care for?"

Student C: "That's what's wrong with this nursing program. We never get to practice like real nurses."

Instructor: "Let's return to Mr. Hall's care and see if we can consider the alternatives for organizing to provide the care we think he needs in the most efficient and effective manner possible. Ms. Solberg seems to be asking for help with this problem. Is that right?"

Supporting. Throughout any effective discussion, the instructor must play a supporting role by providing encouragement, involving reticent members, and relieving tension. Students will shy away from participation if they perceive the discussion as threatening or are punished while participating. Probably the best means of being supportive, without being overly compliant and appeasing, is to practice the basic communication skills of active listening, I-messages, and no-lose negotiation, along with providing praise of student's efforts when such praise is deserved. Those afraid of giving praise too freely should remember that most of us do not provide praise nearly as often as we should. The following examples indicate how a clinical instructor can discreetly inject praise and solicit participation in a problem-solving discussion:

Instructor: "Ms. Solberg raised a good point earlier about the adverse effects of frequent suctioning—let's go back to her concern for a minute." (Praise)

Or

Instructor: "It is easy in a discussion such as this to get off the track but all of you have done a good job of listening to each other and in moving the discussion toward the accomplishment of the task." (I-message; praise)

Or

Instructor: "Jan, I was glad to see you express your feelings today. Was this a positive experience for you?" (Active listening; praise)

Instructor: "Robert, you've looked really interested in this entire discussion. Is there something you would like to add?" (Active listening; praise)

Closing. Instructors frequently overlook providing closure at the end of a discussion, restating the key points of the discussion and launching the group into its next activity. This is probably because effectively closing a discussion requires substantial progress during the discussion and a clear notion of where the group is headed in the future. Thus, the closing is really an indicator of both success and direction and is a procedural benchmark in the life of an ongoing discussion group. Preferably, an instructor should close a discussion when participants have achieved their stated goal, but closure may be necessary when allotted time expires or discussants experience attention lapses. Because of the time and work demands encountered in clinical settings, the clinical instructor should become adept at conducting and closing discussions before they cut deeply into time needed by students for their clinical responsibilities. The following example shows how a clinical instructor might close a problem-solving discussion:

Instructor: "You've done an excellent job of formulating a priority nursing diagnosis with appropriate interventions. Tomorrow let's try to discuss and finalize the evaluation aspects of Mr. Hall's plan of care."

Problem-solving discussions are only one type of discussion. The clinical teacher will conduct a variety of other types as well. Hyman describes four typical types of discussion other than problem-solving discussion.[49] These include policy, explaining, predicting, and debriefing. All of the skills just described are appropriate for these types of discussion. In addition, it is not necessary that four or five people be present to constitute a group discussion. The skills can be adapted for use in the smallest possible group, that of the instructor and a single student.

SUMMARY

Effective clinical teachers need to use particular teaching skills to transmit knowledge, shape attitudes, and develop the psychomotor abilities of students in the clinical setting. These instructional process skills include communicating enthusiasm, providing organization and clarity while demonstrating nursing skills, lecturing and communicating to groups as well as individual students.

Communicating enthusiasm, both verbally and nonverbally, for the nursing profession and all that it entails, although difficult to define, measure and practice, is an important attribute to the clinical instructor and should be cultivated and consistently used to stimulate student learning.

Organization and clarity are important conditions for learning. Techniques for providing organization and clarity while lecturing and teaching psychomotor skills in the clinical setting can be learned.

Since clinical teaching involves group as well as one-on-one teaching episodes, it is important for clinical instructors to know and use principles and techniques of group communication. Such skills include use of active listening, I-messages, and no-lose negotiation, as well as introducing, questioning, contributing, crystalizing, focusing, supporting, and closing techniques.

PROFESSIONAL SKILLS

The professional skills category is used as an organizing framework to address the impact on clinical teaching effectiveness of the clinical instructor's knowledge, clinical competence, and role-modeling abilities. The direct clinical teaching strategies described under the categories of supervisory skills and instructional process skills are effective for improving clinical instruction only if the instructor already possesses professional skills. Unfortunately, faculty development efforts and graduate nursing programs have traditionally over-emphasized the educational process and often have neglected to recognize the impact on student learning of individual faculty nursing expertise. If a clinical instructor is not knowledgeable, competent, and able to demonstrate abilities, then he or she cannot possibly be an effective facilitator of student learning.

Knowledge

Nursing is an emerging, evolving scientific and professional discipline. While all disciplines have experienced a knowledge explosion in the last 20 years, none surpasses that which has occurred in nursing. For instance, doctoral programs in nursing have grown from 4 in 1956 to 24 in 1982.[50] The number of nurses holding the earned doctorate has increased from 504 in 1969[51] to 3650 in 1983.[52] Nursing research conferences, almost nonexistent in 1970, now proliferate on the local, state, and national scene, and new scholarly nursing journals appear yearly in phenomenal numbers. Nursing is rapidly changing, not only because of the discovery of new nursing knowledge, but also because of new health care delivery systems and revised health care policies. The introduction of computer technology in processing client information and advances in medical treatment have revolutionary implications for nursing practice and, consequently, for nursing education.

Most newly appointed nursing faculty, fresh out of graduate school, possess current nursing knowledge. Quite soon, however, these neophyte teachers discover that their faculty responsibilities often include a number of diverse and time-consuming activities. Responsibilities may include teaching several courses for several levels of students, serving on course, departmental, school, or institutional committees, providing professional community service, teaching continuing education courses, and—depending on institution philosophy—conducting research and publishing or engaging in professional practice. Faculty who possess good organizational and leadership skills may also acquire administrative responsibilities as chairs of committees or coordinators of courses. Given such demands, it is difficult to find time for one's own professional development such as updating one's nursing knowledge. Thus, this activity must become a personal priority. If a clinical instructor does not have a commitment to maintaining a current knowledge level, he or she will have a severe knowledge deficit within five years or less. Therefore, every faculty member should devise a personal plan for professional development.

Of course, such a plan will differ for each individual, depending on institutional expectations and each nurse's own area of expertise, long-term professional goals, and level of education. Nevertheless, each clinical instructor might benefit from the following suggestions for maintaining up-to-date knowledge.

First, identify a particular area of expertise. Accept the fact that it is impossible to be an expert on everything. Every clinical instructor must maintain a minimally current knowledge level in content related to the course or courses taught. One or two areas of nursing knowledge should also be identified for continual in-depth study. In nursing programs that emphasize research, these areas should be the basis for a program of research.

Second, set aside time each week for professional reading. At least three nursing journals should be read regularly. Clinical instructors are well advised to consider reading at least one nursing research journal, one nursing practice journal, and one nursing education journal. Professional reading should not be limited to nursing journals. To be an effective clinical instructor, one must be able to teach nursing within a current societal context. Thus the clinical instructor should also spend some time reading material that focuses on the supporting sciences, contemporary fiction and nonfiction, and items discussing daily news events.

Third, join a relevant professional nursing association. Association newsletters are a constant source of current issues and insights related to one's area of expertise. Professional association meetings provide an opportunity to exchange ideas with others with whom one shares a common interest.

Fourth, plan to attend at least one research or scholarly conference annually. Clinical instructors should avoid attending continuing education conferences that are designed for nurses with less educational background than their own. Review carefully the credentials of presentors. Choose continuing education opportunities deliberately. Research conferences are most likely to present the latest information on a topic. They are also a source of intellectual stimulation because of the critique-and-debate format used at most of these meetings.

Irby points out that knowledge is inferred from the clinical instructor's ability to discuss current developments in a specialty, direct students to useful literature, and discuss other's points of view.[53] Clinical instructors who do not systematically and conscientiously plan for their own professional growth will quickly find they are unable to meet students' learning needs.

Clinical Competence

According to Donald Wolfe, competence always has an environmental context, is rooted in a knowledge base and in analytic skills, is inevitably interdependent with a value system and (like experiential learning) involves the whole person.[54] The competence of a clinical nursing instructor should, therefore, be defined within a specific environmental context, such as an intensive care unit, an ambulatory clinic, or a client home. Clinical nursing instructors should not be expected by their students or colleagues to be clinically competent in every context. A clinical instructor who maintains a current knowledge base in an area of expertise will have the prerequisite cognitive skill for clinical competence. The extent of this cognitive base will also greatly influence the value system of the clinical instructor and will provide a required framework for mastering psychomotor skills. Since competence involves the whole person, the competent clinical instructor should be highly skilled in the cognitive, affective, and psychomotor learning domains. In addition, like all teachers, the clinical instructor should know teaching and learning theory and principles and be able to apply this knowledge to clinical teaching.

Irby notes that instructor clinical competence includes objectively defining and analyzing patient (client) problems, effectively performing procedures, establishing rapport with patients and working effectively with health care team members.[55] The mechanism for maintaining clinical competence in nursing is currently a controversial issue. A preponderance of the contemporary nursing literature, however, tends to support a practice role for nurse faculty. Anderson and Person recently surveyed faculty who were engaged in practice and who taught in National League for Nursing-accredited baccalaureate programs.[56] The faculty participating in their study indicated three primary reasons for maintaining a practice: (1) to enrich their teaching, (2) to maintain clinical skills, and (3) for personal satisfaction. In addition, 95 percent of the respondents believed students thought positively about their professional practice.

Several models exist for maintaining faculty clinical competence through practice. These include: joint appointments, dual appointments, "moonlighting," outside practice without compensation, and summer employment. The extent to which a clinical instructor maintains a practice will depend on institutional policies and on personal philosophy. Whether or not one practices in the true sense of the word, a mechanism should be found to periodically test the currency of one's own clinical competence. Only through such an approach can effectiveness as a clinical instructor be achieved.

Role Modeling

If a clinical instructor is knowledgeable and clinically competent, he or she will generally be an effective role model. Effective role modeling is an important means of promoting the professional socialization and competence of nursing students. Bragg defined socialization as a "process by which individuals acquire the values, attitudes, norms, knowledge, and skills needed to perform their roles acceptably in the group or groups in which they are, or seek to be."[57] Nursing students, especially in their initial socialization process, require behavioral role models in order to learn desirable professional behaviors. In addition to being knowledgeable and clinically competent, therefore, clinical instructors should consciously identify those professional characteristics that they wish to model. These might be: ethical behavior, self-confidence, empathy, respect for clients and colleagues, or a willingness to admit errors. If a clinical instructor is unable or unwilling to model positive professional behaviors, students may imitate and identify with other professionals observed in the clinical setting. These other role models may or may not demonstrate professional behaviors consistent with the nursing curriculum objectives. If they do not, students will experience counterproductive socialization.

SUMMARY

The professional skills of the clinical instructor are the most crucial elements leading to effective clinical teaching. Administrative faculty responsible for appointing and reappointing these people must assure that they are knowledgeable, clinically competent, and able to serve as professional role models. Nurse faculty who do not concentrate some effort on personal professional development and maintenance of clinical skills will all too soon find they have lost much of their effectiveness as clinical instructors. This includes keeping up with current research, clinical procedures, educational methodologies, and technology. A commitment to teaching, research, practice, and lifelong learning is a basic necessity for all clinical instructors.

FUTURE DIRECTIONS FOR CLINICAL INSTRUCTION RESEARCH

On the whole, it appears that research related to clinical teaching has largely been neglected. Although some good studies have been carried out, many more are needed. In nursing, as in other health-related professions, clinical instruction holds numerous, exciting possibilities for research. While useful guidelines exist for distinguishing effective from ineffective clinical teaching, there still are many unresolved questions about how to best promote clinical problem solving, how to structure effective clinical experiences, and how to teach skills most efficiently when faced with the daily press of work demands on a nursing unit. Indeed, the best clinical teaching strategies may have to be tailored specifically to the particular types of units on which instruction occurs.

There is a need to clearly identify the most important distinguishing features in the clinical learning environments of the different nursing specialties and to specify the behaviors related to effective and ineffective nursing instruction in these settings. In this manner, the recorded behaviors of the more effective teachers can be used to posit optimal models for particular settings. Of course, such models might also be supplemented or altered by the addition of creative new teaching ideas, and these need to be investigated immediately.

Once models are formulated, the major question remains as to whether or not a large number of nursing instructors can be trained to emulate the models. To answer this question, it is necessary to devise clinical faculty development programs and to evaluate their impact rigorously. Efforts such as these will have to be replicated in a wide variety of settings to give a true indication of the potential of clinical instructor education.

The areas described here alone constitute an impressive agenda for nursing instruction researchers, and these are likely to be only a small portion of the total existing possibilities. Out of creative research efforts, creative teaching recommendations will flow.

CONCLUSION

It may seem that excellent clinical teaching requires a highly refined blend of skills that demand an intense level of commitment by the instructor. This is indeed the case. Excellent teaching always is a demanding profession, but the outstanding clinical teacher must strive for excellence in two areas, that of clinician and that of teacher. One may view this requirement as intimidating, or one may see it as an exhilarating challenge.

The key to accepting this challenge is to find ways to make these professional roles more manageable. A wholehearted effort to improve one's supervisory, instructional, and professional skills within a short period of time is quite likely to overwhelm most people. On the other hand, by focusing on specific skills at particular times of the year, or during particular phases in one's career, steady progress can be made. It takes a long time to become an outstanding teacher, and there are always bound to be some disappointments and setbacks along the way. Still, there is no reason why the road to excellence has to be a tortuous one. By setting realistic, manageable goals and creatively experimenting with different teaching strategies, we can reap a great deal of satisfaction as we grow into the clinical teaching role. Remember, experiential learning is powerful. As we evolve as clinical teachers, perhaps our greatest thrill will be monitoring and directing our own experiential learning.

POSTTEST

MULTIPLE CHOICE

DIRECTIONS: Select the *best* answer for each item.

1. What are the three general dimensions of clinical teaching under which Weinholtz and Ostmoe have grouped Irby's seven clinical teaching factors?
   a. Writing skills, problem-solving skills, intellectual skills
   b. Supervisory skills, diagnostic skills, intellectual skills
   c. Supervisory skills, instructional process skills, professional skills
   d. Instructional process skills, writing skills, professional skills
   e. Intellectual skills, supervisory skills, problem-solving skills
2. Why should a clinical instructor develop a clinical education guide for students?
   a. To provide the students with necessary information and efficiently communicate faculty, curriculum, and agency expectations
   b. To promote more effective problem solving in various clinical settings
   c. To enhance higher level learning and more efficient transfer of information
   d. To facilitate recall and reinforce key concepts
   e. To promote use of cost-effective techniques
3. What is a variable that instructors applying situational leadership theory must assess to determine their selection of leadership style?
   a. Learner intellect
   b. Learner sensitivity
   c. Learner aptitude
   d. Learner perseverance
   e. Learner maturity
4. Why should clinical instructors practice formative evaluation by providing feedback to students throughout the clinical learning experience?
   a. To fulfill legal responsibilities
   b. To assist student learning
   c. To ensure judgment of most student behaviors
   d. To meet departmental requirements
   e. To guarantee compliance with NLN guidelines
5. Which of the following behaviors is *not* one of the guidelines for effective lecturing offered by Holcomb and Garner?
   a. Knowing the subject thoroughly
   b. Following an organized logical sequence
   c. Illustrating main points with appropriate examples
   d. Embedding probing questions
   e. Summarizing the main points while closing

6. To how many key points do Weinholtz and Ostmoe recommend limiting lectures?
   a. 1 or 2
   b. 2 or 3
   c. 4 or 5
   d. 6 or 7
   e. 8 or 9

7. Which of the following best summarizes the skill of active listening?
   a. Asking frequent questions while listening to someone
   b. Demonstrating appropriate body language while listening to someone
   c. Restating in your own language the message expressed by the person to whom you are listening
   d. Speculating about the actions to be taken by the person to whom you are listening
   e. Developing solutions to the problems experienced by the person to whom you are listening

8. For what purpose do Weinholtz and Ostmoe recommend that the I-message be used?
   a. Demonstrating authority over rebellious students
   b. Ensuring that communication remains a two-way process
   c. Probing alternative solutions to problems
   d. Exercising creative initiatives in previously ignored areas
   e. Expressing personal insecurities

9. Which of the following phrases most accurately describes no-lose negotiation?
   a. A conflict resolution technique focusing on joint problem solving
   b. An arbitration technique for resolving teacher/labor disputes
   c. A method for specifically addressing differences in client-care plans
   d. A method for contracting for student grades
   e. A behavior modification technique

10. Which of the following items is *not* an instructional advantage of group discussion pointed out by McKeachie?
    a. Enables application of principles
    b. Promotes practice thinking using subject matter
    c. Promotes evaluation of logic of one's own positions
    d. Transmits information efficiently
    e. Motivates for further learning

11. Which of the following is *not* a suggestion offered by Weinholtz and Ostmoe for maintaining an up-to-date knowledge base?
    a. Identify a particular area of expertise for continual in-depth study
    b. Attend at least one research or scholarly conference annually
    c. Set aside time each week for professional reading

d. Join a professional nursing association
e. Enroll in courses from other disciplines—for example, business education

12. Which of the following professional characteristics is *not* one that Weinholtz and Ostmoe indicate that clinical instructors might consider modeling for students?
    a. Research competence
    b. Ethical behavior
    c. Empathy
    d. Respect for clients and colleagues
    e. Willingness to admit errors

SHORT ANSWER

DIRECTIONS: Supply the correct answers to the following items.

13. What are the seven factors that Irby's research indicates best differentiate effective from ineffective clinical teachers?

14. What are the four types of leadership behaviors prescribed by situational leadership theory?

15. What are the last three procedures (extraordinary steps) in Michael Gordon's guidelines for assessing students' affective behavior?

16. What are the four steps suggested by Foley and Smilansky for ensuring the organization and clarity of skill lessons?

17. List four of the "roadblocks" to effective active listening described by Thomas Gordon.

18. What are the three basic components of an I-message?

19. What are the six steps of no-lose negotiation?

20. What are the seven discussion-leading skills described by Hyman?

POSTTEST ANSWER KEY

1. c
2. a
3. e

4. b
5. d
6. c
7. c
8. b
9. a
10. d
11. e
12. a
13. Approach to clinical supervision, enthusiasm, organization and clarity, group instructional skills, knowledge, clinical competence, modeling of professional characteristics
14. Telling, selling, participating, delegating
15. Determine potential seriousness of problem, inspect performance, take administrative action
16. Performing a skill analysis, modeling the skill, facilitating students' practice, providing supervision and evaluation
17. You could have listed any 4 of the following 38 behaviors: ordering, directing, commanding, warning, admonishing, threatening, moralizing, preaching, imploring, advising, giving suggestions or solutions, persuading with logic, lecturing, arguing, judging, criticizing, disagreeing, blaming, praising, agreeing, evaluating positively, buttering up, name calling, ridiculing, shaming, interpreting, analyzing, diagnosing, reassuring, sympathizing, consoling, supporting, probing, questioning, interrogating, distracting, diverting, kidding
18. Behavior, feeling, effect
19. Identify and define the problem, generate alternative solutions, evaluate alternative solutions, make a decision (choose preferred solution), implement decision, evaluate solution
20. Introducing, questioning, crystalizing, contributing, focusing, supporting, closing

SUGGESTED APPLICATION ACTIVITIES

1. Reflect on the behavior of two clinical teachers who taught you sometime during your career as a nursing student, one who struck you as very effective and one who seemed considerably less effective. Analyze the teaching of each using the seven factors described by Irby. Write down and compare the apparent strengths and weaknesses of both teachers according to each factor.
2. Develop an outline for a clinical education guide that you could distribute to students that you might supervise on a specific nursing unit.
3. Create a clinical teaching plan containing a sequenced set of activities designed to result in student nurses performing a skill or several skills without need for supervision. Then justify your plan according to situational leadership theory.

4. Review Michael Gordon's affective assessment model and specify both the strengths and problems related to each step in the eight-stage process.
5. Develop a checklist or rating scale for the set of lecture guidelines offered by Holcomb and Garner. Compose and deliver a ten-minute lecture, videotaping yourself while you lecture. Replay the tape and evaluate your performance using the instrument that you developed to establish a personal profile.
6. Using a clinical nursing skill with which you are quite familiar, develop a skill analysis checklist that you could use to evaluate student performance.
7. Pair up with a fellow student and practice the skill of active listening by having each of you active-listen while the other presents a two-to-three-minute monologue of hypothetical personal problems. After each monologue, exchange views on how you felt in your roles.
8. Working with your partner from the active-listening exercise (or another partner), deliver five I-messages (each) in which you both communicate your distress over hypothetical situations. In each situation the person receiving the I-message may respond by active-listening.
9. Dream up a potentially awkward situation that might occur between a nursing student and a clinical instructor. With a partner playing the role of the student, adopt the role of the teacher and initiate the no-lose negotiation process. Develop another situation, exchange roles, and repeat the process.
10. Using the general leadership skills described by Hyman and the specific problem-solving steps offered by Foley and Smilansky as your guides, lead a nursing problem-solving discussion with several fellow students as participants. After completing the discussion, solicit feedback on your performance.
11. Using the criteria presented in the professional skills section of this chapter, write a list of your strengths and weaknesses in each of the following areas: knowledge, clinical competence, and role modeling of professional characteristics. For each weakness that you identify, generate a strategy that would help you overcome the weakness.
12. Choose one or more of the contrived or indirect teaching strategies from Chapter 3 and determine how they might be used in clinical teaching to promote a particular clinical outcome.

REFERENCES

1. Rogers C: Freedom to Learn. Columbus, OH, Charles E. Merrill Publishing Co., 1969, p. 5.
2. Coleman JS: Differences Between Experiential and Classroom Learning. In M Keeton (ed): Experiential Learning: Rationale, Characteristics and Assessment. San Francisco, Jossey-Bass Inc., Publishers, 1976, pp. 49–61.
3. Reichsman F, Browning FE, Hinshaw J: Observations of Undergraduate Clinical Teaching in Action. Journal of Medical Education 39:147–153, 1964.
4. Schweer J, Gebbie K: Creative Teaching in Clinical Nursing, ed 2. St. Louis, C.V. Mosby Co., 1976, pp. 3–4.

5. Ostmoe P, Denehy J, et al.: Nursing Education: Process, Roles and Strategies (graduate course). University of Iowa, College of Nursing, 1980.
6. Daggett CJ, Cassie JM, Collins GF: Research in Clinical Teaching. Review of Educational Research 49:151–169, 1979.
7. Irby DM: Clinical Faculty Development. In CW Ford (ed): Clinical Education for the Allied Health Professions. St. Louis, C.V. Mosby Co., 1978, pp. 95–105.
8. Hersey P, Blanchard K: Management of Organizational Behavior, ed 3. Englewood Cliffs, NJ, Prentice-Hall Inc., 1977, pp. 4–5.
9. Mager RF: Preparing Instructional Objectives, ed 2. Belmont, CA, Fearon-Pittman Publishers, Inc., 1975, pp. 5–17.
10. Brown AF: Clinical Instruction. Philadelphia, W.B. Saunders, Co. 1949, p. 511.
11. Guinee KK: The Aims and Methods of Nursing Education. New York, Macmillan, Inc. 1966, pp. 10–12.
12. Schweer J, Gebbie K: Creative Teaching in Clinical Nursing, ed 3. St. Louis, C.V. Mosby Co., 1976, p. 72.
13. Quinn FM: The Principles and Practice of Nurse Education. London, Croom Helm, 1980, pp. 80–92.
14. Daggett CJ, Cassie JM, Collins GF: Research in Clinical Teaching. Review of Educational Research 49:162, 1979.
15. Weinholtz, D: A Study of Instructional Leadership During Medical Attending Rounds. Unpublished doctoral dissertation, University of North Carolina, 1981, pp. 101–102.
16. Ford CW: The Clinical Education Guide. In CW Ford (ed): Clinical Education for the Allied Health Professions. St. Louis, C.V. Mosby Co., 1978, p. 173.
17. Ibid., p. 175.
18. Stritter FT, Flair MD: Effective Clinical Teaching. Bethesda, MD, National Medical Audiovisual Center, 1980, p. 7.
19. Houle CO: Continuing Learning in the Health Professions. San Francisco, Jossey-Bass, Inc., Publishers, 1981, pp. 76–123.
20. Hersey P, Blanchard K: Management of Organizational Behavior, ed 3. Englewood Cliffs, NJ, Prentice-Hall, Inc. 1977, pp. 159–188.
21. Blake RR, Mouton JS: The Managerial Grid. Houston, TX, Gulf Publishing Co. Book Division, 1964.
22. Hersey P, Blanchard K: Management of Organizational Behavior, ed 3. Englewood Cliffs, NJ, Prentice-Hall Inc., 1977, p. 161.
23. Ibid., p. 161.
24. Ibid., p. 163.
25. Lawrence R, Lawrence S: Clinical Evaluation of Students of Nursing: A Step Toward Quality Nursing Practice, Image 12 (2):46–48, 1980.
26. Wood V: Evaluation of Student Nursing Clinical Performance: A Problem That Won't Go Away. International Nursing Review 19:336–343, 1972.
27. Morgan MK, Irby DM (eds): Evaluating Clinical Competence in the Health Professions. St. Louis, C.V. Mosby Co., 1978.
28. Daggett CJ, Cassie JM, Collins GF: Research in Clinical Teaching. Review of Educational Research 49:162–163, 1979.
29. Gordon M: Assessment of Student Affect: A Clinical Approach. In MK Morgan, DM Irby (eds): Evaluating Clinical Competence in the Health Professions. St. Louis, C.V. Mosby Co., 1978, pp. 69–88.
30. Morgan B, Luke C, Hebert J: Evaluating Clinical Proficiency. Nursing Outlook 27: 540–544, 1979.

31. Richards A, Jones A, et al.: Videotape As An Evaluation Tool. Nursing Outlook 29: 35-38, 1981.
32. Dunn MA: Development of An Instrument To Measure Nursing Performance. Nursing Research 19:502-510, 1970.
33. McKeachie WJ: Teaching Tips, ed 7. Lexington, MA, D.C. Heath & Co., 1978, pp. 77-78.
34. Holcomb DJ, Garner AE: Improving Teaching in Medical Schools. Springfield, IL, Charles C. Thomas, Publisher, 1978, p. 44.
35. Foley RP, Smilansky J: Teaching Techniques: A Handbook for Health Professionals. New York, McGraw-Hill Book Co., 1980, pp. 84-85.
36. Irby, DM: Clinical Faculty Development. In CW Ford (ed): Clinical Education for the Allied Health Professions, St. Louis, C.V. Mosby Co., 1978, pp. 99-100.
37. Gordon T: Leadership Effectiveness Training. New York, Wyden Books, 1977.
38. Ibid., pp. 60-62.
39. Ibid., pp. 101-103.
40. Ibid., p. 178.
41. McKeachie WJ: Teaching Tips, ed 7. Lexington, MA, D.C. Heath & Co., 1978, pp. 35-36.
42. Hyman RT: Improving Discussion Leadership. New York, Teachers College Press, 1980, pp. 64-83.
43. Foley RP, Smilansky J: Teaching Techniques: A Handbook for Health Professionals. New York, McGraw-Hill Book Co., 1980, pp. 49-50.
44. Ibid., p. 50.
45. Hyman RT: Improving Discussion Leadership. New York, Teachers College Press, 1980, pp. 74-75.
46. Ibid., pp. 50-55.
47. Skelly F, Hooaday M, et al.: The Effectiveness of Two Preoxygenation Methods to Prevent Endotracheal Suction Induced Hypoxemia. Heart and Lung 9:316-323, 1980.
48. Hyman, RT: Improving Discussion Leadership. New York, Teachers College Press, 1980, pp. 55-59.
49. Ibid., pp. 22-27.
50. NLN Data Book 1982. New York, National League for Nursing, 1983, p. 79.
51. American Nurses' Association Staff: Facts About Nursing. Kansas City, MO, American Nurses' Association, 1980, p. 5.
52. Galliher JM: Directory of Nurses with Doctoral Degrees. Kansas City, MO, American Nurses' Association, 1984, p. 3.
53. Irby DM: Clinical Faculty Development. In CW Ford (ed): Clinical Education for the Allied Health Professions. St. Louis, C.V. Mosby Co., 1978, p. 99.
54. Wolfe DE: Developing Professional Competence in the Applied Behavioral Sciences. In ET Byrne, DE Wolfe (eds): Developing Experiential Learning Programs for Professional Education. San Francisco, Jossey-Bass, Inc., Publishers, 1980, p. 2.
55. Irby DM: Clinical Faculty Development. In CW Ford (ed): Clinical Education for the Allied Health Professions. St. Louis, C. V. Mosby Co., 1978, p. 101.
56. Anderson E, Person P: An Exploratory Study of Faculty Practice: Views of Those Faculty Engaged in Practice Who Teach in an NLN-Accredited Baccalaureate Program, Western Journal of Nursing Research 5:129-140, 1983.
57. Bragg AK: The Socialization Process in Higher Education (ERIC/HE Research Report No. 7). Washington, DC, American Association for Higher Education, 1976, p. 6.

BIBLIOGRAPHY

American Nurses' Association Staff: Facts About Nursing. Kansas City, MO, American Nurses' Association, 1980.

Anderson E, Person P: An Exploratory Study of Faculty Practice: Views of Those Faculty Engaged in Practice Who Teach in an NLN-Accredited Baccalaureate Program. Western Journal of Nursing Research 5:129–140, 1983.

Blake RR, Mouton JS: The Managerial Grid. Houston, TX, Gulf Publishing Co. Book Division, 1964.

Bragg, AK: The Socialization Process in Higher Education (ERIC/HE Research Report No. 7). Washington, DC, American Association for Higher Education, 1976, p. 6.

Brown AF: Clinical Instruction. Philadelphia, W. B. Saunders Co., 1949.

Carpenito LJ, Duespohl TA: A Guide for Effective Clinical Instruction. Rockville, MD, Aspen Systems Corp. 1981.

Coleman JS: Differences Between Experiential and Classroom Learning. In M. Keeton (ed): Experiential Learning: Rationale, Characteristics and Assessment. San Francisco, Jossey-Bass, Inc., Publishers, 1976.

Daggett CJ, Cassie JM, Collins GF: Research in Clinical Teaching. Review of Educational Research 49:151–169, 1979.

Dunn, MA: Development of An Instrument to Measure Nursing Performance. Nursing Research 19:502–510, 1970.

Foley RP, Smilansky J: Teaching Techniques: A Handbook for Health Professionals. New York, McGraw-Hill Book Co., 1980.

Ford CW (ed): The Clinical Education Guide. In CW Ford (ed): Clinical Education for the Allied Health Professions. St. Louis, C. V. Mosby Co., 1978.

Galliher JM: Directory of Nurses with Doctoral Degrees. Kansas City, MO, American Nurses' Association, 1984.

Gordon M: Assessment of Student Affect: A Clinical Approach. In MK Morgan, DM Irby (eds): Evaluating Clinical Competence in the Health Professions. St. Louis, C. V. Mosby Co., 1978.

Gordon T: Leadership Effectiveness Training. New York, Wyden Books, 1977.

Grace, HK: Nursing. In CH McQuire, RP Foley, et al.: Handbook of Health Professions Education. San Francisco, Jossey-Bass, Inc., Publishers, 1983.

Guinee KK: The Aims and Methods of Nursing Education. New York, Macmillan Inc., 1966.

Hersey, P. Blanchard K: Management of Organizational Behavior, ed 3. Englewood Cliffs, NJ, Prentice-Hall, Inc., 1977.

Holcomb DJ, Garner AE: Improving Teaching in Medical Schools. Springfield, IL, Charles C. Thomas, Publishers, 1973.

Houle CO: Continuing Learning in the Health Professions. San Francisco: Jossey-Bass, Inc., Publishers, 1981.

Hyman RT: Improving Discussion Leadership. New York, Teachers College Press, 1980.

Irby DM: Clinical Faculty Development. In CW Ford (ed): Clinical Education for the Allied Health Professions. St. Louis, C. V. Mosby Co., 1978.

Lawrence R, Lawrence S: Clinical Evaluation of Students of Nursing: A Step Toward Quality Nursing Practice." Image, 12(2):46–48, 1980.

Mager RF: Preparing Instructional Objectives, ed 2. Belmont, CA, Fearon-Pittman Publishers, Inc., 1975.

McGuire CH, Foley RP, et al.: Handbook of Health Professions Education. San Francisco: Jossey-Bass, Inc., Publishers, 1983.

McKeachie WJ: Teaching Tips, ed 7. Lexington, MA, D. C. Heath & Co., 1978.

Morgan, B, Luke C, Hebert J: Evaluating Clinical Proficiency. Nursing Outlook 27: 540–544, 1979.

Morgan, MK, Irby DM (eds): Evaluating Clinical Competence in Health Professions. St. Louis, C. V. Mosby Co., 1978.

NLN Data Book 1982. New York, National League for Nursing, 1983.

Quinn FM: The Principles and Practice of Nurse Education. London, Croom Helm, 1980.

Reichsman F, Browning FE, Hinshaw J: Observations of Undergraduate Clinical Teaching in Action. Journal of Medical Education 39:147–153, 1964.

Richards A, Jones A, et al.: Videotapes As an Evaluation Tool. Nursing Outlook 29:35–38, 1981.

Rogers C: Freedom to Learn. Columbus, OH, Charles E. Merrill Publishing Co., 1969.

Schweer JF, Gebbie K: Creative Teaching in Clinical Nursing, ed 2. St. Louis, C. V. Mosby Co., 1976.

Skelly BF, Hooaday SM, et al.: The Effectiveness of Two Preoxygenation Methods to Prevent Endotracheal Suction Induced Hypoxemia. Heart and Lung 9:316–323, 1980.

Stritter FT, Flair MD: Effective Clinical Teaching. Bethesda, MD: National Medical Audiovisual Center, 1980.

Weinholtz D: A Study of Instructional Leadership During Medical Attending Rounds. Unpublished doctoral dissertation. Chapel Hill, NC, University of North Carolina, 1981.

Wolfe DE: Developing Professional Competence in the Applied Behavioral Sciences. In T Byrne, DE Wolfe (eds): Developing Experiential Learning Programs for Professional Education. San Francisco, Jossey-Bass, Inc., Publishers, 1980.

Wood V: Evaluation of Student Nurse Clinical Performance: A Problem That Won't Go Away. International Nursing Review. 19:336–343, 1972.

5

Selecting and Using Teaching Strategies, Resources, and Materials for Client Education

Martha J. Craft

OBJECTIVES

Upon completion of this chapter you will be able to:

1. Identify the role of the nurse in client education.
2. Compare teaching clients to teaching academic students on five dimensions.
3. Identify variables influencing the effectiveness of client learning.
4. Select appropriate, feasible teaching strategies, resources, and materials to improve client welfare.
5. Identify contributions of nursing research to client teaching and relate these to the selection and use of teaching strategies, resources, and materials.

INTRODUCTION

Nurses are responsible for increasingly complex and exciting dimensions of client teaching. Consider the following scene. It is Thursday afternoon in the pediatric clinic. In the waiting room a nurse demonstrates equipment and then encourages children to play with replicas of the equipment that will be used for examinations. In another room children and parents are watching a televised puppet show on cardiac catherization. A nurse elaborates on the topic and answers questions. The consultation room is being used for the weekly oncology parent support group with a nurse as the facilitator and professional resource person. Carrie is about to have a lumbar puncture in the treatment room, where a nurse is using puppetry and a stuffed dog to show four-year-old Carrie what to expect. At the clinic door another nurse is gathering up a group of children for a tour of the pediatric inpatient area, where they are to be admitted the next day. She is teaching these children and their parents what it will be like to stay at the hospital.

Nurses have always been teachers. One of our first nursing leaders taught others how to maintain health and deal with the effects of illness.[1] Nurses today continue to expand this tradition; teaching remains an essential function of the professional nurse, and client education is an integral part of any nursing process. Definitions and dimensions of client teaching and related variables to successful teaching need to be understood for nurses to be effective teachers.

Teaching can be defined as a professional discipline based on a body of theoretical knowledge composed of processes and actions that are planned, implemented, and evaluated with the purpose of guiding the learning of individuals and groups. Teachers impart knowledge and instruct by precept, example, and experience.

Educators (teachers) work to increase learning through use of strategies, resources, and materials by which they help students learn. The terms *teaching* and *education* are sometimes used synonymously. The goal of both teaching and education is learning. The focus of this chapter is on client teaching and the role of the nurse in client education; however, the trend in educational research and practice is to look more critically at the learning dimension of teaching.[2] Teaching and learning must be addressed simultaneously. Learning has many definitions, but it is most easily measured by performance or behavioral changes as a result of experience.

The teaching-learning process is similar to the nursing process in which client welfare is the focus. Learning is directed toward increase of control, use of coping skills, and health-promoting self-care behaviors. Learning goals and objectives focus on changing behavior or the way in which clients can or will behave. In this chapter, nurses who teach students will be called academic teachers and nurses who teach clients will be called client teachers. Client teaching is defined as the purposeful, systematic activities or processes that result in desired changes in clients. Specific changes and processes used to reach goals may differ from those used in academic settings because of the diverse nature and circumstances surrounding the client learner.

COMPARISON OF CLIENT AND STUDENT LEARNING ON FIVE DIMENSIONS

In clinical settings the learner population is diverse. Learning needs and objectives vary widely, depending on individual characteristics and circumstances. Learner characteristics are generally unknown. On the other hand, in academic settings, learner characteristics are usually known. In addition, academic settings require certain prerequisites, and some data about learners' past performance is available. This data can be used to predict future performance and to establish expectations. Client teachers generally assess and develop objectives for individuals or small groups with similar needs, whereas academic teachers spend more time working with large groups of homogeneous learners. The objectives for clients focus on a variety of topics and tasks. For example, the acute-care client will need to be oriented to the hospital and to the roles of health professionals and will need to know the ramifications of the illness, as well as how to use coping strategies. The client will also need to be prepared for diagnostic tests and for discharge. It is important to note that content is often presented when clients are in a state of crisis, when physical and emotional resources are low.

Learner Characteristics Dimension

Assessment of client learner characteristics is difficult because of the wide range of client knowledge and abilities. Clients may be mentally handicapped, speak a foreign language, be young or old, or be too depressed to care. Assessment of knowledge and ability is often inexact. Various resources can be used, however. Some data can be obtained from clients, family members, or other health professionals. Also, previous teaching by nurses should be documented; however, this is not done consistently. Absence of data in patient records can be interpreted two ways. It can mean lack of teaching or lack of documentation. Because of these gaps in data, many nurses assess prior learning by questioning clients and their families; however, such questioning may not be systematic.

Generally, client teachers do not have tools for assessment or are not aware of available tools and how to use or adapt them to specific needs. Methods used to assess academic students tend to be more objective, standardized, and complete than techniques used to assess clients. Until systematic assessment tools are used, client teachers will continue to rely on limited data, sensitivity, intuition, and personal judgement.

In both academic and clinical settings competent teachers individualize objectives, resources, strategies, and materials to match prior learning and other learner characteristics. Student and client learning needs are similar in some respects but differ markedly in others. For instance, client readiness to learn is affected by variables such as health concerns, illness, and reaction to hospitalization.

Dealing with readiness to learn is a challenge to client teachers. Academic teachers assume students have some desire to learn. This may be a false assumption, but students or parents are paying tuition and students walk into classrooms of their own volition. They are considered to be physically and mentally ready to learn. People who come to hospitals, health clinics, and agencies with health problems are in a very different situation, however. Some clients are physically stable, highly motivated, and ready to learn, while others are very ill or completely unmotivated. Great differences in learning readiness are apparent, for altered health poses a threat to well-being or perhaps life, with cognitive, emotional, and physical effects having an impact on learning.

Readiness to learn is modified by emotions. Like motivation, emotional responses to illness will vary a great deal. A few variables affecting response to illness include the nature of illness, perceived threat, length of illness, coping mechanisms, developmental level, and available support systems. Normal adaptation to illness is a continuing process that begins with an inability to acknowledge the presence of illness. Denial is a common reaction, frequently accompanied by anger. Denial, shock, and anger are stages of preadaptation in which clients are not ready to learn.[3] Nurses must detect cues of preadaptive behavior and offer support to clients as they work through their feelings. These cues are not discrete and are difficult to detect in some instances. Further, length of preadaptive behavior is individual and cannot be predicted. Unfortunately, emotional effects on learning are less well understood than physiological effects.

Physiological effects of illness are usually more apparent. For example, neurological impairment or injury to extremities will have an obvious negative effect on psychomotor learning. Fatigue and concentration difficulties that occur from illness, pain, surgery, general anesthesia, and childbirth seem to be easily identifiable.

It is relatively easy to demonstrate that emotional and physiological effects of illness do alter readiness to learn. It follows then, that client status should determine optimum timing for learning; however, client teachers have less control over this aspect of teaching than academic teachers.

The Timing of Learning Experiences Dimension

Clinical realities present barriers to effective teaching. Clinical teaching seems to be conducted according to professional convenience instead of learner readiness. Even the most careful planning cannot overcome constraints of clinical learning situations in many instances. Several problems are common. First, trends toward short hospital stays and ambulatory care mean clients are sometimes taught when still in denial and shock. Furthermore, acute-care clients are frequently discharged by physicians who do not communicate the discharge to nurses ahead of time, leaving nurses to teach people who are not concentrating because they are eager to go home. While academic teachers can predict when learners are available to teach, client teachers must use opportunities when clients are there, without much consideration of readiness to learn. It is difficult to follow sound principles of learning in such situations.

Nurses face difficult problems related to learner characteristics and readiness to learn. In addition, readiness to learn is affected by factors somewhat beyond the control of nurses who teach clients with an extreme diversity in abilities and prior learning, which is usually undocumented. These problems are further complicated by lack of space, privacy, adequate preparation time, and resources.

The Setting and Preparation Time Dimension

Academic teachers usually have space for teaching individuals and large and small groups of learners. Psychomotor skills are usually taught in a well-equipped laboratory. Unfortunately, such facilities may not be available in ambulatory or acute-care settings. Instead, a great deal of teaching is done in the presence of other clients, families, and other health care professionals. Excessive noise and interruptions are common. Utility, treatment, and nursing report rooms are sometimes available for teaching but do not provide needed privacy. Also, needed equipment may not be easily transported to the room. For example, consider a situation where a client must learn use of suction and oxygen equipment. The only private areas in which to teach are treatment and utility rooms, and the one available place with suction and oxygen equipment is the treatment room, which is being used. Therefore, it may be impossible to teach as planned unless an empty client room with suction and oxygen is located. This scenario is not uncommon.

Both academic and client teachers are unable to plan adequately in clinical settings because of a broad range of learning needs and implementation constraints and complications. Possibilities for implementation shift suddenly, with teachers changing plans as existing conditions dictate. Creativity and flexibility are assets to nurses who face such challenges.

The Safety Dimension

Client safety is a major concern of the client teacher, making teaching in the clinical setting exacting. Clinical teaching requires a broad base of knowledge and expertise that can be retrieved and applied readily for sound decision making. Academic teachers in the clinical setting must decide if it is safe to leave some students unsupervised while teaching others. They must judge student capabilities for administering safe care. Similarly, nurses teaching clients must make safety judgments. They must also evaluate client self-care ability. These demands require client teachers who are competent, patient, and comfortable with making rapid decisions based on sound judgment. Teaching must be individualized to meet client safety needs.

The Dimension of Teacher Influence Over Learner Behavior

All nurses face obstacles when teaching in the clinical setting, but there is a difference in amount of influence over learner behavior. Academic students must meet certain grade requirements. Because grades are given, academic teachers' expectations strongly influence student behavior. In contrast, client teachers have little or no control over learner behavior. If clients do not listen or listen politely and then totally disregard what they hear, there is little recourse except to make recommendations regarding prolonged hospitalization or follow-up teaching and community nurse supervision. Client teachers must provide reward and reinforcement conditions.

The difference in influence experienced by academic teachers and client teachers is also related to opportunities for evaluation of learning. Because grades are given to students, evaluation is an integral part of educational planning and implementation. Effective client teaching should also include an evaluation component. In many instances, however, nurses working in acute-care settings lack opportunities to evaluate client learning. One remedy is to ask other nurses to evaluate learning. For example, nurses in clinics and acute-care settings can collaborate with community health nurses to obtain follow-up evaluation. Too often such an evaluation is inadequate or completely lacking, with clients applying learning independently in their homes without guidance. If they are unsuccessful, they return to the clinic or acute-care setting. In many cases this is unnecessary.

Difficulties in evaluation provide hurdles for client teaching not seen in academic settings. There are advantages to client teaching as compared to academic teaching, however. Client teaching situations can foster positive teacher-learner relationships. First, communication styles are often two-way information-sharing episodes. Second, teaching can be done with family members as co-learners and evaluators. Both features can facilitate learning and are rewarding for the client teacher.

Teacher-learner relationships in clinical settings are unique. Some clients will perceive nurses as authority figures, but for other reasons than fear of grade reduction, as may be the case in academic teaching.[4] Use of a more informal, personal, information-sharing communication strategy may lower barriers and facilitate learning when nurses are not perceived as authority figures.

Presence of family members during teaching can be advantageous. Young clients and those who are anxious or ill need another person to hear information. Family members or close friends can verify and clarify information and increase client motivation for learning and compliance.

Some nurses perceive teaching students and teaching clients as very different. Certainly, goals and evaluation methods do differ. Also, learner characteristics and teacher influences are different to some extent. Similarities do exist. Recognition of the differences and similarities will assist nurses to identify, select and use teaching resources, strategies, and materials as they plan learning events to influence achievement of learning outcomes.

SUMMARY

Like academic teachers, client teachers assess and diagnose learning needs, establish expectations, and plan, implement, and evaluate learning experiences designed to help learners obtain learning outcomes. The nature of the setting for client education and differences in client learner characteristics, however, impose demands and constraints that make this kind of teaching especially challenging.

Assessment of client characteristics and readiness to learn is often inexact and, indeed, actually lacking in most cases. It is difficult to plan and implement sound learning experiences because of constraints of time and space imposed by the setting. Often the client teacher has difficulty evaluating learning because of such circumstances as lack of time and influence. Concern for client safety is paramount, requiring sound judgment and decision-making practices on the part of the client teacher, who must be very skilled.

Like academic teaching, client teaching can be rewarding, particularly when effective, two-way communication strategies result in positive achievement of goals and objectives that enhance the well-being of the client.

THE ROLE OF THE NURSE IN CLIENT EDUCATION

Nurses practicing in any setting have a unique opportunity and responsibility to teach. They function in several capacities as primary and secondary educators. Clinical nurses are frequently primary educators. That is, nurses are usually the first health professional to recognize individual or group teaching needs. They independently assess, diagnose, plan, implement, and evaluate an educational program for a particular target population. In addition, nurses have always been secondary educators, because they act to clarify, validate, and reinforce what others teach or communicate. In the past decade another dimension has been added. Nurses have increasingly become responsible for education in multidisciplinary health teams. Several examples can be found in every health care setting. For instance, a health care team that works with people who have renal problems often teaches clients about their illness and how to live with it. A similar situation exists with oncology and cardiology teams and infant apnea programs. Nurses with infant apnea programs spend hours teaching families to use infant apnea monitors, to assess infant respiratory status, and to perform cardiopulmonary resuscitation. The nurse's role in client teaching, then, is to establish realistic objectives that assist clients to maintain or improve their health status, to determine ways to help clients to meet these objectives, to evaluate achievement of the objectives, and to determine future learning needs.

Nurses functioning within a multitude of roles teach a variety of content (information), which seems to fit into several major categories. These categories include medications (actions, administration, and side effects), diet, desired level of activity, skills (such as dressing changes), self-care activities, adapting illness constraints to preferred life-style, coping strategies, prevention measures, available community resources, and symptoms indicating need to seek out a health professional. Also, continued health professional supervision such as visiting nurse care is planned as necessary.

While the beginning nurse-teacher frequently views teaching as "telling" clients what they need to know, experience soon reveals that teaching is much more. For example, a nurse who begins telling parents how to draw up a medication dose in a syringe to administer to their child soon discovers that prior planning of the teaching episode should have included assessment of readiness, setting objectives, task analysis, selection of strategies, resources, and materials, and actual practice of drawing up the medication, as well as evaluation of learning. Teaching, then, is a professional discipline requiring knowledge of learning and teaching theories, principles, and skills, and the ability to apply them.

Variables Influencing Teaching Effectiveness of Client Teachers

Learning is a process involving perception, motivation, sensory and information processing, and memory. Hundreds and perhaps thousands of scientists in psychology and education have spent their entire careers investigating the phenomena of learning, while many professionals like nurses strive to apply their guidelines and recommendations. Client teachers generally target teaching efforts on health maintenance, restoration, and promotion behaviors, but the probability that change will occur is related to numerous variables. Teaching responsibilities like the selection of activities, resources, strategies, and materials should be based on consideration of these variables.

Many of the factors that influence teaching effectiveness fall into four basic categories. These categories are: (1) the critical tasks or the kinds of outcomes used to evaluate the degree of learning, (2) characteristics of the learner, (3) the nature of the content to be learned, and (4) learning activities—the kinds of strategies, resources, and materials teachers use and learners experience when presented with content to facilitate achievement of critical tasks. These basic categories are illustrated in Figure 5-1, which shows a useful organizational framework for exploring the teaching process. It is adapted from a model presented by Bransford and Jenkins.[5]

Determining Critical Tasks and Measuring Learning Outcomes for Effective Teaching. The planning of any teaching event in client education begins with identification of critical tasks—those tasks teachers view as essential for the learner to achieve. Selected testing criteria for critical tasks reflect different assumptions about what teachers mean by learning and are used to evaluate the degree of learning.[6]

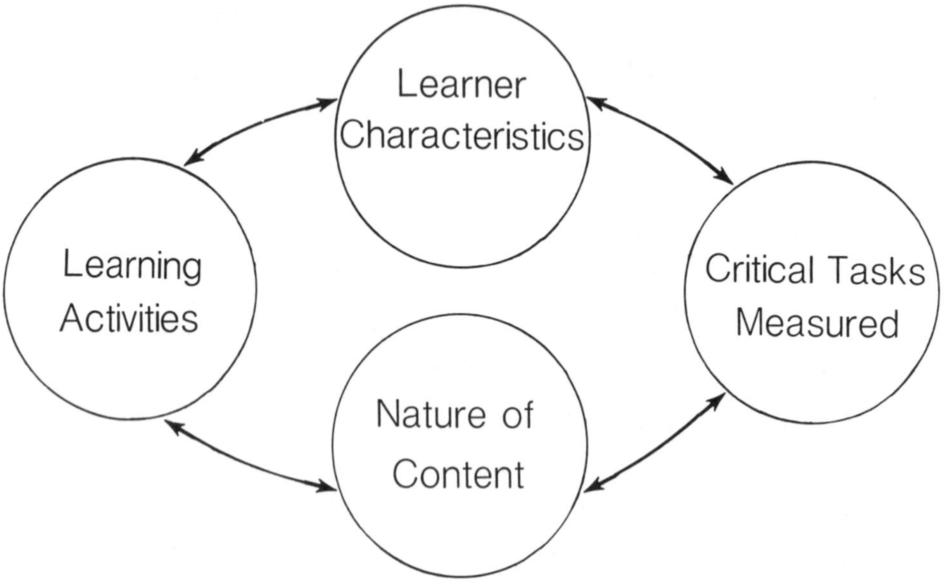

Figure 5-1. Variables related to client learning. (*From Bransford JD: Human Cognition. Belmont, CA, Wadsworth Publishing Co., 1979, p.8.*)

Logically, the critical tasks also guide choices of content and teaching strategies, resources, activities, materials, and means of evaluation.

Assumptions about critical tasks and the nature of learning are defined and communicated by learning objectives. Objectives aid both teachers and learners. Teachers use objectives to formalize realistic expectations and to measure learning. Thus, measurement of learning is facilitated by behavioral objectives narrowed to critical tasks of interest; that is, cognitive critical tasks are written according to a cognitive domain, such as Bloom's taxonomy of educational objectives.[7] Similarly, affective and psychomotor objectives follow appropriate taxonomies. Bloom's taxonomy is used in a pyramid fashion, with the learner mastering level one (knowledge) and two (comprehension) before going on to application (Figure 5–2). This taxonomy can be readily used in any teaching situation. To illustrate, nurses teaching diabetic clients self-care might start by teaching the relationship between diet and blood sugar before expecting clients to plan a menu.

Learning usually involves affective and psychomotor domains as well as the cognitive domain. Like the cognitive domain, both affective and psychomotor domains proceed from the bottom up, requiring learners to exhibit a prerequisite behavior before proceeding upward. Krathwohl's affective taxonomy shows how learners must first be able to receive information through demonstrating an aware-

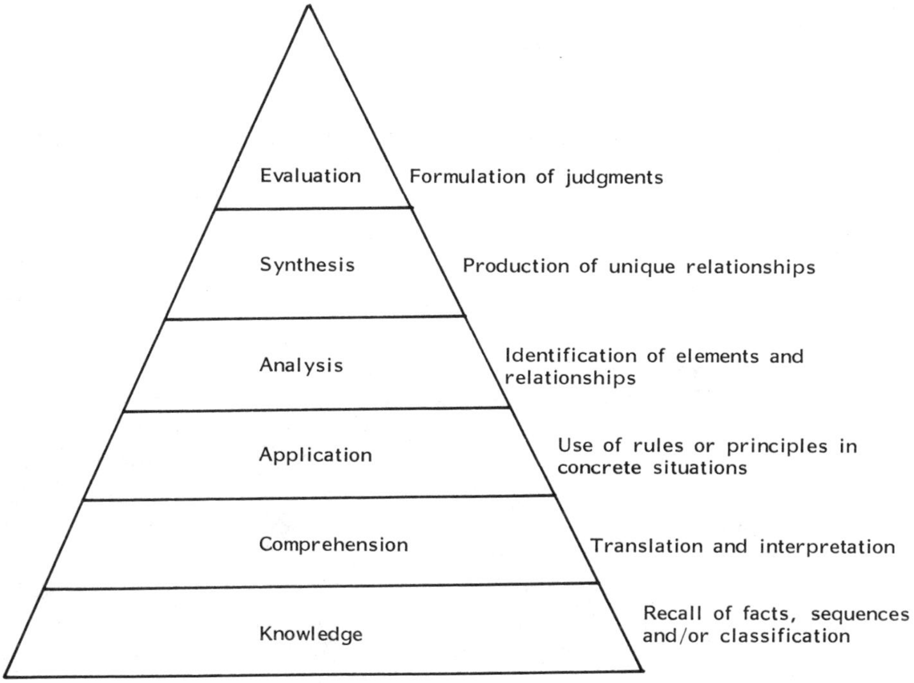

Figure 5–2. Taxonomy of the cognitive domain.

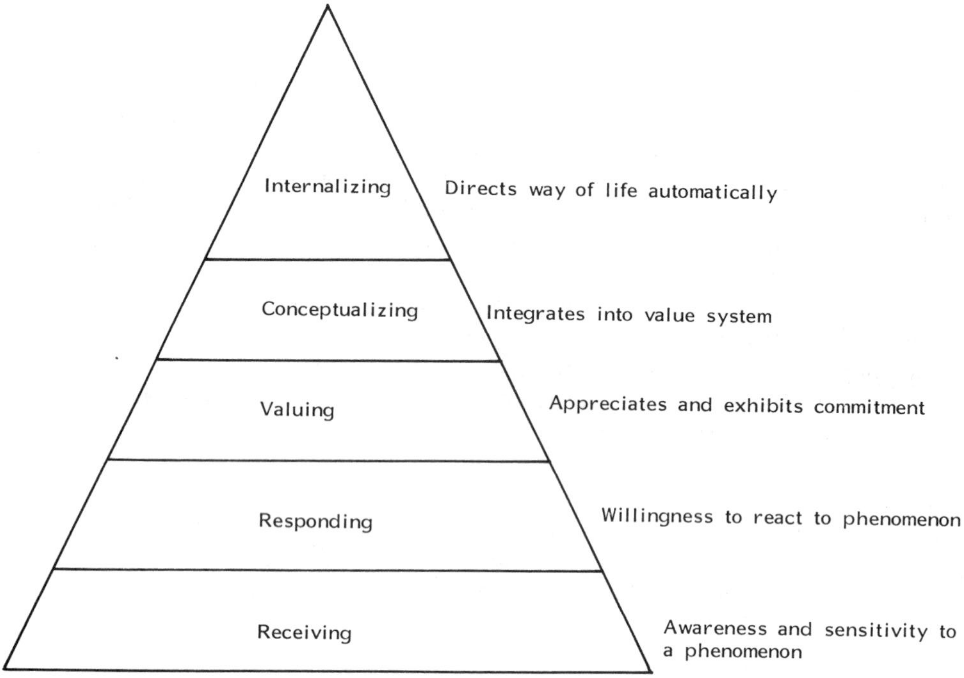

Figure 5-3. Taxonomy of the affective domain.

ness of phenomenon.[8] For example, a client with a new colostomy must be able to look at a stoma site before accepting the importance of colostomy self-care. Initial objectives include statements like "Client looks at stoma." (Figure 5-3).

In a parallel fashion, beginning objectives in psychomotor skills address Simpson's steps one and two.[9] Nurses encouraging clients to turn in bed after surgery could not expect cooperation or guided response until perception and set were evidenced (Figure 5-4). Realistic client expectations or objectives are best established through use of all three domains as appropriate.

Learning objectives convey the behaviors that nurses expect clients to exhibit upon completion of teaching. But taxonomies make it clear that learning is continuous and hierarchical. Objectives also serve as a feedback mechanism for both teacher and learner. Formative or short-term objectives may be the most appropriate for several reasons. First, such objectives enable nurses who teach and clients who learn to evaluate mastery throughout the learning process. Second, use of objective statements with embedded questions to evaluate learning progress can make difficult learning tasks much easier.[10] Learners are assisted through formative statements or short-term objectives because they aid in setting realistic objectives. Realistic objectives are essential from the standpoint of fairness to both learner and teacher. Consider the postcoronary experience. Clients learning to manage a coronary illness

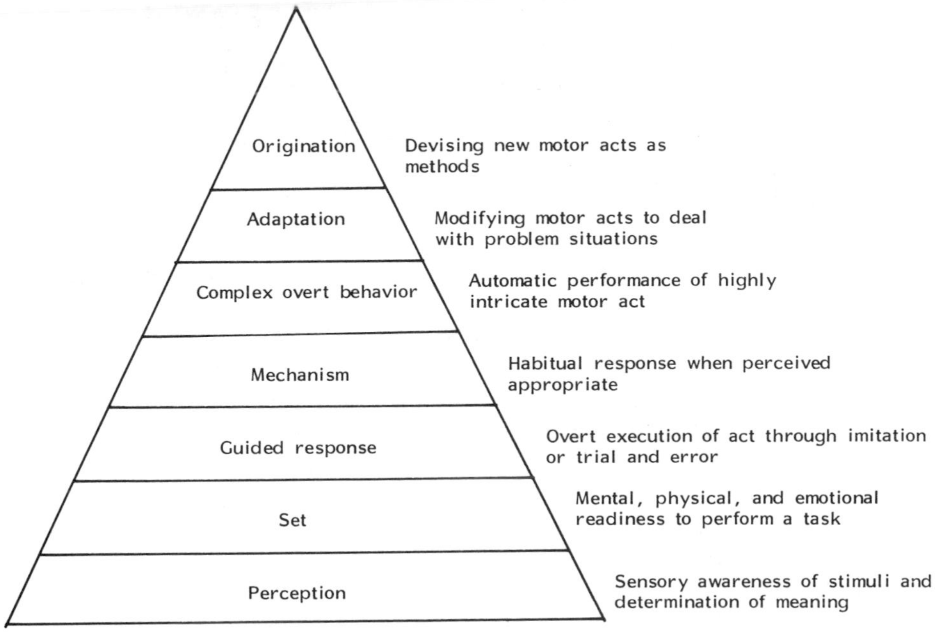

Figure 5-4. Taxonomy of the psychomotor domain.

cannot be expected to reach stage 5 of the affective and cognitive domains during their brief stay in the hospital.

Both clients and their client teachers become frustrated when attempts, although well-meaning, are made to reach unrealistic objectives. Nurses in acute care settings can, however, realistically establish responding (stage 2) objectives of the affective domain and comprehension objectives of Bloom's cognitive domain, leaving higher level objectives to be met after discharge through carefully planned follow-up strategies. Summative objectives can then be used to measure change in client behavior by clinic and community health nurses.

Testing context is a crucial consideration for client teachers, since estimates of learning will vary as a function of the testing context and retrieval environment.[11] Nurses frequently measure learning in the wrong context. Many learning outcomes, such as those relating to compliance, would be more valid if data were collected in homes. Currently, acute-care nurses do not have opportunities to collect this kind of evaluation data but can plan with community-based or ambulatory nurses to evaluate learning in the appropriate setting. To illustrate, acute-care nurses who teach wound-care procedures to clients and families can request evaluation data from community-based nurses.

Measurement of other outcomes is possible in acute-care settings. Such outcomes have been used as dependent variables by nurse researchers investigating the effects of teaching. Only selected examples will be discussed here. Felton and colleagues looked for differences in frequency of postoperative complications, ventilatory function, manifest anxiety level, and patient's perceptions of psychological well-being.[12] Lindeman and her fellow researchers have studied these outcomes as they relate to preoperative teaching methods: (1) postoperative ventilatory function, (2) length of hospital stay, (3) postoperative need for analgesics, (4) length of learning time, (5) preoperative and postoperative level of anxiety, (6) mode of emergence from anesthesia, and (7) number of postoperative physiological problems [13-15]. Other reported measures of teaching effects are postoperative pain, stress-related physiological measures, such as pulse and respiration rate, and blind observer assessment of operation.[16-18]

Outcomes are measured with a variety of instruments. Some instruments are very precise, such as Bartlett's use of performance on an incentive spirometer for measurement of pulmonary functions after teaching.[19] Evaluation of teaching effects is more difficult in practice settings, though, where nurses cannot easily isolate variables through use of experimental and control groups or systematic measurement.

In clinical settings, objectives are helpful to measure learning, even though outcome measurement is imprecise. Clinical situations present a diverse range of learning objectives. Nurses who do preoperative preparation frequently identify objectives that demonstrate decreased postoperative complications. Nurses who prepare couples for labor and delivery often establish objectives to measure reduction of delivery complications. Interpretation of results is difficult. Realistically, objectives in these two situations may not be met because of other intervening variables. Conversely, objectives could be met regardless of teaching. The issue of compliance and knowledge illustrates this dilemma. Even though much effort in client teaching is directed toward increasing health maintenance and health promotion actions, evaluation studies in health education document that knowledge is rarely a sufficient basis for actions.[20]

Teaching is only one variable related to client response, but nurses who teach need to know whether teaching makes a difference. If it does not, the reason needs to be detected. Attainment of objectives should be evaluated through careful analysis of client records and integration of pathophysiological knowledge and teaching-learning principles to determine why the objective was or was not met. The following scenerio is presented for illustrative purposes. Suppose Nurse Jones taught administration of oral phenobarbital and phenytoin to parents of Jason, a profoundly retarded 20-year-old. Suppose a week later Jason was admitted to the hospital in status epilepticus. What happened? Was there a problem with the teaching? Maybe Nurse Jones taught too much content in a hurry, without assessing parental abilities. Perhaps Nurse Jones did not carefully evaluate learning before sending the parents out on their own. These possibilities must be explored, but other explanations are possible. What about the possibility that Jason spit out the medication, or perhaps his serum levels did not rise according to dosage? Jason may have needed more medication than predicted according to body size. Further, what if Nurse Jones did not realize that Jason was cared for part of the day by another person who had not learned about medication administration. Lastly, more serious explanations must be examined. It is possible that Jason had a serious infectious process operating, such as encephalitis, or had a brain lesion. All of these possibilities must be explored. Such careful scrutiny requires adequate time, analytical ability, and honesty, but such critical self-monitoring is required if nurses are to increase teaching effectiveness.

Objectives unrelated to physiological outcomes may be less difficult to appraise, but opportunities to collect data for outcome evaluation must be planned as critical tasks are determined. For example, nurses working with babies who are at high risk for sudden infant death syndrome usually establish at least two critical tasks for parents. First, parents must demonstrate correct use of an apnea monitor that will be used in the home. Second, they must demonstrate correct cardiopulmonary resuscitation techniques. These critical tasks include objectives at various levels of the cognitive, affective, and psychomotor domains and require planned data collection to determine whether the objectives have been attained or not. Table 5-1 illustrates critical task identification, objectives, strategy options, and test items for this situation.

Nurses who teach have a variety of methods available for outcome data collection, but observation and questioning are used most frequently. Nurses may observe parents responding correctly to the apnea monitor in the hospital. These observations are most useful if recorded in anecdotal note form so that patterns or inconsistencies can be identified. While anecdotal notes are suggested for observation, problems of limited sampling and observer bias must be recognized.

Reliability and validity of observational data are increased by use of peer impressions and observational tools, such as checklists. For example, a nurse might ask other nurses for their observations or ask them to purposefully observe parental use of the apnea monitor to see if agreement can be reached. Such peer validation increases the usefulness of observational data. Rating scales are also helpful in formative evaluation because they summarize a series of trials and describe levels of attainment.[21] Such scales are a means of showing progress. In our example, the parents might consistently place monitor leads on their baby incorrectly, proceed to a point when leads are placed incorrectly occasionally, and reach the point where leads are rarely placed incorrectly before taking their baby home.

Psychomotor skill attainment can be difficult to evaluate unless broken down into components. Checklists aid in such evaluation. Each step in the skill is listed to avoid making subjective judgment of performance. For instance, the critical task of parental performance of cardiopulmonary resuscitation can be systematically evaluated through observation and notation on a checklist.

Observational data collection can be expanded through the use of oral and written questioning. Oral questioning is used commonly, but not always effectively. While use of oral questions seems easy, it is difficult to formulate questions that will obtain needed data without giving the answer away. For example, asking if it is important to leave monitor alarms on while the baby is sleeping will elicit the answer "yes." But open-ended questions such as, "Describe how you will prepare your baby for sleep," will better explore knowledge of the importance of keeping alarm buttons on. In a similar fashion, written measurement is a complex process,

TABLE 5-1. OBJECTIVES, TEACHING STRATEGY, AND TEST ITEMS FOR APNEA MONITOR TASK

Critical Task	Objectives	Strategy	Test Items
Parents will demonstrate correct use of the apnea monitor.	Parents will: 1. Visually identify parts of the monitor and explain the function of each part. 2. Apply monitor leads and turn on the monitor. 3. State, in order of priority, the steps to be taken when alarm sounds. 4. Demonstrate actions to be taken when alarm sounds. 5. State when the monitor should be used and when it is safe not to use it.	1. One-on-one discussion with use of pamphlets and other written materials. 2. Viewing and listening to videotape or film showing correct use of apnea monitor in the home. 3. Actual demonstration of monitor use. 4. Actual demonstration of steps to be taken when alarm sounds. 5. Several return demonstrations with immediate feedback and reinforcement. 6. Daily phone calls to the home following client discharge, decreasing in frequency as family becomes more independent. 7. Collaboration with community nurses.	Parents will: 1. Point out each part of the apnea monitor and explain the function of each part. 2. Apply monitor leads and turn on the monitor. 3. Explain the actions to take when the alarm sounds, in order of priority. 4. When the alarm sounds, exhibit correct actions. 5. Tell when to use the monitor and when it is safe to leave the child off the monitor.

and questions asked will probably determine data obtained. Measurement of knowledge and comprehension levels in the cognitive domain is less difficult than higher levels. Valid test item construction requires knowledge and continual practice. Effective client teachers will want to use literature from educational psychology and measurement for assistance in preparing written questions. [22,23]

Data collection techniques and data collected for evaluation flow from critical tasks and objectives. Techniques and setting used for data collection are selected to provide an answer to the question "Were the objectives met?" or "Did clients learn tasks I wanted them to learn?"

Nurses are accountable for client learning, including client preparedness for self-care. Government regulations, patient care standards set by hospital accrediting bodies, and standards of practice for professional nurses make client teaching mandatory.[24] Hospital accrediting bodies, such as the Joint Commission for Accreditation of Hospitals, expect people to be prepared for self-care prior to discharge. Therefore, it is necessary to document teaching with evaluation of its effectiveness. The following is a hypothetical example:

> Parents taught CPR and demonstrated correct performance. See attached checklist #172. Pamphlet on "Care of Babies at Risk for SIDS in the Home," #312, sent home with parents. Parents told nurse would call them daily for two weeks. Nurse page telephone number given to parents, who were encouraged to call with any questions.

It is clear that teaching is a responsibility of nurses for which they are held accountable. This responsibility encompasses five dimensions: (1) identifying critical learning tasks, (2) delineating appropriate objectives, (3) selecting appropriate content, (4) selecting and implementing activities that will facilitate objective attainment, and (5) evaluating success in meeting objectives. Although teaching effectiveness is traditionally controlled by client teachers, it is important that the client's perspective be considered as well.

Client and nurse perspectives of teaching effectiveness do not always agree. Adam and Wright asked nurses and patients to respond to identical comments regarding perceptions of teaching.[25] One comment presented to patients was "I obtained information from others in this group." Nurses were given a similar comment, "I have observed patients giving one another information during group sessions." Nine comments were presented, with a perception percentage difference between nurses and patients ranging from 13 to 43 percent, illustrating that teachers and learners can see things quite differently. Learner perceptions need to be identified and used to increase teaching effectiveness. Perceptions can be obtained through use of formal learning contracts, evaluations, and informal approaches such as asking "What questions do you have?" or "What other information would you like?" and giving them options to choose from. Assessment of client perception demonstrates respect for individuals. Learner differences affect all aspects of teaching and learning, as shown in Figure 5–1.

Considering Learner Characteristics for Effective Teaching. Critical tasks are based on learner needs for health maintenance or restoration, health promotion, and individual differences in clients. Nurses will want to consider these differences when selecting resources, strategies, and materials: (1) learning ability or disability, (2) cognitive development, (3) prior knowledge and skills, (4) readiness for learning, and (5) relevant psychological and sociocultural factors. Like nursing process models, the teaching process includes assessment and diagnosis of clients. Client characteristics will lead to modification of objectives, content, and activities, as teaching is individualized and personalized through determination of an educational diagnosis.[26]

Ability. Variance in ability to learn is the first learner characteristic that becomes obvious to every teacher. Abilities and aptitudes affect level of mastery and rate of learning. At one time it was hoped that all learners could be brought to one level of learning through individualized self-paced learning programs, but research has shown this goal to be idealistic. People with superior ability tend to increase abilities, with "the-rich-get-richer" phenomenon occurring.[27]

People vary in learning ability as in all other human traits. Objectives, content, learning activities, and methods of evaluation and measurement are planned with these differences in mind. For instance, it would *not* be realistic to expect an individual with severe learning disabilities to calculate insulin requirements based on a daily chemstrip bG analysis, nor would it be wise to use a very low-level instructional program when teaching a person of high ability about home hyperalimentation. The first person would probably be overwhelmed and health would be jeopardized, while the second person would be frustrated and bored.

Assessment of learning ability can begin with client records. In fact, when teaching children, nurses frequently determine whether the child is in the appropriate grade according to age. A word of caution is warranted, however. Age and grade level do not always correspond because of a number of factors. For example, some children with severe reading problems are promoted with their class; hence, reading ability cannot be predicted by school grade alone. Similarly, grade completed in school can be helpful in assessment of adult learning ability but may not give an accurate picture. People graduate from high school without attaining expected reading and writing levels, so nurses have to make additional individual assessments. Reading ability should be diagnosed by having clients read passages. Also, the length of the time interval since formal education can influence predictions of future performance. Consider a situation where a client states he was a straight-A student in high school. He may or may not have trouble comprehending information dealing with management of chemotherapy side effects, depending on the amount of time that has elapsed since high school and his use of cognitive abilities since that time. Factors such as the use of technical medical language and jargon can throw the best of us.

All kinds of differences in aptitudes and abilities exist from person to person. Learners lacking verbal skills needed for reading comprehension and writing may be strong in perceptual motor skills and prefer hands-on learning activities. The same people who have trouble comprehending an abstract explanation of how a ventilator works might excel in managing a ventilator for their children at home. Teaching strategies for such individuals will have to include a hands-on approach, with learners seeing how each part affects others so that lungs are expanded. Real challenges to client teachers lie in diagnosing client's strengths and weaknesses so that the strengths can be utilized for effective learning. Until predictive assessment tools are available, nurses will have to assess carefully, try various approaches, get feedback, and modify actions accordingly.

Cognitive Development. Cognitive developmental stages also affect learner abilities. It is easiest to see differences in cognitive development as they exist in children. Young children process information through their senses. They learn through active exploration.[28] A concrete, hands-on experience is the teaching strategy of choice for such children. Toddlers and preschoolers are helped to cope with diagnostic tests and procedures by seeing, touching, and feeling equipment ahead of time. Demonstrations with dolls, puppets, and stuffed animals are also helpful. After demonstration, children should be encouraged to carry out procedures using safe, realistic equipment, maximizing their normal use of fantasy and play as they work out their feelings. During procedures, sensation preparation and stress-point preparation assist children and people of all ages to maintain control.[29,30] Young children learn best through use of auditory, visual, and tactile materials that assist them to attend to the situation, make associations, and process information.

Interestingly, these same methods are suggested to teach non-English-speaking clients when no interpreter is available and also clients who have difficulty learning. For instance, it is possible to teach parents from India how to prepare formula and perform infant-care techniques through demonstration and gestures. Further, clients who are highly anxious may benefit from concrete demonstrations more than abstract discussions.

As young children reach school age and progress through elementary school, their cognitive abilities expand to higher-level verbal or semantic processing. Most can verbalize questions and answers readily. While this development of verbal skill facilitates teaching, children remain more context-dependent for learning than adults because of their lack of real-life experiences.[31] Learning is episode-related, and difficulty with abstraction is common.

In early adolescence, the ability to hypothesize and think abstractly appears, enabling teens to see cause-effect relationships and consequences of action. Presence of verbal skills and abstract cognitive abilities make it possible to teach this age group through relatively abstract written materials and complex examples. Their own awareness of the importance of the information also aids teaching and learning.

Developmental differences are readily apparent in vocabulary usage. Children use words that are hard to distinguish as well as define. Words such as *owie* may refer to a suture line from a thoracotomy or a finger stick for blood specimens. Also, school-aged children and adolescents pick up and use slang. Imagine hearing phrases such as "like totally" and "gross me out the door" for the first time. Similarly, clients at the opposite end of the age span use colloquial terms that may be foreign to young nurses, such as the "woof and warp" of a situation. Vocabulary is ever-changing, making communication challenging, although frustrating at times. Since vocabulary is frequently learned at home, family members are the best interpreters. Keep in mind that the language you use, either directly or indirectly, may seem a foreign language to your clients.

Time Perspective. Orientation to time also differs according to developmental level. Children under seven years of age have a different time perspective, as do many clients at the opposite end of the life-span. They are unable to comprehend surgery "two weeks from now," making lengthy preparation far in advance inadvisable. Clocks and calenders should be used to explain time instead of verbalizing about it. Toy stores and educational materials supply houses have clocks with movable hands that a child can easily manipulate, as well as reusable calendars that can be written on. Also, a clock can be readily constructed using a paper plate, markers, and construction paper. At the beginning of each new year, many businesses give away calendars free of charge.

Attention Span. Another major difference between children and adults is difference in attention span. Normally, children have a shorter attention span than adults. It is not unusual for preschool children to need a change in activity about every ten minutes or less. Concentrated learning for a period as long as one hour cannot be expected until the individual is into adolescence. Even then, learning activities should be divided into 15-to-20-minute segments. The 15-to-20-minute rule holds true for adults as well.

Dependency. Children are physically, emotionally, and legally dependent on adults. Adults must often learn to care for them. Of course dependent clients of all ages require caretakers. Examples of such clients include infants, young children, and paralyzed and comatose persons. In such cases, nurses should address family members or other caretakers as learners. Teaching activities are carried out to assist families and caretakers to meet the client's needs. Of course, for those who view families as systems, a responsibility to teach family members always exists. One member of the system affects all others. Information will promote a sense of control for all family members. This sense of control will decrease anxiety. And, in the long run, clients will benefit from the decrease in anxiety and increase in knowledge of family members. Dependency factors such as these from social psychology have been only partially studied by nurses. More nursing research is needed on family interaction and client anxiety.

Prior Knowledge and Skill. Clients come to learning situations with diverse levels of knowledge and skills. Clients with a new illness may have little prior knowledge about their situation. On the other hand, those who have lived with a chronic illness for years often possess a great deal of knowledge about it. In the former case, it is easy to present inadequate information when teaching and in the latter case, too much content can be presented. Consequently, clients may either not recieve enough information to manage their health problem, or they may be insulted with redundancies. Confusion is a possibility, too, for health professionals commonly teach conflicting content.

It is important for client teachers to assess existing knowledge and skills of clients during the planning stage of teaching. Since nurses have little data on past learning, they must resort to on-the-spot assessment. Pretesting is one way to assess present knowledge and skill. There are many ways to pretest. For instance, nurses teaching diabetic clients might develop a written pretest for administration to all persons with a new diagnosis of diabetes. During interviews nurses can ask clients or family members open-ended questions. Questions such as "What do you know about ______?" encourage clients to share existing knowledge. Skill level can be assessed by having clients perform necessary skills if equipment or replicas are available for teaching purposes. If equipment, models, or mock-ups are not available, a verbal description of procedure can be elicited by asking something like "Would you please tell me how you did ______ at home?" Of course, verbalizing does not necessarily mean the skill can be done, is done, or is done accurately. A sense of confidence can be promoted by asking "How do you feel about doing this procedure?" Oral questioning during interviews or conferences is a method all client teachers can use, although it may be less precise than a structured written test or actual demonstration as a pretest. Assessment is difficult, and a margin of error exists regardless of the method used.

Validation of assessment is possible through use of established objectives. Consider the following scenario: A 4-year-old child is admitted to an acute-care setting with a two-year history of cystic firbrosis and hypoxia problems. Parents have been caring for the child at home and say they perform chest percussion four times a day and will continue to do so during their child's hospitalization. Nurses determine that a critical task to be met before client discharge is parental performance of chestphysiotherapy (CPT) or chest percussion. Consequently, prior to client discharge the parents are each asked to demonstrate correct performance of CPT. Both parents omit half of the steps in the skill. Their lack of skill went undetected up to the evaluation stage of teaching. Development of systematic assessment procedures is recommended. For example, the same checklist used for evaluation can be used as a pretest during the assessment stage. This case illustrates how evaluation is used to validate assessment. It is, however, an expensive way to deal with insufficient assessment data.

One skill that must be assessed carefully for all clients who will be expected to read information is the ability to read and comprehend. Reading comprehension is necessary when nurse-teachers choose to use print materials such as books, worksheets, pamphlets, and so on as teaching strategies. Literacy cannot be assumed. In 1957, the United States ranked 14th in the world literacy level, but today our country ranks 49th. At least 23 million Americans lack skills required to write checks, complete a job application, or take a written driver's license examination. At least another 40 million people function at or below a level of marginal literacy.[32] Many people go to great lengths to conceal lack of reading ability.

Assessment of reading skills is possible through use of formulas, such as the Cloze method, which removes every fifth word and asks the reader for completion.[33] Another formula, called the Fry formula, provides a chart for computation of the grade level of print materials.[34] To calculate the reading level of an item, three 100-word passages are randomly selected. The average number of syllables and words per sentence are plotted on a graph to determine readability level (Fig. 5-5). Grade level of the material can be determined and compared to the grade level attained by clients. Grade level attainment is only a gross estimate of reading ability, however, and further assessment is indicated. For instance, a sixty-year-old female who left school at the eighth grade and seldom reads would probably have different

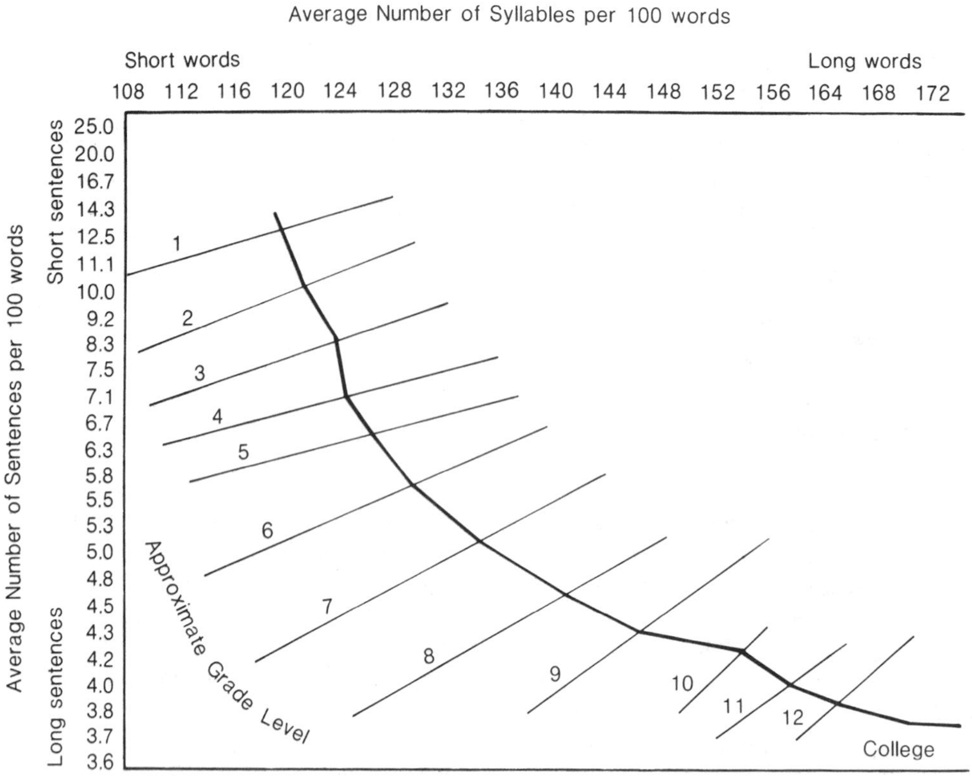

Figure 5-5. Estimating readability. *(From Fry EE: A Readability Formula That Saves Time. Journal of Reading 11:513-516, 575-577, 1968.)*

reading skills from those she'd have if she read four books a week. Grade levels are only one criterion and must be used in conjunction with other client data.

Client teachers should consider using readability formulas when developing or purchasing written materials. The Minnesota Educational Computing Consortium (MECC) has produced a program for the Apple computer called "MECC School Utilities, Volume 2," which allows one to enter any text passage and calculate the readability level in seconds. The program will analyze passages using any or all of the Spache, Fry, Dale-Chall, Raygor, Flesch, and Gunning-Fog readability formulas.

Precise data on reading ability can also be obtained simply by asking clients to read from the material you will expect them to read. In addition, clients who are uncomfortable when reading benefit when nurses help them read. A client teacher might say "You read one line and I'll read the next line," or "You read the first paragraph and I'll read the second" in a relaxed, accepting manner. One method of assessing comprehension is to use open-ended questions such as, "What does that passage mean to you?" or "What did you learn from reading that paragraph?" These methods provide accurate, rapid data.

When clients exhibit difficulties with written materials, other teaching strategies must be used. Less difficult written materials may be available. If not, client teachers must switch to more concrete sensory strategies. For example, a client who cannot read and comprehend an explanation of how urine goes from the kidneys to the bladder might benefit from a simple drawing or model and oral explanation or short film or video program that can be both seen and heard. Methods used to teach must be adapted to learner abilities and characteristics to be effective.

In ideal teaching situations, prior knowledge and skills will articulate with new information so that growth occurs in a systematic fashion. Such a situation happens rarely in client teaching for several reasons. Assessment is complex and difficult. More importantly, client cognitive and emotional regression results from the illness crisis. A client's readiness to learn is affected by physiological and emotional variables that impact on teaching and learning.

Readiness to Learn. Readiness to learn is a multidimensional concept referring to learning receptivity. Receptivity is crucial for optimum learning, and teaching efforts will have fullest impact when clients are ready to learn when teaching occurs.

The term readiness has been defined in various ways. Pohl writes that readiness is a person's physical and mental ability to learn viewed in terms of neuromuscular development.[35] Redman includes two facets in her definition of readiness: motivation and experience.[36] Motivation is expressed as a perceived lack of needed knowledge for self-protection or enhancement and desire to avoid future threat. Still another component of the concept of readiness must be addressed by all client teachers. That component is physiological readiness.

Physiological variables will significantly affect readiness to learn. Clients who are acutely ill should become stabilized before any teaching plans are implemented. The fact remains, however, that prolonged physiological effects of illness will remain during periods in which nurses do a great deal of teaching. Surgical clients offer a primary example of this dilemma. Effects of general anesthesia last for approximately six weeks. Throughout this period, clients have a lower attention span, have trouble concentrating, and cannot always engage in prolonged activity. They are easily distracted, as are clients experiencing pain. Both general anesthesia and pain are experienced by many clients who need to learn something. Further, generalized fatigue follows general anesthesia and accompanies most illnesses. Fatigue decreases the desire and energy to learn. Other common types of pathology also interfere with learning. These include hearing and vision deficits, which inhibit information processing unless appropriate modalities are used. Various physical problems like paralysis, arthritis, or amputation will alter skill attainment. Lastly, grief responses that accompany many aspects of illness and health, such as body-image changes and poor prognosis have both physical and emotional ramifications for learning.

Altered body image is common during illness. Changes range from weight loss to loss of a body part. These changes are thought to produce a grief response that affects client reaction to illness.[37] Similarly, clients with deteriorating physiological status and threat to life respond with a grieving process. Manifestations of grieving processes are shock, numbness, denial, anger, weeping, despair, feelings of unreality, guilt, and helplessness. Acute stages of grief are thought to last one to two months, but total duration is much longer.[38] Obviously, these clients are not in a state of readiness for learning, but nurses too often must teach in spite of these conditions. Consider situations in which women have mastectomies and are told they have metastatic cancer. Nurses must and do teach several topics during the postoperative period to these women.

The exact effects of client physiological status on learning outcomes are largely unknown. Physiological effects on learning are reported in the psychology literature to some extent, but most research has been conducted in the laboratory under carefully controlled conditions. Nursing research in naturalistic client-care settings is needed to answer critical questions like the effects of pain on learning. Just think of women who are taught infant care while sitting on painful stitches as one example. It would be fascinating to compare learning outcomes of a group of women who had no stitches with those who had painful stitches and see if this condition makes a difference in learning. Nurses need to know to what extent physiological variables modify learning to use their time and energies efficiently as well as to maximize client benefits from teaching efforts.

Readiness to learn is continuously modified by interacting physiological and emotional variables. Emotional variables stem from several theoretical frameworks, such as: (1) health-illness models, (2) nature of illness, (3) sick role behavior, and (4) learned helplessness. Furthermore, individual differences in locus of control, values and beliefs, and other relevant psychological and sociocultural factors will affect client readiness to learn.

Health-illness models address client perception of health or illness. The premise is that perception affects reaction to illness. Is health perceived as a state of balance with illness a state of imbalance? Is illness perceived as a punishment? To what force or circumstances do clients attribute illness? These questions demonstrate a relationship between health-illness models, attribution theory, and motivation to learn. Wu presents five health-illness models with their relationship to potential client response.[39] First, the primitive model places illness as an attacking force, with client response being passive acceptance of whatever fate has to offer. The equilibrium model, however, presents illness as a disruption of normal homeostatic mechanisms. Interventions are directed toward turning disequilibrium back to a state of equilibrium through support of homeostatic mechanisms. The third model, called the ecological model, addresses agent-host reactions, with response focused on strengthening of host conditions. Illness is a result of causative agents in the medical model. Once causative agents can be identified and managed, illness will disappear. Client response is predicted to be one of cooperation in identification of causative agents and treatment regimens. Lastly, a sociological model outlines illness as an interference with obligations or social roles. Client responsibilities include getting well and staying healthy in order to function according to social norms.

Each of these models can affect motivation to learn. Use of health-illness models and attribution theory in predicting client response to illness offer exciting research opportunities. In addition, it is useful to use health-illness models to determine client motivation incentives. For example, comparing clients with primitive health-illness models and passive responses to clients with medical or equilibrium models reveals extreme differences. In addition, nurses will want to be aware of their own model to recognize communication barriers between themselves and clients. For instance, nurses operating under a medical-model framework may not communicate well with clients operating under the primitive model of health-illness.

Client readiness is affected by health-illness models because causality is associated with a sense of control. Other models related to readiness are nature of and adaptation to illness. Nature of illness refers to meaningfulness. Clients' perception of the nature of illness can be elucidated by questions such as the following ones. First, do clients see illness as a threat to life? Are illnesses such as mental disorders regarded as a stigma, or do many friends have a similar problem? How noticeable is the problem? Can it be mostly ignored or is it impossible to forget, such as constant pain? To what extent does the illness interfere with current life-style? Is it possible to continue life as usual, because the illness is not interfering with walking, talking, or mental functioning? In addition, what is the operating cost/benefit ratio? Is a lengthy wait in a physician's office, X-rays, and a fifty-dollar fee likely to alleviate the problem? Or, are outcomes of an X-ray exam likely to generate discomfort, embarrassment, and danger of radiation exposure? Such perceptions are one aspect of individual differences, like knowledge base, support systems, and health-illness models, all of which should be considered before implementing teaching strategies.

Nature of illness, health-illness models, and adaptation models attempt to predict client adaptation to illness. The adaptation model addresses individual response to illness. It outlines a sequence of emotions that occur in a rather unsystematic fashion but serve to guide client teachers as they look at timing of teaching-learning situations.[40] Timing of teaching is a crucial factor for learning. Clients who have just been told they will be paralyzed are certainly not ready to learn self-catherization, but these same people may be ready to learn in two months. What happens in these two months? Not only is physiological status stabilized, but the clients have gone through preadaptation and, it is hoped, have reached a stage of adaptation to circumstances. Preadaptation emotions include shock, denial, anger, realization, defensive retreat, and acknowledgment. The last step, adaptation, follows the painful step of acknowledgment. Adaptation includes a willingness to accept reality, to part with the old self but appreciate worth of the new self, and to try out new roles. During the adaptation stage is the ideal time to learn. Behavior indicating adaptation is a helpful determinant for timing of actual teaching, but characteristics of adaptation can be altered by sick role behavior and learned helplessness.

Normal sick role behavior includes four responses: (1) attention is drawn to body functions, (2) withdrawal from usual role responsibilities, (3) regression, and (4) compliance and dependency. Variables related to sick role behavior are: (1) type of illness, (2) societal expectations, (3) role of significant others, and (4) health care system culture.[41] In other words, our society accepts withdrawal, regression, and dependency during illness. Illness may lead to a sense of helplessness, as shocking, painful, and inescapable events occur independent of client response. This phenomenon is described in Seligman's theory of learned helplessness.[42] The theory is presented in three stages. In the first stage, clients learn probabilities of their ability to control situational outcomes. Second, expectations are formed that situational outcomes occur independently of client response. The third stage describes behavior changes. Motivation is diminished and emotions are characterized by high anxiety, fear, and passivity. Anxiety and fear can be reduced if control is encouraged. If clients do not perceive a sense of control, they are likely to enter a state of helplessness, futility, passivity, and depression. Expectations that outcomes are independent of responses reduces motivation to control outcomes. Such expectations interfere with learning that responding controls outcomes. Thus, motivation to learn and accept self-care decreases. This complex process is further complicated by individual differences in locus of control, values and beliefs, and sociocultural factors.

Locus of control is a social learning theory that addresses a personality variable related to client motivation.[43,44] Internal locus of control is characterized by an individual's actions to affect the environment, such as seeking and using information. Clients who have an internal locus of control believe they can control or alter circumstances. Experts often say these people are intrinsically motivated. On the other hand, clients who have an external locus of control perceive little or no control over their environment. They are controlled externally, or simply react to circumstances. While little is known about the origin of this personality variable or how to modify it once it exists, realities of illness and health care systems produce some interesting paradoxical situations for this aspect of personality.[45] Thus, clients with internal locus of control may be unable to modify circumstances or their environment. Realistically, they find themselves in situations beyond their control. Control might have to be relinquished. Effects of this relinquishment are unknown, but frustration would be an expected outcome. Clients with external locus of control, however, are likely to comply with authority. Their compliance could be more adaptive than that of an intrinsically motivated person with internal locus of control. In summary, a personality variable that is adaptive in some situations, such as in academic or certain other occupations, can be handicapping in health care environments. Perhaps a balanced internal-external orientation is the ideal therapeutic goal.[46]

Measurement of locus of control is not difficult because of available standardized tools for this purpose. Generalized expectancies of internal-external control (I-E Scales) have been measured and validated. Rotter, or locus of control, scales have also been developed for children. Scales are being used to study various aspects of client behavior and offer promise in determining what motivates people.

Client teachers often try to change well-established practices that have proven detrimental to health. The probability of changing client behavior is likely to depend on beliefs and values in addition to knowledge. Clients need to believe they can have an impact on their health status before becoming active participants in change. Furthermore, they must value health or an improvement in health status. It is possible for people to be knowledgeable, aware of their contribution to health, and demonstrate internal locus of control, but still to avoid changing life-style patterns. They might not value health or have competing values and needs with greater priority. For some clients the need to avoid alcohol, cigarettes, fatty foods, and excessive calories conflicts with perceived rights to social acceptance, pleasure, gratification, and tension reduction.[47] Classic examples are teens who begin smoking for peer approval, even though the dangers of smoking are well known. Asking clients to change habits and patterns of behavior challenges deeply held values that permeate lives. Abilities, integrity, and autonomy are threatened by proposed behavior changes. Clients need help in substituting one value for another.[48] A new value must be equally as rewarding as the one replaced if behavior is to be changed.[49]

The beliefs and values of clients are affected by complex sociocultural variables, such as religion, cultural heritage, and socioeconomic status. All of these factors influence readiness to learn and, hence, teaching practices. Religious beliefs affect health practices. Direct effects are seen in clients who practice health habits recommended by their religion. For example, people of the Mormon faith are taught to avoid alcohol, tobacco, and coffee. Jehovah's Witnesses refuse blood transfusions. When the human body is regarded as a "temple of God," healthful self-care habits and practices predominate. In contrast, religious beliefs can lead to carelessness in health care practices, because some beliefs place God in total control. Such beliefs place responsibility for health in God rather than individuals.[50]

Cultural heritage affects health practices in America, although the impact is sometimes difficult to detect in such a pluralistic society. Therefore, nurses need to know the health beliefs, values, and practices operating in their setting. Cultural health practices can be persistent and ongoing within a health care environment. For instance, Tripp-Reimer reports that an immigrant Greek population has retained ethnomedical beliefs and practices related to the configuration surrounding the evil eye over a four-generation period.[51] Such cultural beliefs may be limited to one culture or may spread to other groups. Identifying the cultural heritage is a part of the assessment component of the teaching process. Learner characteristics such as this should be assessed to determine critical tasks and appropriate teaching interventions. The effects of religious and cultural beliefs on client learning have been studied less then the effects of socioeconomic status on client learning.

Socioeconomic status seems to be a major variable in determining health behavior. It relates to other variables such as sex, age, educational level, and family structure, all of which affect health beliefs and practices and readiness for learning critical health tasks. The lower socioeconomic group has been studied more than others, perhaps because the views of this group about health deviate most from those of the health professionals who care for them. The lower stratum of society is characterized by indifference to symptoms until poor health interferes with lifestyle and independence.[52] The individual's view of life includes a sense of powerlessness, meaninglessness, and isolation.[53] Isolation includes isolation from middle-class knowledge of health and need for preventive measures, such as administration of vaccines to children.[54]

Does the high cost of health care affect the health practices of individuals in lower socioeconomic groups? Today, people at all socioeconomic levels are examining health care costs and benefits, because physician, hospital, and other related costs continue to increase. During the economic recession of 1982–1983, anecdotal comments of health professionals indicated a decrease in preventive health care. People who were seen were more frequently acutely ill. Low-income families continue to be most severely affected by reduction in federal assistance from Medicaid and Medicare.[55] Few families, however, can afford the devastating costs of illness and must rely on health insurance. People who are without a job lose this insurance. These dilemmas, along with the spiraling costs associated with illness, have increased public interest in illness prevention and health maintenance. These themes are familiar to all nurses, and current economic trends are providing opportunities for nurses to direct teaching efforts toward maintaining and promoting the health and fitness of clients.

Nature of Educational Content and Teaching Effectiveness. Like critical tasks and learner characteristics, the content, or subject matter, to be learned by clients is also diverse. Some content areas can, however, be generalized to most clients and are becoming a part of consumer expectations for health-illness education. These areas include health maintenance and health restoration. Specific topics like orientation, preparation for diagnostic tests and procedures, coping with anxiety and stress, and self-care practices evolve from these broad areas of content.

Health Maintenance. Health maintenance, or assisting people to stay well, is as old as the nursing profession itself. Currently, nurses provide clients with accurate information about habits and life-styles that are conducive to maximum function of body and mind. Health maintenance measures throughout life are also addressed. Client teachers teach topics such as family planning, prenatal care, preparation for birth, parenting, and health needs of infants and children to assist families to bear and rear healthy children. Children are taught responsibility for their own health in classes provided by nurses in preschools, day care centers, and public schools. Topics include dental care, need for proper diet and exercise, and dangers of drug abuse, including alcohol abuse, all of which promote healthful life-styles. Content provided on anatomy and physiology increases grade school children's knowledge of body complexity and the need to take care of their bodies. Information to assist children to cope with life stressors has been added to the curriculum by some school nurses. Examples of these stressors include school exams, peer rejection, divorce, and death. Of course, many adults face similar stressors. Stress interventions are just as appropriate for health maintenance teaching as is exercise, dangers of smoking, and early detection of cancer.

Finally, increased life-span has a multitude of implications for client teachers. Nurses play an important role in sharing knowledge with geriatric clients that will enhance their quality and quantity of life. Topics like the importance of exercise, a well-balanced diet, and socialization are just as appropriate for people of 70 years of age as they are for people of other ages.

Health Restoration. While content on health maintenance is taught with increasing frequency in a variety of health care settings, information in the area of health restoration still consumes the largest share of the client teacher's time. One of the initial topics addressed under this heading is orientation. Orientation may involve helping the client to become familiar with a hospital unit, the physician's office, a particular clinic, or what to expect from a visiting nurse. Clients need to be oriented to the basic physical setup of any setting in which they use health services. They have a right to know the names of the health professionals who will be providing care, their roles and functions. All health professional's expectations or "rules" for clients should be explicit and clearly communicated. It is important for people in any setting to know to whom they can go with questions or needs and what procedure to follow.

Since anxiety is high prior to all new experiences like undergoing diagnostic tests and procedures used to manage illness, clients should be taught strategies to decrease anxiety and use of coping skills. Sensation preparation is one method used to reduce anxiety and lessen the discrepancy between what clients expect and what actually occurs. Informing people of the sensations they will experience ahead of time has been shown to alleviate anxiety.[56] Preparation immediately prior to a stressful event, called stress-point preparation, has also been helpful.[57] For instance, the client teacher might say, "Now you will feel a sharp stick. Squeeze my hand hard." Notice that the nurse was honest but also taught a coping strategy to deal with the stress. Distraction and relaxation techniques are also effective in reducing stress. Furthermore, peer groups can be used for education and support. Strategies to cope with anxiety, pain, and even upcoming death are taught as fairly new dimensions of health content. Sensation and stress-point preparation are well supported by research. A data base is being developed for relaxation and imagery; however, many basic nursing relaxation measures, such as back rubs, need to be investigated through controlled research to document effectiveness for reducing anxiety and relieving stress.

Two major assumptions are inherent in such approaches. One assumption is that honesty conveys trust. Nurses expect or trust that clients will cope effectively with the ramifications of their illness. This expectancy is likely to increase the probability that clients can cope.[58,59] The second assumption is that knowledge increases the client's sense of control. Increasing client knowledge not only reduces anxiety but promotes a sense of situation mastery. An increase in client knowledge about health status and management, then, is likely to promote a sense of control and responsibility. It is hoped this sense of responsibility will enhance the probability that the client will return to good health.

Acute care nurses, either directly or indirectly, do teach clients what can be done to improve or remain in optimum health and how to help themselves get well. For example, prior to surgery, people are taught through direct or contrived strategies how to cough and deep-breathe or get out of bed while protecting their incision. After surgery, these same people may be informally encouraged to "drink a lot of fluids because body temperature is up" or "be sure to tell us when you're starting to have pain." Furthermore, nurses who administer new medications teach clients and family members the side effects that may occur from the medication, as well as other factors relating to the drug therapy. If medications or procedures are to be followed at home, appropriate teaching interventions can prepare the client for discharge. People who come to a hospital ill are not ready to go home until they and their family members are knowledgeable about and comfortable with required home care. Client teachers are responsible for choosing appropriate content, tasks, and direct or contrived strategies to restore, maintain, or increase health status and prevent future illness.

Selecting Learning Activities for Effective Teaching. Learning activities are designed to assist clients to achieve critical tasks or learning outcomes. They are the strategies, resources, and materials planned, selected, and used by the client teacher that are appropriate for client characteristics and content delivery and that provide the necessary conditions for learning. In addition, effective learning activities are based on sound learning principles and feasibility for use.

Learning Principles. One major learning principle already mentioned is that learning activities evolve from a client outcome, objective, or critical task to be accomplished. Second, progression from simple activities and content to more complex is recommended. Present thinking along this line emphasizes the importance of marshalling available client knowledge and skills so that learners make content more meaningful.[60] This is the theory of associationism. It is dependent upon the cognitive level of the client and what is to be learned. Building upon prior learning also prevents interference of old learning with new (forgetting). A third principle relates to context. Learning is context-dependent, and promotion of transfer needs to be built into activities. To illustrate, consider a client, Mrs. Jay, who has experienced a stroke and is learning how to bathe, carry out oral care, and shampoo her hair. She can do these tasks well while in the hospital, but what will happen when she goes home? Learning activities in the hospital need to replicate or closely simulate the equipment and routines Mrs. Jay will use at home.

Last, the use of feedback and reinforcement to promote change in behavior is essential. Behavioirists use the term reinforcement when referring to reward, but others view it as a type of feedback that provides a sense of direction. In this context, careful instructional planning can insure that every opportunity is used to provide feedback. For instance, envision planning a group presentation on postcoronary self-care. We can begin the presentation by preparing participants for *what* is to be presented and *why* it is important. Theoretically, such introductory statements establish a mind-set and present an organizing framework (advance organizer) that assists learners to link new information with existing knowledge. Establishing set also lets learners know what to expect as learning activities.[61] In addition, we can insert summary statements throughout the presentation to provide feedback. These statements allow learners to determine whether what they heard was what was intended. A final closure or summary statement at the end of the presentation would serve a similar purpose. Planned activities, such as follow-up questions and group or independent activities would further insure application and transfer of learning.

Feedback and reinforcement should be included as a condition for learning in all teaching events, whether direct, indirect, group, or one-on-one. It is important to let learners know what they are expected to know or do and then to provide ongoing feedback on how well they are meeting the expectations. Assisting clients to monitor their own learning is also an important teaching strategy toward this end.

Feasibility. Feasibility for the use of learning activities involves several issues. The issue of cost is paramount, for all costs incurred in client teaching are indirectly borne by health consumers. Cost-effective strategies, resources, and materials should be based on the circumstances of the situation and a thorough analysis of all variables. Several considerations warrant special mention. First, nurses are becoming increasingly aware of costs to clients. Cost of materials used in teaching clients can be very high, running close to $50,000 per year in large departments.[62] Second, nurses usually avoid purchasing expensive audiovisual equipment because of its cost, but they fail to recognize the dollar value of their own time, knowledge and skill.[63] Direct teaching takes time, and time is money. All efforts that maximize teacher time are cost-effective. When nurses find themselves explaining the same or similar content over and over, it's time to explore other means of content delivery. Options include use of audiovisual programs, written materials, and other technologies.

Last, materials should be durable and easy to adapt. For example, written materials can be prepared using a word processor or a microcomputer so that revision can be done quickly. Methods should be used to preserve materials so that they can be used repeatedly by a number of clients. Again, this approach saves time and materials, and time and materials are costly.

On the other hand, use of audiovisual teaching strategies involves use of equipment. Therefore, funding staff training sessions, hiring specialized personnel, providing for storage, and maintaining equipment are special cost considerations. Staff who use expensive equipment need to be knowledgeable about operation or have access to experts when needed. In addition, equipment has to be available for client teaching when needed but yet have secure storage. These needs can be a problem. Suppose, for example, an evening nurse wants to use a video program on cardiac catheterization, but the video player is stored some distance away from the unit where it is needed, say three floors away. Our nurse would have to leave the unit twice, once to pick up the equipment and a second time to return it to storage. This would be impossible if there were several acutely ill people to supervise at the same time. Planning for use of audiovisual strategies requires long-range planning, including allocation of storage space for required equipment to make it easily accessible. Lastly, sophisticated equipment, such as computer, video, closed-circuit television, or teleconferencing systems should be purchased only if programing and servicing is available. When equipment is unavailable for extended periods of time because of lack of programs, maintenance, or repair, it is not practical or cost-effective.

Advantages and Limitations of Learning Activity Options. There are a multitude of direct and contrived strategies, resources, and materials that can be used for client learning experiences. Currently there is less research data available than needed to guide the selection process. Therefore, it is valuable for client teachers to know the advantages and limitations of options to make intelligent decisions.

Perhaps the most familiar and widely used strategy by client teachers is the one-on-one interview and teaching episode (Fig. 5–6). The primary advantage of the one-on-one teaching strategy is its unique opportunity for personalized and individualized teaching. It is ideal for shy or anxious clients who might not ask ques-

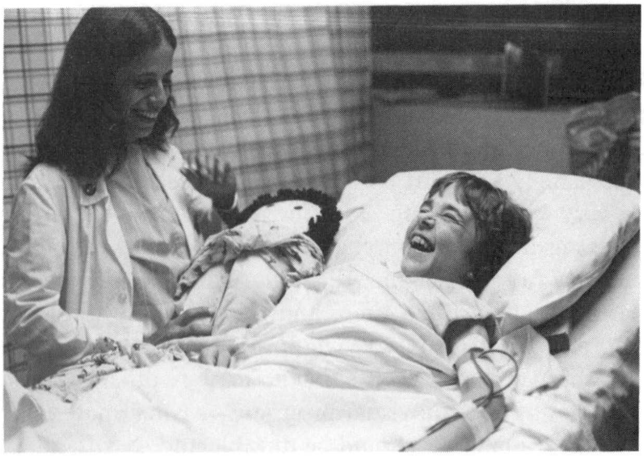

Figure 5-6. A one-on-one teaching strategy.

tions in groups, or for clients with unique health problems. A one-on-one exchange is sometimes threatening or uncomfortable for some clients, however. Furthermore, this approach is very time-consuming and therefore costly.

Group teaching is becoming more popular when content applies to many clients. Advantages of group teaching include client socialization and mutual support as well as delivery of content to a number of clients at the same time. Recorded demonstrations and films are appropriate for group teaching, as are learning centers designed for specific topics. Group teaching is also more cost-effective than one-on-one teaching. On the other hand, this approach may not be appropriate for complex, emotion-laden content in which client reaction needs to be assessed individually, nor is it appropriate for unusual topics that do not apply to more than one or two clients. Other disadvantages are space requirements and equipment needs. For example, it is possible to show one client a picture, graph, or chart in a book, but a transparency and an overhead projector, chalkboard, or other device is needed to convey the same information to large groups of clients.

Role modeling can be an excellent learning activity. For example, clients can attend to nurse's attitudes through observation of verbal and nonverbal nurse behaviors. As one father commented, "We just could not give up! We knew our boy would make it, because those nurses never gave up. They just kept working away to make him live. They gave us hope." Certainly, it is possible to alter attitudes through role modeling, and role modeling is operating every time clients see nurses. Nurses may observe that family members seem unsure of how to respond when their parents have experienced a massive stroke and can only vocalize grunting noises. Modeling acceptance, respect, and warmth through use of touch, smile, explanations, and encouragement can evoke affective behavioral change. Similarly, live or recorded demonstrations and films better prepare clients to perform skills because the client can visually and aurally attend to actions and emulate the model. It can be more beneficial to watch someone perform a task than to jump in immediately and attempt the task.[64] Some critical tasks will require contrived role modeling because of the safety factors involved.

Print materials, such as pamphlets, handouts, books, and journal articles, have several advantages. First, they are portable and they appeal to all ages. They can be read at the client's convenience, whether it be in the comfort and security of the home or in a waiting room (Fig. 5-7).

Second, oral instructions may be less definitive and retained briefly, but written instructions can be referred to often.[65] Third, print materials can contain visual cues such as pictures, charts, and graphs that may facilitate understanding of complex, abstract information. Last, print materials can be prepared in all languages for all ages. The limitations of print materials include potential readability problems and need for frequent revision. There is also a chance that client-teacher-presented content and written content are inconsistent. In this case, the options are to teach what is in the print materials or discuss discrepancies with clients.

Quality and design of print materials, and all other types of teaching materials for that matter, can influence client learning. Use of instructional objectives and inserting relevant questions provide opportunities for self-evaluation of content mastery.[66] Also, use of topic sentences and organized passages can improve recall.[67] Clear, logical organization of information enables learners to relate current information to relevant facts presented earlier in a passage. Failure to organize content clearly and logically decreases learner ability to make inferences.[68] Disorganization also reduces speed of comprehension and memory for statements that refer to previously experienced events.[69] In addition to clear, logical organization, use of relevant examples can also have powerful effects on ability to learn from textual information. Client teachers can increase the probability that clients will learn from print materials by ensuring readability in terms of appropriate language and reading level, use of feedback mechanisms for learners, purposeful, and logical organization, and use of realistic, concrete examples.

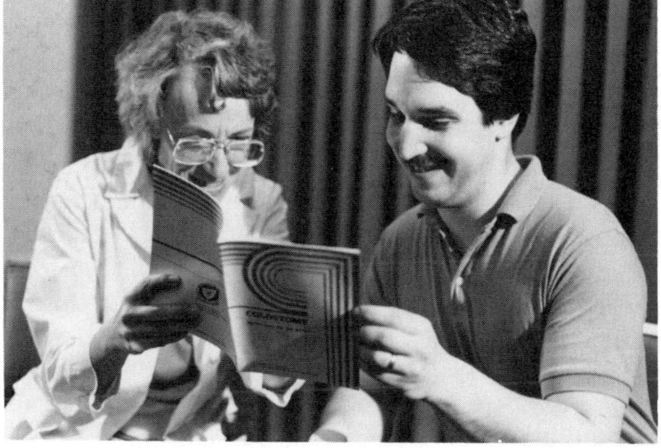

Figure 5-7. A print teaching strategy.

Client teachers wishing to obtain already prepared print materials can choose from various resources. Libraries are a primary source of books, magazines, pamphlets, and other materials. Government publications are listed and available through most libraries. Also, a brief letter to government agencies will place your name on mailing lists. Drug and formula companies and commercial suppliers are other avenues to explore. Salespeople are an additional source of valuable information. Possibilities for publishing originally created materials can also be explored with sales representatives.

Print programed instruction employs many principles from behavioristic psychology with a goal of mastery learning. When first introduced, educators hoped this strategy would enable all learners to reach a similar knowledge level. Research on programed instruction has progressed to a point where an evaluation of the basic approach is fairly clear. The conclusion, so far, seems to be that no method of individualization yet invented removes all effects of prior differences in abilities.[70] There is some evidence that less able learners are more likely to be assisted by programed learning, while more able learners may become bored and frustrated when a low-level, stimulus-response approach is used. In addition, not all clients prefer programed instruction for learning. Certainly, programed instruction has application, depending on learning objectives, learner characteristics, and content. Importantly, development of programed instruction requires knowledge of learning theory along with an extensive time commitment. Nurses who want to use this technique are advised to explore already prepared programs that are published in nursing journals like the *American Journal of Nursing*. Or they can be purchased from commercial publishers and distributors (*see* the Appendix). If desired programs are unavailable, qualified consultants should be sought for guidance and suggestions.

Programed instruction in computerized form is relatively new on the client education scene. The potential for this technology has not been realized, but the advantage in terms of individualized, personalized client learning is a challenge for client teachers. In fact, state-of-the-art technology introduces teaching possibilities unheard of ten, or even five, years ago. Nurses have long used real objects or their models, chalkboards, overhead projectors and transparencies, filmstrips, pictures, posters, slides, and film. But new strategies are now possible because of technological advancement. For example, discharge information can be recorded on audio- or videotape and sent home with clients because many homes now have audio and video players. In the future, most homes will have computers, which will be linked as computer networks, perhaps even with hospitals and other health care agencies. Many will have videodisk systems. Disks with all types of information can be taken from health care setting to home and back again, or just broadcast over telephone lines.

The new technologies exist in most health care settings. Computers and closed-circuit and cable TV systems are examples. Such technologies are used for several purposes, including orientation and ongoing in-service and continuing education for both staff and clients. Many acute-care settings have video players and closed-circuit cable television in client rooms. Teaching can be carried out for individuals as well as groups using these media. Imagine a setting in which clients waiting to be seen in clinics watch a video presentation on what to expect during their clinic experience. In a learning center, clients about to have a diagnostic exam view and listen to a sound filmstrip about the test. At the same time, a man admitted for coronary bypass surgery watches surgery on his television screen while it is actually being done in the operating room, and two hundred nursing students at a distant site view the same surgical procedure on TV screens in a lecture hall as they ask and respond to questions through the interactive system. It is all possible, but the full potential for client teaching is yet to be realized.

SUMMARY

Client teachers function as primary and secondary educators in a variety of settings. They apply the theories and principles of learning and teaching, either independently or as a member of a multi-disciplinary team, to plan, carry out, and evaluate learning experiences and clarify, validate, and reinforce what others teach.

Client teachers assume a multitude of responsibilities, which include diagnosing learner characteristics and needs, determining critical tasks and objectives, identifying appropriate content, determining appropriate learning activities, and evaluating learning outcomes. Teaching effectiveness is reflected and made observable through these basic categories of responsibility.

Critical tasks are those behaviors deemed necessary for clients to learn. Achievement of such tasks is made observable and measurable by stating objectives in behavioral terms according to cognitive, affective, and psychomotor learning domains. Alternative teaching activities and test items, designed to promote and measure learning, are selected on the basis of critical tasks and objectives. These teaching actions, along with thorough documentation of teaching events, ensure that client teachers are accountable for client learning.

Individual differences in learning ability, cognitive development, time perspective, attention span, dependency, prior knowledge and skill (including reading level), readiness for learning, and other relevant psychological and sociocultural variables do influence learning. The assessment of learner characteristics is a major component of the teaching process, and it is prerequisite to planning appropriate content, activities, and critical learning tasks (*see* Fig. 5–1). Many times, inadequate assessment of the client's background, beliefs, and values results in ineffective teaching and deficits in learning.

Readiness for learning is associated with a number of complex variables. Physiological, emotional, and sociocultural factors continually interact to influence when a client is ready to learn a critical health task. Several models can be used to interpret observations and determine readiness to learn. Nurses should be able to recognize cues that indicate when a client is most receptive to teaching interventions. Common behaviors indicating readiness are client-initiated questions about condition and treatment, statements indicating anxiety about the situation, and willingness to respond to inquiries.[71]

Client teachers determine critical tasks and relevant content necessary for clients to learn so as to promote, maintain, or regain health. Although specific topics of information to be communicated depend on individual needs, characteristics, and circumstances, basic content areas include health maintenance and health restoration. Professional nurses should take advantage of every opportunity to teach in these critical content areas either formally or informally. Teaching and learning activities are selected on the basis of identified learning outcomes, content, and the advantages and limitations of activities—the particular strategies, resources, and materials used to promote behavioral change.

All activities used to facilitate learning should be based on sound learning principles. Activities are appropriate when it can be demonstrated that they are selected on the basis of critical tasks, learner characteristics, content, and feasibility.

Learning principles to be considered when determining teaching strategies, resources, and materials for critical tasks include: (1) organizing content from familiar to unfamiliar and simple to complex so that clients can cognitively associate old with new information, (2) building in conditions for feedback so that clients know what is expected and why, and (3) teaching for transfer.

Feasibility questions always enter in when one is determining what resources and materials to use for particular learning experiences. Client teachers need to thoroughly examine cost-benefit factors in terms of time and money, and explore issues relating to durability, adaptability, and accessibility for each alternative. Such factors will influence the final decision and ultimate outcome of the learning experience.

The various direct and contrived activities used to promote client learning have particular advantages and limitations that may make a difference in achievement of critical tasks depending on the circumstances of the teaching-learning event. Client teachers should be knowledgeable about the multitude of options available and take advantage of their unique attributes.

Advances in modern technology are changing the way client teachers teach by providing alternatives to direct one-on-one and group teaching approaches. Transcending the audiovisual and teaching aids of the past, these new technologies help the client teacher to design complete learning systems that facilitate management of learning for both individuals and groups and provide the feedback, reinforcement, practice, control, and other conditions necessary for promoting optimum client learning.

STRATEGIES TO PROMOTE ACTIVE CLIENT LEARNING

Teaching may not be effective unless clients are actively participating in learning and assuming the responsibility for learning. Some researchers in cognitive psychology believe ability to plan and coordinate learning strategies is an important aspect of intelligence.[72,73] New areas of research in metacognition and possibilities of learning-to-learn place increased responsibility on teachers to select activities that increase learner self-regulation of learning.[74] Several strategies have been found to be useful in this regard. First, learners will learn more and transfer information better if tasks are taught in an accurate contextual framework, or in the context in which the knowledge will be actually used. Since this is not always possible, client teachers can ask clients to imagine the real context, such as a home setting. Learners who are provided a contextual framework or learning set prior to introduction of the topic will learn more. For example, the client teacher might say, "If you're in the living room and you hear your baby coughing in the bedroom, you are going to have to be able to get your equipment together fast to suction his tracheostomy. Let's talk about how to arrange equipment to help you work fast." Second, learning will be further enhanced if clients comprehend content meaning. For instance, do clients appreciate the importance of nutrients to health? An active search for meaning by the client is essential for learning.

A third strategy addresses the problem of interference that results from inaccurate learning or current learning of conflicting information. In other words, clients may be hearing many things from many people, which confuses learning. Problems of interference can be minimized by offering information through novel situations. If clients remark that they are getting confused, the client teacher can say, "Well, let's think of it in another way" offering another context and new examples. In addition, clients often suggest appropriate analogies or situations that assist in their own learning. Teachers need to minimize confusion during the initial stages of learning. Research by Nitsch shows that confusion in early learning is reduced by using content examples and transfer is enhanced by using varied-context examples.[75] Application of this approach can be illustrated by situations in which client teachers teach women to breast-feed. Based on findings from Nitsch, nurses would be wise to assist mothers with feeding at the bedside first and then go on to breast-feeding techniques for use at home and in public.

A fourth strategy relates to practice. Because nursing is an applied science, client teachers value practice as a strategy for learning. Various types of practice have different effects, however. Not all types of practice will facilitate transfer of learning. When we are tempted to say "practice makes perfect," we must ask, "perfect with respect to what?" Mastery of psychomotor skills requires repeated practice in appropriate context. Antecedents to mastery are a brief cognitive phase and an organizing phase in which skills become automatic.[76] The last stage, or the perfecting stage, separates experts from novices. Experts simply spend more time practicing and refining their skills.

Another way to get clients actively involved in learning is to take advantage of their preferences and interests. Use of more than one learning activity has merit because of individual preferences, abilities, and potential reinforcement effects. People have a range of preferences and learning modes. Some clients elect or are more able to learn by listening, while others prefer reading or doing. Preferences are probably related to habits established throughout life or to situational variables. Contrast the preferences of an engineer who uses mathematical formulas and abstract forms of representation with those of a mother of young children who is accustomed to frequent interruptions. Depending on the purpose, the first learner might prefer abstract print materials with complex diagrams and charts, while the second might choose simple visual or auditory materials like pictures or audiotapes that can be put down or turned off and then continued later.

Multisensory approaches offer still another option. Such strategies have the potential for incorporating active response, reinforcement, and feedback. For example, clients learning home hemodialysis can acquire knowledge and comprehension through reading or watching a film depicting home hemodialysis, take a self-test, and then actually demonstrate hemodialysis.

Simultaneous activities, such as taking notes while listening to what someone is saying, or using a microcomputer to complete a learning program, are likely to facilitate understanding and retention because of the multisensory nature of the imput and the active overt response required. The value of particular activities such as these will depend on the nature of the information, learner attributes, including learner knowledge,[77] as well as the match between input and output requirements (Fig. 5-8).

Learning contracts are yet another strategy to consider, particularly for self-directed clients. They may be used in conjunction with self-instructional learning activity packages or modular instruction. Implementation varies widely, but some generalizations are valid. First, learning contracts provide a vehicle for mutual planning between nurse and client. Learners actively take part in diagnosing their own needs, formulating objectives, identifying resources, choosing strategies, and evaluating accomplishments. Throughout these processes, clients develop a sense of commitment and control over learning. Contracts are appropriate for clients from school age years through adulthood. To be effective, learning contracts need to be complete and easy to follow. The following eight steps are recommended when developing a contractual agreement[78]:

1. Mutual diagnosis of learning needs
2. Specification of learning objectives
3. Specification of resources and strategies

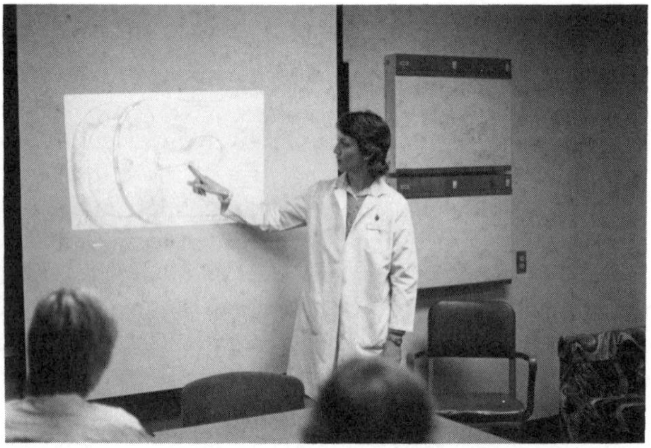

Figure 5-8. Manipulation of control and experimental group variables.

4. Identification of evidence of accomplishment with avenues for validation
5. Periodic, mutual review and revision of contract
6. Implementation of contract by learner
7. Evaluation of learning

Client teachers who choose this strategy act as consultants and facilitators to clients rather than information providers. It may sound easier than didactic teaching, but it requires a breadth of knowledge and flexibility.

The primary advantage of contract learning is that it places responsibility for learning on the client's shoulders. Client teachers must be comfortable with this approach for it to work. It will also be important for nurses to touch base frequently with contract learners; thus the time commitment is great. Development of a timetable with scheduled communication opportunities is suggested. Contract learning is appropriate for many client education situations. For example, let's assume a school nurse has a 12-year-old who is not emptying his colostomy bag periodically. The result is the frequent presence of stool on clothing and embarrassment to the student, teachers, and others. The nurse and child together can develop a learning contract to insure that the child has adequate knowledge and reward for carrying out this major responsibility. The school nurse can provide supervision, reinforcement, and feedback on a one-to-one basis. In this manner, learning becomes personalized and humanistic. And, the responsibility for learning and doing is the child's.

SUMMARY

Active participation or self-involvement in learning is an important condition for learning. Client teachers can question, use imagery, novelty, and practice strategies in the appropriate context, while taking advantage of client's learning styles, modes, and preferences to reduce interference and confusion and promote retention and transfer of cognitive, affective, and psychomotor behaviors.

CONTRIBUTIONS OF SELECTED NURSING RESEARCH TO CLIENT EDUCATION AND TEACHING

Nursing research into various aspects of client education and teaching is characterized by diversity in outcomes, client characteristics, methods, and testing criteria. Client populations in such studies have covered the total life-span. Only a few of the many noteworthy efforts will be discussed here.

Type of Content and Approach as Independent Variables

The Lamaze method of preparation for childbirth has been studied by several researchers: Doering and Entwisle conducted a retrospective investigation comparing the Lamaze method to traditional methods and found that Lamaze-prepared mothers used less medication, were better controlled, and cooperative and retained more positive attitudes about their labor and delivery.[79] Data in three reports showed Lamaze prepared fathers to have more positive responses to the event and theirmates.[80–82] Moore studied two methods of childbirth preparation and compared outcomes for marital satisfaction.[83] The two methods were Psychoprophylactic Method (PPM), commonly known as Lamaze, and the Hospital Class Method (HCM). The PPM classes were taught by instructors certified by the American Society of Psychoprophylaxis in Obstetrics, while instructors for HCM had no certification. Class size differed as well, with a maximum of 12 couples for the PPM method and 20 or more couples per instructor for the HCM method. Groups had similar goals, but content of the HCM method varied, while PPM had standard content and taught specific methods for active participation. Moore contrasted HCM and PPM content. HCM taught specific breathing patterns and coaching techniques, while PPM techniques utilized principles. Moore found a significant difference between groups in male total score, with the PPM group showing a lower level of conflict and a higher level of satisfaction. After controlling for initial differences between groups, however, this difference was not significant. Even though hypotheses were not supported, data showed differences between PPM and HCM groups. Labor variables indicated the Lamaze group had a slightly longer labor, but they used significantly less medication and chose rooming-in more often.

There is a large body of research related to the effects of preoperative teaching. Only experimentally designed research will be included in this discussion. Research on the effects of preoperative teaching has developed largely from the work of Lindeman and colleagues, which was reported in the early 1970s. They explored two types of preoperative teaching approaches.

The first approach studied was structured versus nonstructured preoperative teaching, while the second was a comparison of individual versus group teaching strategies. Data from the study investigating structured and unstructured teaching effects on outcomes revealed that structured preoperative teaching was significantly related to improved ability to cough and deep-breathe postoperatively. Furthermore, mean hospital stay was lower. Structured teaching was not, however, found to affect the need for analgesia.[84] Unstructured teaching was characterized by vagueness and inconsistency. Each nurse determined the priority given to preoperative teaching, and no teaching procedure was followed. In contrast, structured preoperative teaching included a teaching plan and skill demonstration using audiovisual strategies. Effects of individual versus group preoperative teaching were also investigated by Lindeman.[85] Group teaching was found to be as effective as individual teaching, with a reduction in required learning time.

Two investigators implemented a structured preoperative teaching program prior to hospitalization and compared postoperative physical, functional capacity, comfort, and satisfaction outcomes to those of a control group up to 33 days postoperatively.[86] Experimental subjects exhibited significantly higher levels of physical function as measured at days 2, 10, and 33 postoperatively. No significant difference in amount of oral analgesics between groups was found, but fewer intramuscular analgesics were used by the experimental group for the first postoperative 72 hours.

Experimental subjects also reported more comfort, though no significant differences were noted on measure of satisfaction or length of hospital stay.

Three alternate approaches to preoperative nursing intervention were investigated by Felton and colleagues.[87] Dependent variables were physiological and psychological outcomes. Subjects were divided into three groups. The control group had preoperative preparation routinely provided by unit nursing personnel. The approach was formalized and made consistent for all subjects. Information presented addressed preoperative physical procedures, statements indicating that it would be necessary to spend an unknown amount of time in recovery or intensive care, what drainage tubes to expect, and the need to move about after surgery. Time for teaching averaged 15 minutes per learner. A second group was identified as a communication group. A nursing intervention called therapeutic communication was used with these subjects. A nurse consciously attempted to positively influence learners by creating an atmosphere in which clients could verbalize feelings and utilize the problem-solving process. Subjects in the experimental group were taught what to expect and what was expected from them with teaching based on their concerns and questions. Pictures and films were used in conjunction with breathing practice. Two hypotheses were supported. Preoperative to postoperative anxiety was significantly decreased in subjects receiving the experimental intervention, and these subjects had higher scores on measures for psychological well-being. No significant differences in postoperative outcomes of ventilatory capacities, length of hospitalization, or postoperative complications were found among groups.

In the early 1970s, Jean Johnson began an extensive program of research aimed at reducing the discrepancy between expected sensations (what is felt, seen, heard, tasted, and smelled) and those actually experienced, in order to reduce distress.[88] Like Carol Lindeman's research, Jean Johnson's work was a step forward in documenting the effects of teaching interventions. Even though studies in the 1960s supported nurse-patient interaction effects on anxiety reduction, interaction processes were ill-defined, making replication or clinical application impossible. Johnson developed specific, testable hypotheses. Her research has stimulated a wide range of research by colleagues and other investigators. One such study explored sensory and procedural information effects on teaching.

Effects of structured teaching alone and structured teaching combined with sensory and procedural information was studied by Johnson, Rice, Fuller, and Endress.[89] Structured teaching was significantly related to fewer doses of analgesics and increased postoperative ambulation. When structured teaching was combined with information about expected sensations, length of hospital stay was significantly less than when patients received no instruction or information. Subjects with high preoperative fear benefited from structured teaching alone and in combination with sensation information, while no significant differences in postoperative mood was found for those with low preoperative fear.

Johnson's hypothesis was explored with children experiencing orthopedic cast removal. In this study, tape-recorded preparatory information was used to systematically vary expectations about physical sensations. Children were randomly assigned to one of three groups: (1) a sensory information group, which heard information on the sensory experience during cast removal, (2) a procedure information group, which received information on the steps in the experience, and (3) a contol group, which heard no tape-recorded information. Data analysis revealed that the procedure group did not differ significantly from the control group, while the mean distress score for the sensation group was significantly lower than the control group.

Hartfield, Cason, and Cason examined types of information about a threatening procedure in a quasi-experimental study to explore the effects on subjects about to have a barium enema.[90] Baseline data on anxiety was collected prior to intervention using the State-Trait Anxiety Inventory (STAI). Dependent variable measures were a postprocedure sensation inventory and the state portion of the STAI. Like Johnson, these investigators presented a recorded message of either sensation or procedural information followed by completion of post-information sensation inventory. Neither in expected sensations (expectations) reported prior to hearing information or responses provided after the procedure (actual experiences) were there significant differences between the two groups. After hearing the information, however, significant differences in reported expected sensations were found. Subjects receiving sensation information reported significantly less anxiety and expectations more congruent with actual experiences than did the control group.

Padilla and colleagues used filmstrips instead of tapes to present four different types of information about an unpleasant experience (nasogastric intubation for gastric analysis).[91] Locus of control theory was integrated with Johnson's work to develop four hypotheses. These were: (1) subjects receiving a filmstrip showing a combination of procedure and coping behaviors for specific, common distressful sensations would perceive increased control and lower distress than subjects receiving procedural information only; (2) subjects viewing filmstrips showing procedure only and procedure as well as common distressful sensations would have lower distress; (3) subjects viewing filmstrips showing most correspondence between information and actual experience (procedure and coping behaviors) would have least distress; and (4) individual differences in desire for control would show several outcomes. That is, subjects wanting control would have less distress than those wanting no control, since any information offers some cognitive control. Furthermore, a combination of subjects wanting control with the filmstrip showing procedures and coping behaviors would lead to least distress, whereas those subjects wanting no control but viewing the filmstrip showing both procedures and coping behaviors would exhibit the most distress. Various dependent variable measures were used, including objective and subjective tools. Data showed that procedure with sensory and coping behavior information was effective in decreasing discomfort, pain, and anxiety for control and no-control preference subjects during and after the procedure, but was most effective in reducing intubation distress for subjects prefering no control. Second, sensory information led to greater willingness to repeat the procedure. Last, perceived control had little effect on distress reduction.

Johnson's research with children was the basis for a related intervention developed by Visintainer and Wolfer. Psychological surgical preparation of children was investigated about ten years ago by Visintainer and Wolfer at Yale University. These researchers introduced the approach called stress-point preparation.[92] The clinical experiment tested variations of psychological preparation and supportive care designed to increase adjustment of children and their parents upon hospitalization for elective surgery. Three treatment groups were used in the study: (1) combination of systematic preparation, rehearsal, and supportive care conducted prior to each stressful procedure, (2) a single-session preparation conducted after admission, and (3) consistent supportive care given by one nurse at the same points as in the first condition, but including no systematic preparation or rehearsal. Stress-point preparation was communicated to preschool children via play and to older children orally. Throughout preparatory communications, a distinction was made between external events and sensations the children would experience to maximize understanding of what was about to happen, how long it would take, and how it would feel. As hypothesized, results demonstrated that children and parents who received condition number one showed significantly less upset and more cooperation as measured by blind ratings of behavioral upset. Postoperative reactions, such as fluid intake, recovery room medications, pulse rates, and time to first void were also significantly better for group number one.

Visintainer and Wolfer have stimulated other research on stress-point preparation. Individual and group preparation for pediatric surgical patients was compared to a control group in a study by McGrath.[93] The dependent variable was child and parent adaptation to hospitalization as indicated on blind observer ratings of subject upset behavior and cooperation with procedures at five potential stress points. It was hypothesized that children and parents who were prepared through group preparation in contrast to individual stress-point preparation and control children would show less upset and better coping and adjustments. Both group and individual interventions were based on a combination of systematic preparation, rehearsal, and supportive care conducted prior to each stressful procedure. Group preparation also included: peer exposure, support, identification, group process, and group teaching. As hypothesized, children prepared in a group showed significantly less upset and more cooperation. In addition, their parents were better informed and more satisfied than for either other group.

Other methods to assist clients to cope have also been investigated. Use of relaxation techniques to cope with painful, unpleasant procedures is becoming more common. Wells used relaxation training in an experimental investigation to determine whether abdominal muscle tension (surface electromyography [EMG]), self-report of pain and distress, and use of analgesics would differ in adult cholecystectomy patients in two treatment conditions.[94] Six patients received relaxation training. The relaxation technique used was a structured program including a mental device to decrease distracting thoughts (concentration on breathing), a passive attitude, decreased abdominal muscle tonus using feedback from the EMG machine, and exercise. Control subjects received preoperative teaching, including objective information, a description of sensations to be experienced, and practice of deep breathing, coughing, and moving in bed. Results showed relaxation training to lower pain distress significantly, without significant main effects on abdominal muscle tone or use of analgesics.

Programs of research on preoperative preparation begun by Lindeman and procedure preparation started by Johnson have initiated a variety of research efforts. Their impact on nursing research and client welfare continues into this decade and beyond.

Teaching Strategies as Independent Variables

Research on the effectiveness of teaching strategies is a fairly new direction. The majority of studies focus on manipulation of teaching strategies. This type of research is difficult because of large numbers of interacting variables. Work is just beginning to provide direction for this line of inquiry.

Research by Felton and colleagues is important for two reasons. The first important contribution is their demonstration of measurements for evaluation of the effects of teaching strategies. Felton, Lotas, and Eastman developed instruments to appraise quality of stoma educational programs.[95] Their research provides a way to examine outcomes or critical tasks in educational programs for ostomates, which can be used as a model for evaluation of other educational programs. Second, their study used type of educational program with qualifications of teachers as the independent variable. Two types of educational programs were used: (1) structured preparation conducted by an enterostomal therapist or prepared personnel other than an enterostomal therapist, called Treatment A, and (2) preparation conducted on an ad hoc or informal basis and not specifically designed for special needs of the ostomate, called Treatment B. Types of teaching methods and tools were used differently at all sites. These included individual, group, and lecture presentations. Educational materials used were pamphlets, pictures, diagrams, books, films, filmstrips, instruction sheets, tapes, and models. Results showed Treatment A patients were more satisfied with information, service, self-care knowledge, follow-up care, and instructions given to families at discharge. In addition, Treatment A patients exceeded B patients in skill achievement for ostomy care and were better able to describe available resources and health maintenance behaviors. Treatment A patients demonstrated more coping behaviors and attained a more optimal health status at discharge as well. This difference between groups persisted after six months, with a higher percentage of group A patients meeting criteria for optimal health. Last, patients in group A spent less money on equipment and supplies and were constrained by fewer limitations when engaging in normal activities. Treatment A patients found the enterostomal therapist to be the most helpful. These authors conclude that structured educational programs lead to more desirable outcomes than unstructured programs.

Effects of repetitive teaching, use of audiovisual strategies, and self-directed learning have also been investigated. Effects of repetitive teaching on knowledge about drugs to be taken at home was investigated by Sechrist.[96] Sechrist found that one repetition of content significantly increased client knowledge about drugs to be taken at home, but one repetition resulted in mastery of information for only 35 percent of the subjects in the repetitive teaching group. Questions missed most frequently were those related to drug names and their side effects. Effects of long-term memory or compliance were not studied.

The effects of audiovisual teaching strategies have been reported in three investigations. Darr and associates used a slide program to teach clients information on bronchodilator medications.[97] Purposes of the investigation were to evaluate the effects of the sound-slide program on patients' short-term and long-term memory and to determine whether any difference exists in learning or retention patterns for different content areas of drug information. Tests were given at three different times after the teaching episode. Scores obtained on the first posttest were significantly higher than pretest scores; however, test score difference between pretest and last posttest (given at a mean of 2.8 months after teaching) were not significantly different. Investigators found content areas of route, administration, directions, side effects, and self-monitoring techniques to be retained at a significantly higher level than medication name. The authors conclude that carefully designed audiovisual programs can effectively impart drug information, but medication counseling must be ongoing because of loss of knowledge over time. Design problems (such as lack of comparison group) and measurement issues (regression toward the mean in comparing pre- and posttest scores) are found in this report, but it is a useful exploratory study.

Sly also used a sound-slide program to teach mothers of children with asthma.[98] Effects of the sound-slide program were compared to direct interview. Both methods were supplemented with specific oral and printed instructions. This investigator found the slide program to be as effective as direct interview. Lack of a control and vague outcome measures are weaknesses in this study.

Direct interview was compared to programed learning guides and audiovisual strategies when teaching about venereal disease to 450 subjects in an investigation reported by Alkhateeb and colleagues.[99] Each teaching strategy was studied using an experimental and control group. While all three methods increased scores significantly, no significant differences were found between the three experimental groups. Client preferences were interesting. Only 17 percent of the subjects said programed instruction was interesting to very interesting. Subject learner characteristics in this study are unknown.

Programed instruction has been further studied by Wiley. An investigation conducted by Wiley examined the effects of a self-directed learning project and preferences for structure on self-directed learning readiness.[100] In this experimental study, Wiley concluded that neither preference for structure nor the experience of the self-directed learning project contributed significantly to variance in posttest self-directed readiness, but interaction of these two variables did contribute. Findings suggest that persons who prefer low structure may benefit more from self-directed teaching strategies than do persons who prefer high structure.

Two investigators explored the effects of formal versus informal teaching with chronically ill patients. Milazzo reports a study comparing health knowledge on heart disease gained through formal and informal teaching.[101] In this experimental study, the strategy used was a lecture and slide presentation. The content took 45 minutes to present and included anatomy and physiology of the heart, the healing process, danger signals, risk factors, angina, physical therapy, sexual activity, and drug therapy. Informal teaching used for the control group is not described. The experimental group demonstrated a significant increase in knowledge gained as compared to control subjects. A second investigator considered teacher qualifications. Murdough notes that teaching efforts conducted by nurses often fail because teaching is not based on teaching-learning principles. The independent variable in Murdough's study was a 12-hour course entitled "Introduction to Teaching-Learning Principles" developed and taught to teachers by the investigator.[102] The group of people receiving instruction from nurses who took this course (experimental group) did significantly better on an examination than those in the control group. This study indicates that knowledge of teaching-learning principles, including the selection and use of teaching strategies, can influence teaching effectiveness.

Client Characteristics as Independent Variables

Research to date has emphasized teacher, strategy, and content rather than client characteristics. Most research on teaching strategies examines the effects of various methods without systematic manipulation of learner characteristics. Learner characteristics are randomized except for the global description of diagnosis. Scott's research on anxiety, critical thinking, and information processing during and after breast biopsy is a departure from the current trend, however.[103] Rather than grouping subjects into a global category of diagnosis, Scott investigated what was happening to these people and their cognitive ability during crisis. In her study, STAI, critical thinking ability (CTA), and judged duration were tested for coping relatedness and change over time for 85 women, 18 to 20 years of age, who were experiencing breast biopsy. Participants were tested before biopsy reports were known and six weeks later. Data showed extremely high anxiety levels prior to biopsy and compromised reasoning ability at a critical time when demands on cognitive functioning are high. Scott's research, then, is a beginning in critical examination of learner characteristics and how learner characteristics affect teaching and learning outcomes.

Directions for Future Research

Nursing research on client education and teaching has a relatively short history. It has proceeded in spite of the existence of severe problems in conducting controlled clinical investigations and of difficult ethical issues. Ethical issues affect research design. For example, it is impossible to eliminate teaching all together to establish control groups, because these clients would suffer. Therefore, it is not possible to study the effects of no teaching. Some control groups are actually comparison groups. Furthermore, nurses have had to develop many tools needed to measure dependent variables. Dependent variables measured in nursing research are extremely complex, making instrument development difficult, to say the least. The

TABLE 5-2. PARADIGM FOR INVESTIGATION OF TEACHING STRATEGY OUTCOMES

Group	Measure	Treatment	Measure
Control	Entry	Unsystematic teaching	Outcome
Experimental	Entry	Systematic teaching	Outcome

complexity of clinical research has fostered use of global and demographic variables, which are not precise or helpful. Many variables used thus far are surrogates for variables that are less well understood and more difficult to measure. In spite of these problems, it is clear that early investigators have made a significant contribution to research. Their work provides a sound basis for future researchers.

Nursing researchers of the future face several challenges. First, teaching activities need to be defined carefully and clearly manipulated. Many investigators use aggregates in experimental groups. These include interviews, self-directed learning strategies, and audiovisual ones. The paradigm used frequently is a familiar one. Researchers determine and measure variables that might affect learning to make sure both groups are comparable. The independent variable manipulated for the experimental group is usually well-planned and systematically implemented teaching. The control group must have some teaching because of ethical considerations. This teaching is an unknown quantity, however, and varies considerably. Finally, group outcomes are compared (Table 5-2).

Several problems exist in this paradigm. Thus far, most investigators have not discussed problems related to regression toward the mean when comparing pre- and posttest scores. Also, effects of teaching activities cannot be isolated. Manipulation of one strategy at a time is recommended to isolate effects. A more complex paradigm may be indicated, as shown in Table 5-3, in which several strategies are explored with control and experimental groups for each.

Such a paradigm was used by Alkhateeb and associates, but interaction effects were not addressed. Furthermore, basic assumptions of this paradigm are not universally acceptable. Nursing research emphasis to date has been on teaching or teachers. The major assumption seems to be that the potential for affecting outcomes rests with teachers and teaching activities rather than on client characteristics. The validity of this assumption can be challenged. First, some experts in education believe that teaching activities account for a small portion of the variance in aca-

TABLE 5-3. PARADIGM FOR COMPARISON OF SEVERAL TEACHING STRATEGIES

Group	Measure	Treatment			Measure
Control	Entry	Unsystematic	Unsystematic	Unsystematic	Outcome
Experimental	Entry	Treatment I	Treatment II	Treatment III	Outcome

demic learning outcomes. Second, an overwhelming body of literature points to individual ability as the major contributor to differences in learning. Few investigators mention this factor. Third, prior learning, learning strategies, styles, preferences, and modes may be highly significant influences in client learning achievement. Thus far, these variables have been unexplored in client education and teaching for the most part.

A new dimension of investigation seems to be warranted. The complexities of client characteristics need to be integrated into research designs in more depth than has been done. Nurse researchers, like Scott, can use or develop measures for client readiness to learn, abilities, aptitudes, learning strategies, and styles. A modification of current research models is suggested, such as: client learning characteristic (X) given teaching strategy attribute (Y) results in outcome (Z). The experimental design paradigm has been used extensively to study the effects of teaching strategies. Its usefulness has to be questioned in light of the complexity of clinical research. Perhaps it is time to reassess its appropriateness as well as variables addressed. Nurses continue to identify and test variables affecting client welfare, but seldom do we consider their relationship to each other. Researchers conscientiously measure length of hospitalization, number of previous hospitalizations, anxiety, and many other variables; however, few discuss variable interaction effects or determine which variables account for the greatest variance in outcome, as is possible with regression or factor analysis models. Furthermore, there have not been multidimensional analysis of variance models, which could also isolate significant variables from a complexity of interacting variables.

It could be that experimental designs limit our perspective. Other variables yet unmeasured might account for a larger percentage of outcome variance than teaching interventions. Also, specific strategy effects and attributes could be isolated. For these reasons, factor analysis, regression and multidimensional analysis of variance statistical models may be preferable, because these methods enable investigators to broaden research paradigms in order to account for more variables in a systematic fashion.

Nursing research on teaching has established an exciting foundation on which to build further research data bases. It has demonstrated to the public that nurses make a difference because nursing interventions alter client welfare. It has also elicited interesting research questions that pose challenges to current and future nurse researchers who choose to study client education.

SUMMARY

Because of the unique nature of client characteristics, educational settings, content, and critical tasks, factors influencing selection and use of teaching strategies, resources, and materials for client education are somewhat different than those of the academic sphere. Decisions are influenced by differences in client experiences, which include health problems, illness, and crisis. The processes and principles of teaching and selection and use of strategies, resources, and materials are the same, however.

Client teachers must be aware of the effects that circumstances and actions can have on learning outcomes.

All teaching strategies, resources, and materials—the activities for client learning—should be appropriate for critical tasks, content, and learner characteristics. They should convey accurate, relevant content and reflect sound learning principles, providing the necessary conditions for cognitive, affective, and psychomotor learning. Factors such as the size of audience, sensory stimuli needed, active participation in learning, and realism must be considered when deciding on the activities for client learning.[104] Thorough analysis of message, environment, response, and learner characteristics will facilitate sound decision making.[105] Nursing researchers continue to pioneer examination of teaching and conditions for learning with the goal of identifying new knowledge that can be applied to client education. The total body of educational literature benefits from nursing contributions on teaching learners with special needs. More importantly, clients themselves benefit as they learn to maintain, increase, or restore health and well-being.

POSTTEST

MULTIPLE CHOICE

1. The *major* difference between teaching academic students and teaching clients is:
   a. Learner characteristics
   b. Timing of learning experiences
   c. Preparation time
   d. Safety factors
2. A client who automatically counts calories after an educational program on weight control is demonstrating which step of Krathwohl's taxonomy of the affective domain?
   a. Conceptualizing
   b. Internalizing
   c. Receiving
   d. Valuing
3. A client fails to recognize the significance of a positive acetone reading while doing a Clinitest on urine. This behavior indicates that the client has *not gone beyond* which step in Bloom's cognitive domain?
   a. Analysis
   b. Application
   c. Comprehension
   d. Knowledge

4. Nurses can best determine client reading ability by assessing client:
   a. Age on admission
   b. Demonstrated reading ability
   c. Highest school grade
   d. Intelligence test results
5. Young children, highly anxious clients, and learners who do not speak English benefit from a similar teaching strategy. What is this strategy?
   a. Abstract discussion
   b. Concrete, hands-on learning by doing
   c. Explanation of principles and rules
   d. Use of examples as explanations
6. Which of the following models most accurately predicts the probability that clients with asthma will take responsibility for their own health maintenance?
   a. Adaptation
   b. Health-illness
   c. Locus of control
   d. Sick-role behavior
7. What is the most effective way for nurses to assist clients to perceive particular content or subject matter as being meaningful to them?
   a. Discuss meaningfulness for future well-being
   b. Give examples of other learners
   c. Share literature reports
   d. Show connections to prior experiences
8. Which of the following strategies would be most likely to alter client attitudes toward content?
   a. Large-group formal lecture
   b. Independent study
   c. Role modeling
   d. Written materials
9. Some research indicates that simple programed instruction and other activities may be boring for which type of learner?
   a. Adult
   b. Less able
   c. More able
   d. Teen-ager
10. Which of the following strategies can most easily be revised to keep content current?
    a. Sound-slide programs
    b. Filmstrip programs
    c. Print word-processed materials
    d. Video programs

11. Identify the most effective strategy to prepare clients for an uncomfortable procedure.
    a. Emotional support
    b. Explanation of procedure
    c. Reassurance of no pain
    d. Sensation preparation
12. What suggestion would be most helpful to the nurse who is just beginning to teach clients?
    a. Determine what clients bring to the learning experience and build on that knowledge.
    b. List problem areas found for other clients with similiar problems and share their solutions.
    c. Select what content clients need to know and present slowly.
    d. Utilize a teaching strategy you would find most useful if you had the same problem.
    e. Establish realistic objectives, critical tasks, strategies, and activities that assist clients to maintain, improve, or regain health status.

POSTTEST ANSWER KEY

1. a
2. b or d
3. d
4. b
5. b
6. c
7. d
8. c
9. c
10. c
11. d
12. a and e

SUGGESTED APPLICATION ACTIVITIES

Analyze each of the following client situations. Describe learner characteristics, critical tasks, appropriate content, teaching-learning activities, and evaluation methods or measures for each case. Justify your teaching plans in a written rationale for each case. Include principles of learning, factors that influence learning, and necessary conditions for learning relevant to each client situation.

1. Mr. Jay is a 63-year-old man who works as an engineer. He is about 40 pounds overweight, smokes two packs of cigarettes a day, and drinks 6 to 12 beers daily. He has followed this pattern for at least 30 years. Following his father's death, he experienced chest pains. He was admitted to a hospital coronary care unit, where his condition was diagnosed as a coronary. Mr. Jay married a second time late in life and has a teen-age daughter living at home. He insists he must work, even though he is in chronic pain from an arthritic hip.
2. Mrs. May is a 50-year-old woman who has been a teacher all her adult life and has raised 4 children. Her husband died ten years ago. She lives with a daughter in a large house. She began having "bone pain" and was unable to sleep at night, so her physician told her to take arthritis medication. The medication did not relieve the pain. She became short of breath but attributed it to anxiety and asthma. When one of her children finally convinced her to see another physician, a large breast lesion was discovered. Physicians told her that she had metastatic breast cancer that had spread to her bones, lungs, and brain. Mrs. May makes the following statements: "I've been such a fool." "I'm being punished because I've always looked down on sick people and called them weak." "I wonder why I have trouble breathing." "It will help to walk more." "Well, at least my heart is alright. I'm relieved to hear that."
3. Tommy is a 4-year-old child who swallowed lye at 18 months of age while with his mother. He came close to death many times immediately after the accident. His father blames Tommy's mother for the incident. Tommy is to have a colonic transplant to make a new esophagus. His father does not want him to know anything about the surgery or hospitalization. Tommy's father states, "It will just scare him." Tommy's mother disagrees, however, and wants him to know all about what's going to happen.

REFERENCES

1. Smith FB: Florence Nightingale: Reputation and Power. London, Croom Helm, 1982, pp. 72–114.
2. Knowles MS: Modern Practice in Adult Education. Chicago, IL, Follett Publishing Co., 1980, p. 19.
3. Wu R: Behavior in Illness. Englewood Cliffs, NJ, Prentice-Hall, Inc., 1973, pp. 136–156.
4. Redman BK: The Process of Patient Teaching in Nursing, ed 4. St. Louis, C.V. Mosby Co., 1980, pp. 1–18.
5. Bransford JD: Human Cognition. Belmont, CA, Wadsworth Publishing Co., 1979, p. 8.
6. Redman BK: The Process of Patient Teaching in Nursing, ed 4. St. Louis, C.V. Mosby Co., 1980, pp. 1–18.

7. Bloom B (ed): Taxonomy of Educational Objectives: The Classification of Educational Goals. Handbook I: Cognitive Domain. New York, David McKay Co., Inc., 1956, pp. 201-207.
8. Krathwohl DR, Bloom B, Masia B (eds): Taxonomy of Educational Objectives: The Classification of Educational Goals. Handbook II: Affective Domain. New York, David McKay Co., Inc., 1964, pp. 192-196.
9. Simpson EJ: The Classification of Educational Objectives in the Psychomotor Domain. In RM Thomas (ed): Contributions of Behavioral Science to Instructional Technology: The Psychomotor Domain. Mt. Rainer, MD, Gryphon Press, 1972, pp. 82-88.
10. Frase LT: Maintenance and Control in the Acquisition of Knowledge from Written Materials. In JB Carroll, RO Freedle (eds): Language Comprehension and the Acquisition of Knowledge. Washington, DC, V.H. Winston & Sons, 1972, pp. 401-436.
11. Bransford JD: Human Cognition. Belmont, CA, Wadsworth Publishing Co., 1979, p. 55.
12. Felton G, Huss K, et al.: Preoperative Nursing Intervention with the Patient for Surgery: Outcomes of Three Alternative Approaches. International Journal of Nursing Studies 13:83-96, 1976.
13. Lindeman CA, Van Aernam B: Nursing Intervention with the Pre-Surgical Patient: The Effects of Structured and Unstructured Preoperative Teaching. Nursing Research 20 (4):319-382, 1971.
14. Lindeman CA: Nursing Intervention with the Presurgical Patient: Effectiveness and Efficiency of Group and Individual Preoperative Teaching—Phase Two. Nursing Research 21 (3):196-209, 1972.
15. Lindeman CA, Stetzer SL: Effect of Preoperative Visits by Operating Room Nurses. Nursing Research 22 (2):4-15, 1973.
16. Egbert LD, Battit GE, et al.: Reduction of Postoperative Pain by Encouragement and Instruction of Patients. New England Journal of Medicine 270:825-827, 1964.
17. Johnson JE, Kirchhoff KT, Endress MP: Altering Children's Distress Behavior During Orthopedic Cast Removal. Nursing Research 24 (6):404-410, 1975.
18. Wolfer JA, Visintainer MA: Pediatric Surgical Patients' and Parents' Stress Responses and Adjustment as a Function of Psychologic Preparation and Stress-Point Care. Nursing Research 24 (4):244-255, 1975.
19. Bartlett RH, Gazzaniga A, Geraghty TR: Respiratory Maneuvers to Prevent Postoperative Pulmonary Complications. Journal of the American Medical Association 224:1017-1021, 1973.
20. Suchman EA: Evaluative Research: Principles and Practice in Public Service and Social Action Programs. New York, Russell Sage Foundation, 1967, pp. 140-146.
21. Redman BK: The Process of Patient Teaching in Nursing, ed 4. St. Louis, C.V. Mosby Co., 1980, p. 196.
22. Green LW: Evaluation and Measurement: Some Dilemmas for Health Education. American Journal of Public Health 67:155-161, 1977.
23. Ebel RL: Essentials of Educational Measurement. Englewood Cliffs, NJ, Prentice-Hall, Inc., 1972, 55-225.
24. Patient Education. New York, Council of Hospital and Related Institutional Nursing Service of the National League for Nursing, 1976, p. 8.
25. Adam D, Wright AS: Dissonance in Nurse and Patient Evaluations of the Effectiveness of a Patient-Teaching Program. Nursing Outlook 30 (2):132-136, 1982.
26. Jenny J: A Strategy for Patient Teaching. Journal of Advanced Nursing 3:341-348, 1978.

27. Snow RE, Yalow E: Education and Intelligence. In RJ Sternberg (ed): Handbook of Human Intelligence. New York, Cambridge University Press, 1982, pp. 493–571.
28. Piaget J: Science of Education and the Psychology of the Child. New York, Orion Press, 1970, pp. 212–215.
29. Johnson JE, Kirchhoff KT, Endress MP: Altering Children's Distress Behavior During Orthopedic Cast Removal. Nursing Research 24(6):404–410, 1975.
30. Wolfer JA, Visintainer MA: Pediatric Surgical Patients' and Parents' Stress Responses and Adjustment as a Function of Psychologic Preparation and Stress-Point Care. Nursing Research 24 (4):244–255, 1975.
31. Bloom L: Talking, Understanding and Thinking, In RL Schiefelbusch, LL Lloyd (eds): Language Perspectives: Acquisition, Retardation and Intervention. Baltimore, MD, University Park Press, 1974, p. 239.
32. Special Supplement: Educational Materials, Ross Laboratories Currents, 1983. Columbus, OH, Abbott Laboratories, pp. 1–3.
33. Klare GR: Assessing Readability. Reading Research Quarterly 10:62–102, 1974–1975.
34. Fry EE: A Readability Formula That Saves Time. Journal of Reading 11:513–516, 575–577, 1968.
35. Pohl ML: The Teaching Function of the Nurse Practitioner, ed 2. Dubuque, IA, Wm. C. Brown Co., Publishers, 1973, pp. 114–115.
36. Redman BK: The Process of Patient Teaching in Nursing, ed 4. St. Louis, C.V. Mosby Co., 1980, pp. 28–61.
37. Bille D: The Role of Body Image in Patient Compliance and Education. Heart and Lung 6 (1):143–148, 1977.
38. Peretz D: Reaction to Loss. In B. Schoenberg, A. Carr, et al. (eds): Loss and Grief: Psychological Management in Medical Practice. New York, Columbia University Press, 1970, pp. 20–36.
39. Wu R: Behavior in Illness. Englewood Cliffs, NJ, Prentice-Hall, Inc., 1973, pp. 5–16.
40. Ibid.
41. Ibid., pp. 157–175.
42. Seligman M: Helplessness. San Francisco, W.H. Freeman & Co., Publishers, 1975, pp. 123–127.
43. Rotter, JB: Generalized Expectancies for Internal Versus External Control of Reinforcement. Psychological Monographs, 80:40–42, 1966.
44. Rotter JB: Social Learning and Clinical Psychology. Englewood Cliffs, NJ, Prentice-Hall, Inc., 1954, pp. 125–135.
45. Phares EJ: The Locus of Control in Personality. Morristown, NJ, General Learning Press, 1976, pp. 205–217.
46. Schillinger FL: Locus of Control: Implications for Clinical Nursing Practice. Image 15 (2):58–63, 1983.
47. Jenny J: A Strategy for Patient Teaching. Journal of Advanced Nursing 3:347, 1978.
48. Ibid.
49. Clark AW: Understanding and Changing Attitudes. In I Erwin (ed): Health Education in Theory and Practice. Geneva, Switzerland, International Union Against Cancer, 1984, pp. 1–10.
50. Femea P: An Exploratory Study of the Relationship Among Religiosity and Preventive Health Attitudes in a Selected Population. Unpublished manuscript, Purdue University, 1982, p. 22.
51. Tripp-Reimer T: Retention of a Folk-Healing Practice (Matiasma) Among Four Generations of Urban Greek Immigrants. Nursing Research 32 (2):97–101, 1982.

52. Dicicco L, Apple D: Health Needs and Opinions of Older Adults. In D. Apple (ed): Sociological Studies of Health and Sickness. New York, McGraw-Hill Book Co., 1960, pp. 15–20.
53. Ireland LM (ed): Low Income Life Styles. Washington, DC, U.S. Government Printing Office, 1975, p. 11.
54. Deasy LE: Socioeconomic Status and Participation in the Poliomyelitis Vaccine Trial. In D. Apple (ed): Sociological Studies of Health and Sickness. New York, McGraw-Hill Book Co., 1960, pp. 35–41.
55. News for Nurses. American Journal of Nursing 83:860–863, 1983.
56. Johnson JE, Kirchhoff KT, Endress MP: Altering Children's Distress Behavior During Orthopedic Cast Removal. Nursing Research 24 (6):410, 1975.
57. Wolfer JA, Visintainer MA: Pediatric Surgical Patients' and Parents' Stress Responses and Adjustment as a Function of Psychologic Preparation and Stress-Point Care. Nursing Research 24 (4):244–255, 1975.
58. Meichenbaum DH, Bowers KS, Ross RS: A Behavioral Analysis of Teacher Expectancy Effect. Journal of Personality and Social Psychology 13:306–310, 1969.
59. Rosenthal R, Jacobson L: Pygmalion in the Classroom: Teacher Expectation and Pupils' Intellectual Development. New York, Holt, Rinehart & Winston, 1968, pp. 230–240.
60. McCarrell NS, Brooks PH: Mental Retardation: Comprehension Gone Awry. Research colloquium sponsored by the John F. Kennedy Center for Research on Education and Human Development, Nashville, TN, September 1975.
61. Ausubel DP: Educational Psychology: A Cognitive View. New York, Holt, Rinehart & Winston, 1964, p. 2.
62. Frederickson JW: Cost-based Pricing for Biocommunications Departments. Journal of Biocommunication 5(5):19–24, 1978.
63. Brett JL: How Much is a Nurse's Job Really Worth? American Journal of Nursing 83: 877–881, 1983.
64. Bandura A: Social Learning Theory. Englewood Cliffs, NJ, Prentice-Hall, Inc., 1977, pp. 10–20.
65. Redman BK: The Process of Patient Teaching in Nursing, ed 4. St. Louis, C.V. Mosby Co., 1980, pp. 117–118.
66. Rothkopf EZ: Structural Text Features and the Control of Processes in Learning From Written Materials. In JB Carroll, RO Freedle (eds): Language Comprehension and the Acquisition of Knowledge. Washington, DC, V.H. Winston & Sons, 1972, p. 21.
67. Danner FW: Children's Understanding of Intersentence Organization in the Recall of Short Description Passages. Journal of Educational Psychology 2 (4):174–183, 1976.
68. Moeser SD: Inferential Reasoning in Episodic Memory. Journal of Verbal Learning and Verbal Behavior 15 (5):193–212, 1976.
69. Haviland SE, Clark HH: What's New? Acquiring New Information as a Process in Comprehension. Journal of Verbal Learning and Verbal Behavior 13 (5):512–521, 1978.
70. Snow RE, Yalow E: Education and Intelligence. In RJ Sternberg (ed): Handbook of Human Intelligence. New York, Cambridge University Press, 1982, p. 569.
71. Jenny J: Strategy for Patient Teaching. Journal of Advanced Nursing 3:348, 1978.
72. Brown AL: Theories of Memory and the Problems of Development: Activity, Growth and Knowledge. In LS Cermak, F Craik (eds): Levels of Processing and Human Memory. Hillsdale, NJ, Lawrence Erlbaum Associates Inc., 1978, pp. 255–257.
73. Flavell JH, Wellman HM: Metamemory. In RV Kail, Jr, JW Hagen (eds): Perspectives

on the Development of Memory and Cognition. Hillsdale, NJ, Lawrence Erlbaum Associates, Inc. 1977, p. 300.
74. Redman BK: The Process of Patient Teaching in Nursing, ed 4. St. Louis, C.V. Mosby Co., 1980, p. 196.
75. Nitsch KE: Structuring Decontextualized Forms of Knowledge. Unpublished doctoral dissertation, Vanderbilt University, 1977, p. 47.
76. Redman BK: The Process of Patient Teaching in Nursing, ed 4. St. Louis, C.V. Mosby Co., 1980, p. 196.
77. Bransford JD: Human Cognition. Belmont, CA, Wadsworth Publishing Co., 1979, p. 8.
78. Knowles M: The Adult Learner: A Neglected Species. Houston, TX, Gulf Publishing Co. Book Division, 1978, pp. 198–203.
79. Doering SG, Entwisle DR: Preparation During Pregnancy and Ability to Cope with Labor and Delivery. American Journal of Orthopsychiatry 45:825–837, 1975.
80. Cronenwett LR, Newmark LL: Father's Response to Childbirth. Nursing Research 23: 210–216, 1974.
81. Gayton R: A Comparison of Natural and Non-natural Childbirth Fathers on State-Trait Anxiety, Attitude and Self-Concept. Unpublished doctoral dissertation, U.S. International University, 1975. In Dissertation Abstracts International 36:1406, 1975.
82. Tanzer DRW: The Psychology of Pregnancy and Childbirth: An Investigation of Natural Childbirth. Unpublished doctoral dissertation, Brandeis University, 1967. In Dissertation Abstracts International, 28:2615, 1967.
83. Moore D: Prepared Childbirth and Marital Satisfaction During the Antepartum and Postpartum Periods. Nursing Research 32:73–79, 1983.
84. Lindeman CA, Van Aernam B: Nursing Intervention with the Pre-Surgical Patient: The Effects of Structured and Unstructured Preoperative Teaching. Nursing Research 20 (4):319–382, 1971.
85. Lindeman CA: Nursing Intervention with the Presurgical Patient: Effectiveness and Efficiency of Group and Individual Preoperative Teaching—Phase Two. Nursing Research 21 (3):196–209, 1972.
86. Fortin F, Kirouac S: A Randomized Controlled Trial of Preoperative Patient Education, International Journal of Nursing Studies 13:11–24, 1976.
87. Felton G, Huss K, et al.: Preoperative Nursing Intervention with the Patient for Surgery: Outcomes of Three Alternative Approaches. International Journal of Nursing Studies 13:83–96, 1976.
88. Johnson JE: Effects of Structuring Patients' Expectation on Their Reactions to Threatening Events. Nursing Research 21:492–499, 1972.
89. Johnson JE, Rice VH, et al.: Sensory Information Instruction in a Coping Strategy and Recovery from Surgery. Research in Nursing and Health 1:4–17, 1978.
90. Hartfield MT, Cason C, Cason GF: Effects of Information About a Threatening Procedure on Patients' Expectations and Emotional Distress. Nursing Research 31:202–206, 1982.
91. Padilla GV, Grant MM, et al.: Distress Reduction and the Effects of Preparatory Teaching Films and Patient Control. Research in Nursing and Health 4:375–387, 1981.
92. Wolfer JA, Visintainer MA: Pediatric Surgical Patients' and Parents' Stress Responses and Adjustment as a Function of Psychologic Preparation and Stress-Point Care. Nursing Research 24 (4):244–255, 1975.
93. McGrath MM: Group Preparation of Pediatric Surgical Patients. Image 11:52–62, 1979.

94. Wells N: The Effect of Relaxation on Postoperative Muscle Tension and Pain. Nursing Research 31 (4):236–238, 1982.
95. Felton G, Lotas M, Eastman D: A Tool for Research in the Clinical Setting: Outcomes of Educational Programs for Stoma Clients. Unpublished monograph, Nursing Research: A monograph for Non-nurse Researchers, The University of Iowa, 1983, pp. 6–28.
96. Sechrist KR: The Effect of Repetitive Teaching on Patient's Knowledge About Drugs to be Taken at Home. International Journal of Nursing Studies 16 (1):51–58, 1979.
97. Darr MS, Self TH, et al.: Content and Retention Evaluation of an Audiovisual Patient-Education Program on Bronchodilators. American Journal of Hospital Pharmacy 38: 672–675, 1981.
98. Sly MR: Evaluation of a Sound-slide Program for Patient Education. Annals of Allergy 34 (2):94–97, 1975.
99. Alkhateeb W, Lukeroth CJ, Riggs M: A Comparison of Three Educational Techniques Used in Veneral Disease Clinics. Public Health Reports 90 (2):159–164, 1975.
100. Wiley K: Effects of a Self-directed Learning Project and Preference for Structure on Self-directed Learning Readiness. Nursing Research 32 (3):181–185, 1983.
101. Milazzo V: A Study of the Difference in Health Knowledge Gained Through Formal and Informal Teaching. Heart Lung 9 (6):1079–1082, 1980.
102. Murdough CL: Effects of Nurses' Knowledge of Teaching-Learning Principles on Knowledge of Coronary Care Unit Learners. Heart Lung 9 (6):1073–1078, 1980.
103. Scott DW: Anxiety, Critical Thinking and Information Processing During and After Breast Biopsy. Nursing Research 32 (1):24–28, 1983.
104. Frantz RA: Selecting Media for Patient Education. Topics in Clinical Nursing 10 (4):77–83, 1980.
105. Stein D: Selecting and Evaluating Media for Patient Education. The Journal of Biocommunication 22 (3):23–25, 1979.

BIBLIOGRAPHY

Adam D, Wright AS: Dissonance in Nurse and Patient Evaluations of the Effectiveness of a Patient-Teaching Program. Nursing Outlook 82 (2):132–136, 1982.

Alkhateeb W, Lukeroth CJ, Riggs M: A Comparison of Three Educational Techniques Used in Venereal Disease Clinics. Public Health Reports 90 (2):159–164, 1975.

Bartlett R, Gazzaniga A, Geraghty TR: Respiratory Maneuvers to Prevent Postoperative Pulmonary Complications. Journal American Medical Association 224 (7):1017-1021, 1973.

Bille D: The Role of Body Image in Patient Compliance and Education. Heart Lung 6 (1): 143–148, 1977.

Bloom B (ed): Taxonomy of Educational Objectives: The Classification of Educational Goals. Handbook I: Cognitive Domain. New York, David McKay Co., Inc., 1956, pp. 201-207.

Bransford JD: Human Cognition. Belmont, CA, Wadsworth Publishing Co., 1979.

Brett JL: How Much is a Nurse's Job Really Worth? American *Journal of Nursing* 83:877–881, 1983.

Cronenwett LR, Newmark LL: Father's Response to Childbirth. Nursing Research 23 (3):210–216, 1974.

Green LW: Evaluation and Measurement: Some Dilemmas for Health Education. American Journal of Public Health 67 (2):155–161, 1977.

Hartfield MT, Cason C, Cason GF: Effects of Information About a Threatening Procedure on Patients' Expectations and Emotional Distress. Nursing Research 31 (4):202–206, 1982.

Jenny J: A Strategy for Patient Teaching. Journal of Advanced Nursing 3:341–348, 1978.

Johnson JE, Kirchhoff KT, Endress MP: Altering Children's Distress Behavior During Orthopedic Cast Removal. Nursing Research 24:404–410, 1975.

Johnson JE: Effects of Structuring Patients' Expectations on Their Reactions to Threatening Events. Nursing Research 21:492–499, 1972.

Johnson JE, Rice VH, et al.: Sensory Information, Instruction in a Coping Strategy, and Recovery from Surgery. Research in Nursing and Health 1:4–17, 1978.

Knowles M: The Adult Learner: A Neglected Species. Houston, TX, Gulf Publishing Co. Book Division, 1978, pp. 198–203.

Lindeman CA, Stetzer SL: Effect of Preoperative Visits by Operating Room Nurses. Nursing Research 22:4–15, 1973.

Lindeman CA, Van Aernam B: Nursing Intervention with the Pre-Surgical Patient: The Effects of Structured and Unstructured Preoperative Teaching. Nursing Research 20:319–382, 1971.

Lindeman CA: Nursing Intervention with the Presurgical Patient: Effectiveness and Efficiency of Group and Individual Preoperative Teaching—Phase Two. Nursing Research 21: 196–209, 1972.

McGrath, MM: Group Preparation of Pediatric Surgical Patients. Image 11:52–62, 1979.

Milazzo V: A Study of the Difference in Health Knowledge Gained Through Formal and Informal Teaching. Heart and Lung 9 (6):1079–1082, 1980.

Moore D: Prepared Childbirth and Marital Satisfaction During the Antepartum and Postpartum Periods. Nursing Research 32:73–79, 1983.

Murdough CL: Effects of Nurses' Knowledge of Teaching-Learning Principles on Knowledge of Coronary Care Units Learners. Heart and Lung 9 (6):1073–1078, 1980.

National League for Nursing. Patient Education (NLN Publication No. 20–1633). New York, The League, 1978, p. 8.

News for Nurses. American Journal of Nursing 83:860–863, 1983.

Padilla GV, Grant, MM, et al.: Distress Reduction and the Effects of Preparatory Teaching Films and Patient Control. Research in Nursing and Health 4:375–387, 1981.

Redman BK: The Process of Patient Teaching in Nursing, ed 4. St. Louis: C.V. Mosby Co., 1980.

Schillinger FL: Locus of Control: Implications for Clinical Nursing Practice. Image 15:58–63, 1983.

Scott DW: Anxiety, Critical Thinking and Information Processing During and After Breast Biopsy. Nursing Research 32:24–28, 1983.

Sechrist KR: The Effect of Repetitive Teaching on Patient's Knowledge About Drugs to be Taken at Home. International Journal of Nursing Studies 16 (1):51–58, 1979.

Sly RM: Evaluation of a Sound-Slide Program for Patient Education. Annals of Allergy 34 (2):94–97, 1975.

Snow, RE, Yalow E: Education and Intelligence. In RJ Sternberg (ed): Handbook of Human Intelligence. New York, Cambridge University Press, 1982, pp. 493–571.

Tripp-Reimer T: Retention of a Folk-Healing Practice (Matiasma) Among Four Generations of Urban Greek Immigrants. Nursing Research 32:97–101, 1983.

Wells N: The Effect of Relaxation on Postoperative Muscle Tension and Pain. Nursing Research 31:236–238, 1982.

Wiley K: Effects of a Self-Directed Learning Project and Preference for Structure on Self-directed Learning Readiness. Nursing Research 32:181–185, 1983.

Wolfer JA, Visintainer MA: Pediatric Surgical Patients' and Parents' Stress Responses and Adjustment as a Function of Psychologic Preparation and Stress-Point Care. Nursing Research 24:244–255, 1975.

Wu R: Behavior in Illness. Englewood Cliffs, NJ, Prentice-Hall, Inc., 1973.

6

Evaluation

Mark A. Albanese and Craig L. Gjerde

OBJECTIVES

Upon completion of this chapter, you will be able to:

1. Relate relevant issues in evaluation to the role of the nurse as evaluator of teaching, learning, materials, and programs.
2. Compare three basic types of evaluation data: needs assessment, formative evaluation, and summative evaluation.
3. Distinguish between normative- and criterion-referenced interpretation of assessment results.
4. Identify specific types of evaluation instruments and test items used to measure learner knowledge, skills, attitudes, and perceptions and their distinguishing characteristics.
5. Compare the characteristics, purposes, advantages, and limitations of multiple-choice items, supply-type items (open-response), simulations, oral examinations, and anecdotal reports.
6. Compare Likert-type and semantic differential items.
7. Identify three methods used to assess skills and their distinguishing characteristics.
8. Identify sources of error in a score derived from a multiple-choice test, an essay examination, an oral examination, and clinical ratings.
9. Distinguish between a checklist and a rating scale.
10. Relate the issue of grading to that of evaluation.
11. Determine how to use evaluation data as a means of providing feedback to the learner.
12. Cite precautions that should be taken in scoring essay tests.
13. Distinguish between a knowledge and an attitude or perception item.
14. Define cumulative assessment, interference, perception, attitude, and program evaluation.
15. Relate the concept of subjectivity to the issue of evaluation.

16. Relate the usefulness of anecdotal records in evaluation of learners.
17. List areas where students are not the best source of teacher-evaluation data.
18. Determine decisions that can be made on the basis of program evaluation.

INTRODUCTION

This final chapter concerns evaluation as it relates to the activities of the nurse-teacher. Evaluation should be an integral part of the nurse-teacher's activities. It is through conducting evaluation that nurse-teachers can determine where to focus their efforts and improve teaching. This chapter is divided into five major sections. The first deals with general issues that cut across all aspects of evaluation. The next four sections deal, in sequence, with learner evaluation, teacher evaluation, materials evaluation, and program evaluation.

GENERAL ISSUES

Before describing the various types of evaluation, it is necessary to address some broad issues. First, various types of evaluation data will be described, followed by a brief discussion of several major issues in evaluation.

Types of Evaluation Data

There are three basic types of evaluation information that can be collected: (1) needs assessment data, (2) formative evaluation data, and (3) summative evaluation data. *Needs assessment data* are collected prior to a teaching or learning experience and are intended to establish the current status of the learner(s) or the educational needs of the learner(s). These data are used either as a baseline against which later evaluation results can be compared or to develop educational experiences that meet learner needs.

Formative evaluation data are collected during the development stages of a learning experience while things are in a state of flux. These data give feedback for improvement, whether it be to a program developer to improve a program, to learners to improve their learning, or to a teacher to improve the instruction provided.

Summative evaluation data are collected after the development of the learning experience is complete. The data are used to judge the relative merit of the outcomes of the learning experience, to judge whether an educational program should be offered again, to assign grades to a learner, or to determine whether a teacher should be promoted.

Major Evaluation Issues

There are three major issues in evaluation that warrant discussion. First, what is the relationship between a score derived from an assessment and the actual quality assumed to be measured? Second, how often and when should assessments be made? Finally, what are the differences between a normative-referenced interpretation of assessment results and a criterion-referenced interpretation of assessment results?

The Relationship Between an Assessment Result and the Actual Quality Being Measured. It is absolutely essential to understand the relationship between a score and the actual quality one is attempting to measure. In most cases, knowledge and motor skills are the main focus. In some cases, however, attitudes, preferences, or even feelings may be of interest. Note that with the exception of motor skills, none of these characteristics are directly measurable. For example, there is no dipstick in a learner's brain that can be taken out to determine whether the learner is sufficiently full of knowledge. Similarly, there is no known kind of meter we can attach to learners that will tell us when they have adopted a particular attitude we wish them to. These qualities are not observable. The only way we know such qualities even exist is by making inferences from the learner's behavior. Unfortunately, in most situations, learners are unlikely to exhibit spontaneous behavior that can be considered as evidence that learning has occurred; and even if they do, it is likely that the nurse-evaluator will not be there to observe.

Because of the lack of readily observable behaviors, one must often *contrive* a situation in which the desired behaviors can be exhibited and assessed. The situation may be a multiple-choice test, an essay examination, a questionnaire, a performance rating, or some other assessment instrument. The important things to remember are that the situation is contrived and that in developing the contrived situation, the evaluator is making certain assumptions. For instance, if a multiple-choice test is administered, some underlying assumptions are that the examinees can read and that they have sufficient eye-hand coordination to either fill in the blanks on the answer sheet or circle the appropriate response. Although the ability to read and low-level eye-hand coordination are important skills, they are not those that are typically of interest on a multiple-choice test. These are prerequisite skills that the examinees must possess in order to have the ability to demonstrate knowledge. Examinees who have not mastered these prerequisite skills will be hampered to some degree in demonstarting knowledge on the test.

With very few exceptions, evaluation procedures require that the learner possess certain prerequisite skills. If learners lack the prerequisites, their performance on an assessment will be impaired and the assessment will be flawed. Thus, an assessment is only a *method of estimating* what a learner has learned, and as with any estimate, it is very often imprecise.

The prerequisite skills required for an assessment can have an impact on the results. Take for instance, the ability to read as a prerequisite to performance on a multiple-choice test. Let's assume two groups of learners who acquired the same amount from a learning experience take a test; however, one of the learner groups happens to be composed of slower readers than the other. Furthermore, suppose that the test is sufficiently long that even the faster readers will have trouble finishing in the time allotted for the test. The slower readers will not be able to finish the test, forcing them to either guess at or leave blank those items not reached. In this instance, the faster readers' test scores will be more representative of their abilities than those of the slow readers because the slow readers did not have sufficient opportunity to demonstrate their ability on all items.

Different evaluation procedures applied to the same event often yield different results. One reason for this circumstance is that different evaluation procedures may depend upon different prerequisite skills. A second reason is that any single assessment provides only a partial picture of what a learner has acquired from a learning experience. Each evaluation instrument contains only a sample of the different kinds of informaton that could be evaluated. It may be, for example, that a learner who knows 80 percent of the content happens to be particularly unlucky and the content selected for the test happens to emphasize the 20 percent he or she does not know.

Not only is the content of an assessment a sample, but the time at which the assessment is made is also only one of many times that could have been chosen for behavior sampling. As a result, an assessment gives only a "snapshot" of what the learner can demonstrate at one particular time. Thus, evaluation results are influenced by factors that may cause them to be faulty, including inaccurate prerequisite skills assumptions, unrepresentative sampling of content, and time of assessment.

Every measurement of learner behavior provides only an estimate of the quality one is attempting to measure. As with any estimate, it is likely to have errors. It should be evident from this brief discussion that every method of measuring a learner's ability has its own unique idiosyncrasies that color the results. The ideal situation would be to have an estimate of learner performance that is not dependent on the method by which the quality is measured. One way of approaching this ideal is to use several different types of measurement. For instance, in addition to administering a multiple-choice test, one might also use essays, oral examinations, case presentations, or simulations. Each of these measures is imperfect and results may be inconsistent, yet a composite of all these measures is more likely to provide an accurate estimate of a learner's true level of achievement than will any single measure.

How Often and When Assessments Should Be Made. Because the timing of an evaluation can have a critical effect on the results, it is important to understand four issues related to time. First, what effect does the time of day or day of the week have on student performance? Second, how often should learners be evaluated? Third, should assessments be cumulative? Fourth, how long after a learning experience should an assessment occur?

Effect of Time on Performance. The particular time of day or day of the week at which an assessment occurs is usually irrelevant to the purpose of the assessment, but it may have a significant effect on student performance. An assessment occurs at one specific point in time—for example, nine o'clock to ten o'clock on a Friday morning—but we are not usually interested in knowing how a learner will perform on a measure at just this particular time. More often, we are interested in how a learner will perform after instruction over a range of times, for instance, one to five days following completion of instruction. The extent to which a learner's performance might vary over time is usually considered as part of the error associated with the measurement. The error associated with a measurement, or error of measurement as psychometricians call it, refers to the multitude of irrelevant factors that can influence an assessment score so that the score represents, in part, factors other than the learner's true achievement level.

Research on learning has documented that forgetting occurs fairly rapidly after many types of learning experiences, unless the information is reinforced. Thus, comparing the performances of two learners who were assessed at different times may show differences that are more related to when the assessment is made than any real difference between the two learners. For example, suppose one learner group is assessed three days after a learning experience and another learner group is assessed five days afterwards. If no opportunity exists for reinforcement, the second group will be disadvantaged because learners have two more days to forget the content. On the other hand, if some form of reinforcement of learning is available, like additional study time, the first group will have only three days to reinforce learning, while the second will have five days. Thus, if the evaluation goal is to compare learners' performance with peers, every effort should be made to conduct assessments at the same time.

Frequency of Evaluation. How often assessments are made depends to a large extent on what is to be done with the results of the assessment. Two types of use are: (1) to give feedback to the learner, and (2) to make decisions about the degree to which the learner has achieved the goals of the learning experience. If the purpose of the evaluation is to give feedback, it will be useful to conduct evaluations at several key points throughout the learning experience. For a semester course this might translate into daily or weekly quizzes or tests given throughout the semester—maybe spaced every three weeks. In a clinical experience this might mean frequent feedback sessions (daily or weekly) with a clinical preceptor. The primary goal of evaluation as a form of feedback is to make constructive suggestions for improvement. The evaluation that is performed should provide the details necessary for the learner to improve performance and should occur throughout the learning process.

It is important to emphasize that for feedback purposes the consequences of measurement error are not usually very serious. Thus, a formative evaluation need not be as precise as a summative evaluation. For example, students may be incorrectly told they do not adequately understand some concept. If the students do understand it, they can ignore the feedback. Of more consequence is the situation where feedback fails to identify a concept the student does not understand and thus the student is led to a false sense of security. This type of error is most likely to occur with multiple-choice items or true-false items, because of the distinct possibility of guessing the correct answer. Also, if many measurements are made during the learning experience, the effects of errors affecting a single measurement will be minimized.

If an evaluation is to be used for the sole purpose of determining whether or not a learner has achieved the goals of a learning experience, it should be very precise. Some decisions that might be based on this type of evaluation include whether or not a learner passes or fails a course, whether or not a learner has to repeat a clinical experience, or whether a learner should continue a program of study. These decisions are very important and will have a substantial impact on the future of the learner. The more important the decision to be made on the basis of the assessment, the more important it is that measurement error be minimized.

Under ideal circumstances, one would measure using many different methods at many different times so as to keep potential errors related to time and method from clouding the evaluation. This is rarely possible, however. For practical reasons, a compromise must be made. For instance, an instructor may decide that such precautions will be taken only on the final assessment at the conclusion of the learning experience. This final assessment might have several parts, such as a written test, clinical ratings, and perhaps an oral examination of some type. Such an assessment is sometimes made in clinical situations.

There are several reasons why the end-of-learning evaluation is the most commonly performed assessment. First, an entire learning experience can be assessed at one time. Second, many clinical learning experiences are of limited time duration, some as short as one or two weeks, and to perform multiple evaluations in such a short time makes many teachers feel uncomfortable with the quality of the evaluations. Third, conducting evaluations is very time-consuming, and most teachers do not like to take time away from teaching and other responsibilities to make evaluations unless the results will be worth the time investment. End-of-course evaluations seem to provide the most valuable data, since one can assess what the learner has achieved from the entire learning experience.

This is not to say that midcourse or interim assessments do not provide useful data for assessing the degree to which a learner has achieved the goals of a learning experience. On the contrary, interim assessments can be extremely valuable. The amount of information that can be assessed at any given time is usually limited. Given the vast amount of knowledge that can be learned in any given learning experience, the amount of time available for a single assessment, even a final one, is usually too limited to do justice to the entire event. Even if there are no administrative limitations on the time allotted for a final assessment, the learner can maintain total alertness for only a limited time before fatigue sets in. Having interim assessments spaced throughout the learning experience allows the nurse-teacher to assess students over more information in a manner that keeps the length of any single assessment sufficiently short so that fatigue is not a debilitating factor. In addition, if properly done, interim assessments can provide feedback to the student as well as estimate what the learner has learned.

It should be noted that using the same assessment to provide feedback and as a basis for assigning grades requires the exercise of care. When learners are graded, they are not likely to do anything that would suggest they do not understand or to admit that they don't know an answer. And assessments of all kinds—fallible as even the best of them are—may not precisely indicate the learner's lack of understanding in a given area. For example, on a multiple-choice test, two students may select the same wrong answer for completely different reasons. One student might have selected the response because of misreading the item, while another may have a fundamental lack of knowledge. Thus, if feedback is to be made as useful as possible, learners should be partners in the learning process. They should be able to ask questions without fear that asking a "dumb" question will be damaging.

While this type of atmosphere can best be established in a nongraded situation, it may be possible to accomplish it under graded test conditions. One way to promote this type of exchange is to use the assessment itself as a forum for discussion. Under the best circumstances this might be done individually with students. Given the time constraints most of us are under, however, it is most likely to be done in groups. The disadvantage of group feedback is that the students who do not do well may be reluctant to enter into discussion for fear of revealing their ignorance. This keeps the feedback from being as meaningful as it could be for the learners who need help the most. A compromise situation might be to have group feedback sessions for all students and individual feedback sessions for only those learners who demonstrate the poorest performance. The individual sessions should be arranged discreetly to avoid any embarrassment to the student.

It is important to remember that the purpose of individual feedback sessions is to benefit the student. The focus should be on the specific behaviors demonstrated by the student. One might say, "You answered question 9 incorrectly; do you understand why your answer is wrong and why the keyed answer is correct?" All generalizations about personal characteristics should be avoided. It would be inappropriate to say, "Your performance obviously suggests you did not study," or, "Your performance indicates you were too lazy to study." Such statements do not promote an open dialogue. It is better to adopt the position that you are on the learner's side and want to help.

Additional factors to consider in determining how many assessments to make and when to place assessments during the learning program include making the assessment fit the information needs. An assessment that does not give you the information you need is worthless. If, for example, the purpose of the learning event is to expose learners to large amounts of content rather than a thorough learning of a more limited amount of information, the evaluation should reflect this purpose. Second, make certain the assessment results are worth the time and effort invested, since class time spent evaluating students is class time during which students are not being exposed to new information. Also, evaluations usually require a substantial amount of time to construct, score, and record. Finally, if the evaluation is going to be instrumental in determining whether or not a student will have to repeat a course or lesson or be prematurely discharged from the educational institution, the measures must be very precise.

Cumulative Assessments. A cumulative assessment covers all content encountered since the beginning of a course of study. Thus, information previously tested would also be covered in subsequent tests. An advantage of a cumulative assessment is that it encourages learners to review throughout the learning experience. Earlier content is reinforced through repeated study. A problem with cumulative assessment is that there may not be sufficient time available to test both review material and new material adequately. As mentioned earlier, even if there is not a definite limit on the amount of assessment time, fatigue will impose limits. It should be noted that in the specific case of clinical rating, cumulative assessments are not recommended, because clinical ratings are a highly subjective assessment that one strives to make as objective as possible. If raters incorporate their previous ratings into subsequent ratings of students, the process would become even more subjective. The issue of how much weight to assign previous assessments in the process of arriving at a new rating is a further complication.

When an Assessment Should Occur. In a classroom experience, it is common for the assessment to occur at the earliest opportunity after the content to be tested is completed. Usually, learners have an opportunity to study information or practice skills before they are tested. A minimum of new material or no new material is covered before the assessment. This type of situation is probably the most desirable. If new content is covered before the assessment, students may either postpone studying the new material or skip classes to study. Even if students conscientiously attempt to keep up with their study of the new content, it may not necessarily be to their advantage because of a phenomenon called interference. In interference, the new material becomes confused with the old material, causing a decline in performance. Interference has been mostly studied in the context of simple recall, so it may not necessarily cause student scores to decline. In fact, if the new information builds on the old, the new may enable student to better understand concepts. It is not always possible to know in advance, however, if the new material will promote better understanding or cause some temporary interference. It is probably safest to assess before proceeding to new content, to avoid the possibility that interference may occur and avoid making students choose between learning new material or preparing for an assessment.

Normative- versus Criterion-Referenced Interpretation of Assessment Results. There are two major approaches to interpreting assessment results. The first approach, norm-referenced (also known as grading on a curve), is probably the most common. Most standardized tests are norm-referenced. A norm-referenced interpretation focuses on how learners' results compare with those of peers. The results of such assessments are usually reported in terms of the percentage of students who received lower scores. In order to enable the assessment to discriminate as finely as possible among the different learners, the assessment instrument is sometimes built specifically to do just that. Once an assessment instrument is used, statistics can be computed that will guide the development of an instrument that is able to make fine distinctions between learners.

Normative assessments work best when used to make fixed-quota decisions. A fixed-quota decision is one in which there are more individuals wishing to be admitted to a program than there are openings. Admission to nursing college is a good example of a fixed-quota decision. The goal of the assessment is then to identify the very best applicants. Normative assessments also work well when discriminations among students must be made to assign grades and there is a desire to give only a limited number of students each grade.

The second approach to interpreting assessment results is the criterion-referenced approach. A minimum competency test is an example of a criterion-referenced interpretation of a test score. In a criterion-referenced interpretation, the focus is on the performance level of the learner. How well a learner's peers perform is not pertinent. One critical element of a criterion-referenced assessment is that some preestablished performance level (sometimes referred to as a cutting score) is set as the criterion for learners to reach. The decisions made on the basis of criterion-referenced assessments usually are of the yes/no variety. Examples of some types of these decisions are competent versus incompetent, satisfactory versus unsatisfactory, pass versus fail. The decisions are very important and are likely to have a major bearing on the future of the learner. Because of this, the accuracy of the cutting score becomes a critical issue.

There are a number of methods for setting cutting scores on a criterion-referenced assessment. Some, like the Nedelsky method, are limited to use with assessment instruments in which the learner must select a response from a fixed number of choices—for example, a multiple-choice test. Others, such as the Angoff procedure, can be used with a broader assortment of assessment instruments. It is beyond the scope of this chapter to deal with these procedures in depth. But it is important to note that there are problems with each of the methods used to set cutting scores. If the decisions to be based on a criterion-referenced assessment are very important or if there is a potential for litigation to result, an experienced measurement expert should be consulted to assist in determining cutting scores.

Which is better, a norm-referenced or a criterion-referenced assessment? This is a controversy that has raged for years. Luckily, there is no absolute reason to adhere totally to one or the other approach, and they can be combined. For instance, a test might have two parts. The first part would consist of items testing fundamental concepts in which a criterion-referenced interpretation could reasonably be made. A pass in this part of the test would guarantee the student a passing grade. The second part of the test would be either mandatory or optional, and would be used to assign grades beyond minimum pass (A's, B's, and C's). Items in this latter part would be more discriminating then items in the first part.

SUMMARY

Evaluation is conducted to ascertain the learner's current level of knowledge and learning needs, to give feedback to improve learner achievement, to improve teaching effectiveness, and to judge learning and teaching outcomes. Because it is difficult to observe most expected behaviors, contrived situations are used for assessment purposes. Contrived evaluative situations presume certain prerequisites, contain only a sampling of information, and are conducted at a particular point in time; hence they are imprecise measurements of the qualities being measured. It is recommended that several different methods of measurement be used to estimate level of achievement accurately.

If learners are to be compared with one another on the basis of an assessment result, they should be assessed at the same time. Differences in assessment time may result in an unfair advantage to some. If the assessment results are to be used for the purpose of giving feedback to the learner, efforts should be made to have such assessments conducted at several key points throughout the learning experience and results should be as rich in detail as possible; errors of measurement, if not exceedingly misleading, are usually tolerable. If the assessment results are to be used for summative evaluation purposes, assessments should be as precise as possible. Practical constraints are likely to result in attempts to use the same assessments for both formative and summative purposes. Care should be exercised under these conditions, as summative assessments are likely to dampen a learner's willingness to openly discuss misunderstandings. Type and timing of assessments should be matched with the purpose for conducting the assessment.

Cumulative assessment measures assimilate both old and new information. It encourages continual review and information synthesis. Time may be a constraint, and fatigue may influence results. Cumulative assessment is not recommended for clinical evaluation ratings.

Learning should be assessed soon after completion of a learning event. Interference may result when new content is introduced before assessment of old content, unless new information builds on previous information.

There are two major approaches to interpreting assessment results. A normative interpretation compares students' scores with peers and is best used when there is a need to limit the number of students receiving a particular grade. A criterion-referenced interpretation focuses solely on the level of performance students exhibit. While a criterion-referenced approach is very appealing for determining whether students have mastered basic skills, there are difficulties in establishing a cutting score. Combining normative- and criterion-referenced approaches may be a better alternative to selecting one or the other for assessment purposes.

LEARNER EVALUATION

Learner evaluation focuses on the learner. Nurse-teachers are basically concerned with four types of learner groups: undergraduate nursing students, graduate nursing students, practicing nurses participating in continuing nursing education (CNE) or staff development, and client education. Each of these groups has unique characteristics that should be considered in the design of any type of evaluation. While reference will be made to specific characteristics of each learner group, we will focus on topics applicable to all learner groups while emphasizing undergraduate nursing students. The reason for targeting this group is that it is one of the largest groups and the approaches and methods used to evaluate undergraduate learners are most diverse.

The goal of learner evaluation is usually to find out to what degree learners have attained the knowledge, attitudes, or skills emphasized in a learning experience. The evaluation can occur prior to, during, or after a learning experience. If it occurs before the learning experience, the results can be used to target the learning experience to meet students' learning needs (needs assessment), or to serve as a base line for contrasting subsequent evaluations. Evaluations conducted during the learning experience can provide feedback to learners on their progress toward meeting the objectives of the learning experience (formative evaluation) or to make judgments, for the record, of the degree to which learners have met the objectives of a learning experience (summative evaluation).

Types of Assessment Instruments/Items

There are various types of assessment instruments and items used to measure learning. The term instrument is used to refer to all the different methods of assessing a learner's achievement. Just as a nurse uses a blood pressure cuff and a sphygmomanometer as instruments to take a blood pressure reading, tests, rating scales, and simulations are some of the instruments used to assess learner knowledge, attitudes, and skills. In discussing each type of instrument, special consideration will be given to its advantages and disadvantages.

Instruments Used to Measure Knowledge. There are many different varieties of instruments used to assess knowledge. Written tests and oral examinations are two.

Written Tests. The most common type of written test used to assess knowledge is the multiple-choice examination. It is used in admissions tests as well as certification procedures for health professionals and is one of the most common forms of evaluation in the classroom. The single biggest advantage of the multiple-choice-test format is that a large amount of content can be tested in a relatively short amount of time. A second advantage is that the test items can be machine scored. Machine scoring is a considerable convenience, since it shortens grading time, improves grading accuracy, and reduces the cost of grading. Also, when items are machine scored, the questions can be graded objectively. Correct answers can be specified in advance, minimizing the possibility of subjective bias entering into the scoring of any particular student's response.

The disadvantages of multiple-choice tests are that, first, a multiple-choice test is a fairly artificial type of assessment for an area such as nursing. The procedure bears relatively little resemblance to the complex tasks nurses will perform. A second limitation is that multiple-choice items require only that the examinee select the correct response from a limited number of options. In actual nursing practice, it is unlikely the nurse will select a course of action in this manner. A third limitation is that good multiple-choice items are difficult to construct. It often takes even professional item writers an hour or more to write one *good* item. Measurement texts offer fairly lengthy lists of guidelines to be followed in constructing multiple-choice test items.[1] These guidelines are based, in part, on extensive research. A final limitation of multiple-choice items is that there is a certain possibility that one will answer an item correctly by guessing. Thus, just because a learner answers an item correctly does not necessarily mean that the correct answer is known.

A second type of written test is composed of open-response or supply-type items. The feature that characterizes these items is that the learner must supply the answer to the item, as opposed to selecting an answer from a list. There are three basic varieties of open-response items: fill-in-the-blank, short answer, and essay. Each of these varieties has distinguishing features. The question part (also referred to as the stem) of a *fill-in-the-blank* item is similar to a multiple-choice item stem. The primary difference between the two is that instead of selecting one choice from a limited number of options, the learner supplies a very short response (one word or two). This type of item could be created from a well-focused multiple-choice item by simply eliminating the options and having students provide the correct answer.

The short-answer essay consists simply of a question to which the learner must provide a written response. The length of the response, however, is restricted—usually to no more than a paragraph. The question for a short-answer essay will usually be broader than that of a fill-in-the-blank item.

The essay is similar to the short answer essay except no restriction is placed on the length of learner's response to the question or issue. Essay questions are usually even broader than those used in the short-answer essay.

The open-response-type item has several strengths. Because the learner supplies the answer, this type of item does not have the built-in chance-success problem that haunts the multiple-choice item. Also, since the student must construct the response, it is possible to obtain an idea of how well the learner can express a thought in writing. Not surprisingly, the supply-type item also has problems. If the learner happens to have poor handwriting, deciphering the response can be troublesome for the scorer. Also, if a learner provides an answer that the nurse-teacher has not anticipated and that may be partially correct, a bit of subjectivity may enter into the scoring system as the response is incorporated into the scoring system. Another problem is that students may not spell words correctly. This may lead the scorer to mark the item incorrectly. If there are words that are very similar in spelling to the correct answer but are incorrect, this can be a serious problem. For instance, a devious student might take advantage of the system and purposefully misspell words in the hope of arguing, after the fact, that the answer was correct. Thus, the scorer can spend a lot of time trying to make difficult handwriting and spelling judgments—a thankless task.

If supply-type items are to be used, it is very important that scoring be as objective as possible. One method of promoting objectivity is to *specify in advance* what responses will be accepted as correct. In the case of partially correct responses, it should be specified in advance how much credit each response is worth. No matter how thorough one is, however, there is always a possibility that there will be other options that students may come up with that will be partially correct and will need to be incorporated into the scoring mechanism.

To minimize problems in scoring supply-type items, it is advisable to have a *prespecified checklist of the responses that will be given credit* and the amount of credit each will receive. This will make scoring easier and reduce the number of subjective scoring errors. In addition, the name of the learner should be covered in advance by someone other than the scorer to reduce the potential for bias. This can be easily accomplished by taping a piece of paper over the name.

Although the different open-response type items have many things in common, they each have unique features that will govern when each is best to use. The primary advantage of the fill-in-the-blank item is that it can be used to sample a range of content approaching the breadth of that sampled in a multiple-choice test. The increased time necessary to write in rather than select the response will reduce the number of items that can be administered in a given time period. Fill-in-the-blank items are also easier to construct than multiple-choice items, because plausible incorrect choices are not needed. Because fill-in-the-blank questions tend to be more focused than essay and short-answer essay questions, they are usually easier to score.

There are times, however, when the nurse-teacher may feel it is very important to learn how well the learner can express a thought in writing. Under these circumstances the essay or short-answer essay is best to use. Although essay and short-answer essay items tend to be easier to construct than fill-in-the-blank items, they are usually more difficult and more time-consuming to score. In addition, the number of items one has in any supply-type item test is usually less than in a multiple-choice item test. This is especially true for essay and short-answer essay tests, because each item requires substantially more time for students to make their responses. Because of the comparatively few items, errors caused by content sampling are more likely to play a part in supply-type tests than in multiple-choice tests. Although it is true to some degree for all supply-type items, essay and short-answer essay tests have also been criticized on the basis that, all other things being equal, the student who is better able to respond in writing is likely to get a better score.

The *written simulation* is another type of written test. Such instruments attempt to come as close as possible to a real-life experience in a written format. While a written format is the easiest and least expensive method of presenting a simulation, computers are often used to present simulated events for testing purposes.[2]

The goal of a written simulation is to be as realistic as possible within the obvious constraints of the written format. In a real-life situation, the problem-solving tasks faced by a nurse rarely require selection of a single isolated response from a small number of options like the task required in a multiple-choice format. Even if the task calls for a single isolated response, there may be more options available than the four or five typically provided by a multiple-choice item. More commonly, a problem-solving situation involves a sequence of events in which the nurse, when faced with a problem, chooses one or more courses of action, sees the results of the action, and then chooses new course(s) of action. This process continues until the problem is resolved. The process is diagramed in Figure 6–1.

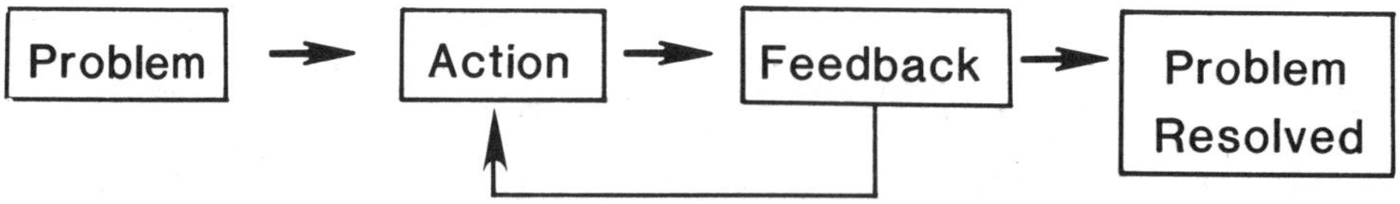

Figure 6–1. A problem-solving process.

The problem-solving simulation scenario begins with a problem. It may be a client who suddenly goes into shock, a coworker who is careless in checking an operative site for bleeding and may be responsible for a hemorrhage going undetected, or a physician who is on call but cannot be reached in an emergency. The common denominator is that the nurse must make decisions and take action to resolve the problem satisfactorily. In the first case, the nurse may decide to initiate treatment for shock and then contact the client's physician. In the second case, the nurse may decide to mention to the coworker that failure to check the operative site frequently for bleeding may have led to the client's going into shock. In the third case, the nurse may give the client oxygen and call the physician's partner for consultation. Once a course of action is taken, the nurse then receives feedback regarding the effects of the action. In the case of a client with symptoms of shock, the symptoms may subside and the physician may order oxygen and blood. In the case of a coworker's negligence, the coworker might reject the insinuation that he/she was in any way responsible for the client's going into shock—forcing further action. In the case of a physician on-call failing to respond when summoned, his partner might resent being disturbed on a day off to take care of the problem.

Once feedback is received, the nurse must then decide on what further action to take. There may be no further action necessary, as in the first and third cases described; however, the nurse might have to make hard decisions, as would be true in the second example. Having failed to resolve the problem by talking to the coworker, the nurse might decide to collect evidence that the coworker is negligent and report observations to the supervisor. Feedback would again be received and a new course of action plotted. The process would be repeated until either the problem is resolved or no further action can be taken.

A written format is not especially amenable to simulations, but it can be done. The most difficult problem with using a written format is determining how to deliver the feedback after a response is chosen. The challenge lies in ensuring that the learner cannot see the feedback prior to choosing a response. Some creative approaches have been used to solve this problem.

One approach is to use a special ink in the printing process that is invisible until it comes into contact with a certain chemical. The chemical is dispensed in a container resembling a marker pen. The "latent image pen," as the containers are called by the manufacturer, A.B. Dick, dispenses a chemical that makes the invisible ink immediately visible. Latent-image simulations can be copied using a commonly available ditto machine.

While the latent-image approach works reasonably well, it has drawbacks. A potential problem is that the image pens and simulations do not store well for long periods of time. Even though the manufacturer suggests the materials can be stored up to two years, it probably is a good idea to store them no longer than a year. Also the pens are relatively expensive. Despite these problems, the latent-image approach is a reasonably simple and easy method for developing a written simulation. There are other methods, such as branching programed instruction, but the latent-image approach is probably the simplest and most intriguing for the developer and the respondent.

While simulations have substantial intuitive appeal, they also have problems. Writing a good simulation requires a lot of thought and careful consideration. Also, there is no consensus on how to score a simulation. Just as there are differences of opinion among nurse-teachers about the appropriate way to handle many situations encountered in nursing practice, there are differences of opinion regarding the way to score simulations. Because of these differences, simulations are better used for formative evaluation than summative evaluation.

Oral Examinations. The second class of tests used to evaluate learners is the oral examination. The format of the oral examination consists of one or more examiners posing questions or issues to an examinee. The examinee's task is to respond verbally to the best of his or her ability. While this is the general format, the actual manner in which it is carried out can vary. One approach is to have the examiner ask a question and then have the learner respond directly to the question. A variation of this procedure is to have the oral examination based upon an earlier written examination. The examinee is then asked to clarify responses to different questions on the written test. Discussion may then proceed to relevant associated topics.

In the clinical arena, the case presentation is similar in many respects to the oral examination. In this case, the learner is asked to describe a patient being cared for and the care that has been provided. The nurse-teacher then asks questions about the patient's problem and care.

The oral examination has the potential advantage of offering realism. For example, a practicing nurse often is called upon to explain the rationale for an action. The response will most likely be made verbally, and perhaps in writing as well. In addition, the oral examination allows the instructor to see how well learners can "think on their feet." To respond to the oral questions, learners must be able to quickly organize their thoughts and express them in a coherent manner. These are compelling reasons to use the oral examination. There are, however, some disadvantages that are probably important to consider.[3]

Difficulty in achieving consistency of ratings between different raters is a major limitation of the oral examination. This problem is called interrater reliability. The rater is the individual who is posing questions, listening to the student responses, and assessing student performance. Difficulty in achieving interrater reliability relates to a situation in which, if two nurse-teachers are independently rating a student's performance in an oral examination, the ratings given by the two may be markedly different. Besides the interrater reliability problem, oral examinations are time-consuming and this has been noted as a disadvantage that should be given careful thought.

The subjectivity of the oral examination is the factor that leads to the most serious deficits associated with the oral examination. Subjectivity is a problem because people's thinking is biased by many factors related to observing and listening to a person speak, including such features as verbal mannerisms, height, weight, and so on. These are not necessarily conscious biases of the rater, but even so, they may influence ratings. Overcoming such subtle biases is not an easy task. One method to minimize these biases is to record the oral examination either on video or audiotape and have independent observers rate the learner by viewing or listening to the recordings. If the raters have never had contact with the learner, this method will eliminate the instructor's biases developed by previous experience with the learner. Video or audiotaping the session will not affect the interpersonal bias generated by speech or physical mannerisms, however. Recording voice only will remove the biasing effects that are caused by the student's physical features. It is important to note that if the raters have had previous contact with the learner, then video or audiotaping may not necessarily eliminate bias. There is a strong tendency for people to want to identify individuals whose identity is being withheld. It becomes something of a game or challenge to make the identification. Thus, it is possible that recognition will occur even when sessions are recorded. Having a record of the examination will, however, enable independent review in the event that a need should arise. It also provides for the possibility of reviewing the examination with the student as a means of feedback.

A final consideration is that the stress associated with taking an oral examination tends to be greater than with other testing formats. Students who do well under other examination methods have been known to get flustered under oral examination. This is probably most true for students who have had little previous experience with oral examinations. Therefore, if an oral examination is to be used, some provision for practice should be provided before it is used in earnest.

Instruments Used to Measure Attitudes and Perceptions. There are times when the goals of an educational program are other than to increase the knowledge of the learner. Just because one increases a learner's knowledge does not necessarily mean that the learner will apply that knowledge. A learner must want to change behavior in order for the new knowledge to be applied. This predisposition to apply new knowledge is an attitude. There are many times when the primary goal of a learning experience is not to increase knowledge but simply to change attitudes.

Learner perceptions are closely related to attitudes. The primary difference between the two is that perceptions reflect how the learner views some experience, whereas attitudes reflect some belief that is held. Course evaluation questionnaires are an example of an effort to assess student perceptions. In this instance, questions should focus on specific characteristics of the course as opposed to belief systems promoted by the course. The measurement of both attitudes and perceptions is usually done with written instruments, although structured oral interviews are also common.

Written Attitude and Perception Instruments. There are several common types of instruments or items used to assess attitudes and perceptions. There are major problems inherent in the assessment of such qualities as well. The *Likert* item, named after a man named Likert in 1932, is one type of assessment method. It is characterized by a statement or stem, followed by several responses from which the learner chooses a response. The following illustrates a Likert-type item:

I like being a nurse.

a. Strongly agree
b. Moderately agree
c. Slightly agree
d. Slightly disagree
e. Moderately disagree
f. Strongly disagree

An item such as the one illustrated is useful for measuring both perceptions and attitudes.

A second type of attitudinal item is the *semantic differential.* A semantic differential item consists of two opposite words or statements placed on a continuum and separated by a series of blanks. There may be seven blanks that separate the two words. The learner is to place an X in the particular blank that reflects his or her attitude. An example of this item follows.

How would you describe your feelings about being a nurse?

rewarding	___	X	___	___	___	___	___	thankless
happy	___	___	___	X	___	___	___	sad
bad	___	___	___	X	___	___	___	good

In this example, the respondent feels that being a nurse is fairly rewarding because the X has been placed nearest to the word "rewarding," however, happiness in the profession is neutral. The semantic differential item is not as useful for assessing perceptions as it is for attitudes.

A third type of attitude item is the *multiple-choice item.* Its appearance is very similar to the knowledge-type multiple choice item. The primary difference between the two is the type of information sought. For example:

How important do you feel the tasks performed by a nurse are?

a. Extremely important
b. Very important
c. Moderately important

d. Somewhat important
e. Unimportant

Items such as this one are useful for measuring both perceptions and attitudes.

Which of these three formats (Likert, semantic differential, multiple-choice) a nurse-teacher uses to assess attitudes depends on how the attitude can best be expressed. The overriding consideration should be clarity of expression. An ambiguous attitude question is *worthless* at best and may even be damaging if the results are used to make faulty decisions. Achieving clarity of expression is a time-consuming and arduous task. Attitude questions should be carefully reviewed by several different nurse-teachers before use and, if possible, tried out with learners who are as similar as possible to those with whom the instrument eventually will be used. A strategy that is usually very helpful is to sit down with several learners individually and ask each of them what they think each question means. In this manner, it can be determined whether learners will interpret the question similarly.

Attitude measures are known to be affected by at least two undesirable elements: the halo effect and social desirability. The *halo effect* refers to the tendency of individuals to rate uniquely different characteristics according to their overall perception. Thus, the ratings on different attitude questions tend to be more alike than they should be. *Social desirability* refers to the tendency of individuals to avoid making a response that they feel would reflect undesirably on themselves. In the case of an attitude instrument, it is often fairly evident what might be the most desirable response to an item. If the results of the assessment are to be used as part of the course grade, it is almost certain that at least a few students will misrepresent their true attitudes in order to improve their grade. There are many other factors that attitude researchers suspect influence attitude results, but they have not been documented in research. Nunnally gives a good summary of this research.[4]

Unlike tests on which, if students do not have the desired knowledge, they are unlikely to deduce the desired response, students can often deduce the desired response on an attitude questionnaire whether or not they hold the desired attitude. The validity of attitude results thus depends on the respondent's willingness to answer the questions openly and honestly. For this reason, we do not recommend that attitude questionnaire results be used as a basis for assigning grades. Attitude questionnaires are of greater use in assessing the effects of an educational program, because in this case students have little to gain from misrepresenting their attitudes.

Oral Attitude and Perception Instruments. The structured oral interview is another way of assessing attitudes or perceptions. It is the most usable format for orally gathering information on attitudes and perceptions. The distinguishing feature of a structured interview is a written protocol to which the interviewer must adhere. The interviewer usually records responses on a standard form. By following a uniform protocol, the data collected can be more easily analyzed and compared among learners than if an unstructured format is followed.

Interviews are useful for collecting in-depth anecdotal information. While questionnaires can be used to survey a large number of students fairly inexpensively, they often do not provide great insight into the reasons for responses. The interview can add richness of detail and meaning to response. We have found interviews with a few students (five to ten) after administering a questionnaire to add a great deal to the interpretation placed on the questionnaire results. Structured interviews are often the best procedure for gathering information from clients, particularly those who have difficulty seeing or reading. While oral interviews can be extremely valuable, they have limitations. They are time consuming to administer and there is a potential for interviewer bias that may color the results.

Instruments Used to Measure Skills. The learning of skills or motor behaviors is a major concern for nurse-teachers. For example, a student who has the desired knowledge but is unable to apply it in the clinical setting is not much better than one who does not have the knowledge. There are many fundamental nursing skills that must be mastered to practice nursing effectively—for example, giving injections, taking vital signs, conducting a physical assessment, inserting a retention catheter, conducting a home visit, and so on. While each of these skills has a knowledge component, the actual performance of the skill is critical.

Skill evaluation may take place either in a simulated situation or in the course of actual client care. Simulations are best used when the need to use a skill is infrequently encountered during the normal course of client care or when the procedure is in any way disagreeable or dangerous for the client. In the latter case, it is desirable that the learner have a high level of proficiency before attempting to perform a procedure on a real client. Cardiopulmonary resuscitation (CPR) is an example of such a critical skill.

A simulation is an attempt to reconstruct as closely as possible a real situation. Resusci-Anne, the manikin used to teach CPR, is a good example of a simulator. Neophyte nursing students often give each other injections before attempting them on clients, a second example of a simulated experience.

Evaluating performance in a simulated situation has the advantage of providing a "cleaner" estimate of a student's ability than would be the case during the normal course of client care. The estimate is cleaner in the sense that the evaluation is uniform for each student. Real clients differ in the seriousness of their illness, their anatomy, complications caused by secondary illnesses, or their reactions to a procedure. These factors can affect how the student performs a skill. For instance, clients react differently to receiving an injection. It is more difficult to give a struggling client an injection than a calm one. While the example is extreme, the point is that differences between clients may make the difficulty of performing a skill very different, depending on the idiosyncrasies of the client and circumstances involved.

It is best to have clean evaluations when learners are just beginning to learn skills. Specific, clear feedback is needed at this time to improve skill performance. On the other hand, it is important for advanced learners to be evaluated during actual client care, because the manner in which skills are performed in spite of extenuating circumstances is an important element to consider.

Skills are usually evaluated using either checklists, rating scales, anecdotal records, or some combination of these instruments.

Checklists and Rating Scales. *Checklists* require yes-or-no responses: either something occurred or it did not occur. If a single skill is being assessed, a checklist can be developed by listing all the steps necessary to perform the skill adequately. Then, as the student performs the skill, the nurse-teacher checks off each step as it occurs. The checklist can be a very precise measure of student performance. If a step is omitted, it is carefully documented. Below is an example of a checklist that could be used to evaluate a learner who is administering an injection.

_____ Informs patient why medication is to be given
_____ Checks mental status ("Is that OK with you?")
_____ Swabs injection site with alcohol
_____ Fills hypodermic needle to appropriate level
_____ Purges air from needle
_____ Informs patient of expectations for discomfort
_____ Inserts needle appropriately
_____ Depresses plunger in a smooth, steady motion using the appropriate fingers
_____ Covers site with an absorbant material (cotton)
_____ Withdraws needle appropriately
_____ Stops the bleeding in an appropriate manner (applies pressure on cotton swab)
_____ Instructs patient in what to do and what will happen next (side effects of medication, next medical procedure, etc.)
_____ Disposes of components safely
_____ Stores instruments and medications properly

A checklist can be misleading. For instance, it may say nothing about the order in which the steps were performed by the learner. Order can make a tremendous difference in whether or not a skill is performed properly. Suppose, for example, one student swabbed the skin with alcohol before penetrating the skin with a hypodermic needle and another did not swab the skin until after the injection. Obviously, the second student made a grievous error, but the two students would appear identical on a checklist evaluation.

Checklists can also be used to document exposure of learners to different types of client care problems considered to be important. In this approach, the instructor develops a logbook that describes the number of experiences and level of involvement students should have for each important type of client care problem. Students carry the logbook with them as they conduct their clinical responsibilities. Each time a student participates in one of the experiences listed in the logbook, he or she must describe it and have a clinical supervisor initial the entry to validate it. In this manner, it can be ensured that all students have at least a minimum set of clinical experiences.

Rating scales are often used as an alternative to checklists. In rating scales, a range of options is used rather than a yes-or-no choice. Thus, a checklist might be transformed to a rating scale by having the rater choose from a range of options reflecting the degree of quality with which each step is performed, rather than a simple yes or no. Table 6–1 shows the preceding checklist transformed to a rating scale.

The rating scale can be more meaningful, because it adds detail about the quality with which a procedure is performed. Thus, a rating scale can indicate not only that a learner has had a particular experience but also can provide an indication of the quality of the experience.

A rating scale can identify problems that a checklist would not detect. For instance, in the previous example, one student wiped the skin with alcohol after the injection was given, but not before. If a rating scale had been used, the rating for the alcohol wipe would have been very low, reflecting its occurrence out of sequence.

TABLE 6-1. RATING SCALE EVALUATING THE ADMINISTRATION OF AN INJECTION

	Poor	Fair	Good	Very Good	Outstanding
Informs patient why medication will be given	1	2	3	4	5
Checks mental status ("Is that OK with you?")	1	2	3	4	5
Swabs injection site with alcohol	1	2	3	4	5
Fills hypodermic needle to appropriate level	1	2	3	4	5
Purges air from needle	1	2	3	4	5
Informs patient of expectations for discomfort	1	2	3	4	5
Inserts needle appropriately	1	2	3	4	5
Depresses plunger in a smooth, steady motion using the appropriate fingers	1	2	3	4	5
Covers site with an absorbant material (cotton)	1	2	3	4	5
Withdraws needle appropriately	1	2	3	4	5
Stops bleeding in an appropriate manner (applies pressure on cotton swab)	1	2	3	4	5
Instructs patient in what to do and what will happen next (side effects of medication, next medical procedure, etc.)	1	2	3	4	5
Disposes of components safely	1	2	3	4	5
Stores instruments and medications properly	1	2	3	4	5

Although very specific rating scales like that in Table 6–1 are in use, it is more often the case that rating scales tend to assess broader and more general qualities than do checklists. Checklists usually provide very precise measurements of a very narrow range of skills, whereas rating scales may provide relatively imprecise measurements of a broad range of skills. For instance, rating scales are often used to measure such subjective qualities as a student's interpersonal skills, his or her ability to establish rapport with clients, or the ability to work well in a team situation. These are very difficult qualities to define precisely. Quite different results can be obtained with such rating scales depending on who completes the form.

There are two major types of rating scales that can be used. The first is the *descriptive graphic rating scale.* In the descriptive graphic approach, each number on the scale is accompanied by statements (descriptors) that describe exactly what type of behavior is reflected by the number. The second variety is the *single descriptor.* In the single descriptor scale, the quality being evaluated is usually (but not always) carefully described, and the rater chooses a number on a scale corresponding to a range from good to bad or excellent to poor. Examples of both of these types of rating scales appear in Table 6–2.

The descriptive graphic approach is very appealing, as each position on the

TABLE 6-2. EXAMPLES OF ANCHORED STATEMENT AND SINGLE DESCRIPTOR RATING SCALES

I. Anchored Statement Scale

		Ability to Establish Rapport with Clients		
A	**B**	**C**	**D**	**E**
Fails to introduce self; appears unconcerned with client; is rude or fails to observe common amenities.	Introduces self in a cursory manner; shows a little concern for client's welfare; occasionally rude or fails to observe common amenities on occasion.	Adequately introduces self; shows concern for client's welfare; observes common amenities.	Is warm and caring toward clients; establishes a good client-nurse relationship.	Is perceived by client as warm and caring; establishes a trusting relationship with clients.

II. Single Descriptor Scale

Is able to establish a trusting relationship with clients and is perceived by clients as warm and caring.

A	B	C	D	E	F
Poor	Fair	OK	Good	Very good	Outstanding

rating scale is accompanied by a statement that describes the indicated performance in comparative detail. A serious problem with the descriptive graphic approach is that a particular learner may not fit neatly under any single description. For instance, suppose a student is frequently guilty of failing to introduce him-or herself but otherwise does a very good job of establishing a trusting relationship with clients. Using the scale in Table 6–2, a rating of A would be deserved for introductions and perhaps a D or E for the other aspects related to rapport. A rater is then in a dilemma as to how to rate the student. The single descriptor variety, on the other hand, usually causes no such confusion. It basically requires the rater to make a global judgment about the quality being assessed. While the rater may be spared some confusion, global assessments may lead to less consistency between various raters.

Some of the inconsistency between raters can be eliminated if the quality being assessed by a single descriptor rating scale is carefully defined. A clear definition of the term will make it more likely that each rater is rating the same quality; however, thorough definitions tend to be relatively long and detailed. This can create a lengthy and unwieldy rating form. Also, as details are added to the definition of a quality, what usually happens is that the quality is made up of multiple components, each of which may be somewhat independent of the others. This can lead to the same dilemma that we encounter with the anchored statement type of scale in which a student may have one rating on some components and another rating on other components. Arriving at a single overall rating then becomes extremely difficult. A compromise that can simplify rater decision making would be to assign a separate rating for each component of the quality being assessed. For instance, rather than having a single rating for the nebulous quality of rapport, one might have several qualities rated that relate to rapport. Table 6–3 illustrates how this might be accomplished. Making each rating more discrete also promotes more consistency among raters.

Two types of rating scales have been discussed. There are others. In any case, the type of scale one uses is a matter of preference. No matter which type of scale is used, there are two important administrative matters related to use that must be considered. First, all raters should be instructed in the use of the rating form. This

TABLE 6–3. RAPPORT WITH PATIENTS

	Poor	Fair	OK	Good	Very Good	Outstanding
Introduces self to client	1	2	3	4	5	6
Observes common amenities	1	2	3	4	5	6
Shows concern for client's comfort	1	2	3	4	5	6
Establishes trusting relationship	1	2	3	4	5	6
Is warm and caring toward client	1	2	3	4	5	6

may range from an orientation session where all raters are introduced to the form and allowed to ask questions, to an extended training session in which raters actually use the rating scales under controlled conditions. The latter type of training session is preferred, but it is not always possible. The more instruction provided to raters, the better will be the results.

The second important point is that the rating form and how it is used should be reviewed on a regular basis, every one to two years. All raters should be asked to comment on the procedures with an emphasis on improvement. An evaluation system, no matter how well conceived, may prove to be unworkable when it is actually implemented. One should always be prepared to make changes.

Anecdotal Records. The final major class of evaluation measures used to assess skills is the anecdotal record. The anecdotal record is basically a narrative report of a student's behavior, which the nurse-teacher has observed and recorded. The richness of detail that an anecdotal record can provide is its greatest strength. The documentation and detailed description of specific behaviors makes this a powerful evaluation tool. This type of evidence is very important when giving feedback to students or when drastic actions must be taken, such as expulsion from a nursing program.

A major weakness of the anecdotal record is that it is time-consuming to complete. Nurse-teachers in one teaching hospital were spending a half hour each week for each of 20 students writing anecdotal reports. Thus over one quarter of their time was being spent writing anecdotal reports. A second major weakness is that such reports reflect the personal biases of the nurse-teacher. Because they are often completely unstructured, these records are likely to reflect the individual nurse-teacher's intrinsic reporting style.

A final limitation is that anecdotal reports are difficult to summarize. Unlike test scores or numerical ratings, comments contained in anecdotal reports cannot be summed or averaged to arrive at an overall performance measure. This is an unfortunate feature of an evaluation mechanism that consumes such a great amount of effort and time. The time necessary to complete anecdotal reports can be reduced to some degree by only sampling behaviors on certain days, rather than doing it on a daily basis. For example, one might choose Tuesday and Thursday one week, Monday and Friday another week, or Wednesday and Friday in another week. Another way of approaching it might be to divide the students into five subgroups corresponding to each day of the week. Anecdotal reports would then be written for members of the same subgroup on the day that group is designated for evaluation. The day on which each particular group is evaluated might then be randomized from one week to the next.

Attempting to reduce the subjective elements of an anecdotal report is a difficult task. The process has subjectivity built in because of its unstructured nature. There are some guidelines, however, that can assist in making the process less subjective. The notes should be limited to describing behavior only and references or inferences related to general personality traits or attitudes should be avoided. For example, a statement like "This student is lazy" should not be used. A better statement would be, "This student failed to complete all tasks that were assigned." Failure to complete the tasks is an observation that can be independently verified. Calling a student lazy is a subjective inference that the student's failure to complete tasks is due to some innate quality of laziness. It is quite possible, that there are other reasons why a student might not complete assignments. It could be because of personal problems, overcommitment to outside employment, or illness. By concentrating on describing behavior, one avoids the subjective interpretation of the cause of the behavior. It also allows one to concentrate on a concrete problem as opposed to diffuse personality traits and minimizes the potential for conflict when discussing the results. It is difficult to argue with documented behavior, whereas inferred personality defects can always be challenged.

If a student demonstrates some especially poor or damaging behavior that may lead to a reprimand or even expulsion, it is advisable to record as many details as possible (date, time, location, others present, and so on). Details add credibility to anecdotal reports as they increase the likelihood that the observation can be independently verified. It is a good policy to always date anecdotal reports. Thus, if one wishes to show student progress, one can go back through the notes to profile change over time.

A final point to remember is that one should comment on the good things a student does as well as the bad. Just as it is important to document the failings of a student who is given poor ratings, it is important to document the successes of a student given excellent ratings. Also, even the poorest student does some things right. To dwell entirely on the negative can brutalize a student's self-concept. To mention some good things a student has done will help keep things in proper perspective.

Perhaps the best use of anecdotal reports is in the support of numerical ratings. The numerical ratings can be statistically manipulated to facilitate administrative needs. Anecdotal reports in support of the ratings add meaning and substance to what otherwise would be an abstraction. This can be very helpful in preparing letters of recommendation.

SUMMARY

Multiple-choice tests have the desirable qualities of (1) being able to assess a broad range of content in a comparatively short time period, (2) objectivity, (3) accuracy, and (4) ease of scoring. Supply-type items are useful when there is interest in how well a student can express a thought in writing or it is important to minimize the likelihood of a student's guessing the correct answer to an item. The task of taking a multiple-choice test is artificial and there is a very real chance of guessing answers correctly, yet the scoring of supply-type items is time-consuming and prone to human error. Written simulations offer an alternative that approximates reality; however, scoring problems limit their usefulness primarily to formative evaluation. The oral examination is a format that corresponds in many ways to nursing practice;

however, it is time consuming to administer, and subjectivity in scoring is difficult to overcome.

Written tests composed of Likert, semantic differential, and multiple-choice items, as well as structured oral interviews, can be used to collect data on learner attitudes and/or perceptions. Likert and multiple-choice items are useful for measuring both perceptions and attitudes, whereas semantic differential is more suitable for assessing attitudes. Approaches are selected according to how the attitude or perception can best be expressed by the learner. It is best to try out items on a sample of the population before actual implementation. Attitude measurements are affected by the halo effect and social desirability. In addition, interviewer bias may cloud the results of oral interviews.

Skill learning is important in both client care and nursing education. Checklists, rating scales, and anecdotal records are some of the instruments nurse-teachers can use to assess attainment of psychomotor skills.

Checklists generally require the evaluator to simply check a yes or no, satisfactory or unsatisfactory response, whereas rating scales usually offer a range of response options and reflect a degree of quality. In addition, items are usually hierarchically ordered on a rating scale. The more discrete the rating instrument, the more interrater reliability increases. Training in use and periodic review are important aspects in the use of checklists and rating scales.

Narrative anecdotal records provide detailed documentation of performance. They are valuable sources of information for teaching, learning, and administrative feedback; however, they tend to reflect the subjectivity of the writer, are time-consuming to prepare, and are difficult to summarize or average to arrive at an overall performance measure.

LEARNER GROUPS

Just as one should attempt to tailor educational programs to meet the needs of the learners, the evaluation procedures should flow from the objectives of the program and also consider the idiosyncrasies of the learners. An evaluation system that does not relate to the educational program's objectives and purposes is useless. Failing to consider the learner group involved in the program can have the same result.

The four types of learner groups of which nursing is concerned, undergraduate nursing students, graduate nursing students, practicing nurses, and clients, can be contrasted along two dimensions related to evaluation: (1) decisions to be based on the evaluation results, and (2) learner motivation.

Decisions to be Based on the Evaluation Results

As previously mentioned, evaluations must provide information to make necessary decisions if the results are to be useful. These decisions tend to vary depending on the particular learner group that is participating in the educational program. For undergraduate and graduate students, the decisions are very similar. The primary summative decision that is always being considered is whether or not the student has learned material to the point where he or she is ready to proceed to the next level of education or graduate. The process of assigning grades is an elaboration of this process in which those students who are capable of proceeding onward are given different grades, depending on merit. In severe cases, the decision may be whether or not the student will continue on in the educational program.

In most continuing education programs, the only summative decision to be based on learner evaluation is whether or not to award continuing education credit each year in order to maintain licensure. In many instances, it is a foregone conclusion that if the learner simply "shows up," the credit will be awarded. There is no formal testing of learning gained from the experience.

In client education programs and daily teaching interventions, the primary consideration is whether the client's knowledge, attitudes, or skills are sufficient to enable participation in self-care. Instruction is provided until proficiency is achieved. It is important that the evaluation procedures used provide the information necessary. If one needs to know whether a person with diabetes has the ability to check blood sugar level and administer the appropriate dose of insulin, a written test would not provide the best information. Observation as the client actually performs the task would provide better evidence. Similarly, in the case of in-service or staff development programs, where goals relate to understanding new information, performing new procedures, or updating existing knowledge and skills, the primary summative decision pertains to proficiency.

Learner Motivation

Learner motivation to perform well is essential if an accurate assessment is to be made. An unmotivated learner may not perform up to potential. Learner motivation to do well on an evaluation is again similar for undergraduate and graduate students. In both cases, learners are concerned with doing well in order to pursue career goals. The more students invest in career goals, the more likely they are to be motivated to do well on evaluations.

In continuing nursing education, the motivation to participate is provided by the need to renew one's license periodically, the intrinsic motivation to learn, the desire to do the job to the best of one's ability, and the desire to appear competent to one's peers. Some individuals have a high degree of internal motivation, while others do not.

Unfortunately, rigorous learner evaluation is rarely practical in continuing education. The licensing agencies do not require it, offerers of continuing education rarely demand it, and participants often balk at completing even short course-evaluation questionnaires. Administration of cognitive tests to assess learning at continuing education courses has encountered substantial resistance. Thus, while there is merit in the concept of making the amount of continuing education credit awarded contingent on demonstrated learning through test performance or actual performance, it will remain impractical unless there are substantial changes in the manner in which continuing education is structured.

There is one continuing education program, however, that perhaps could serve as a model for developing effective learner evaluation systems. The program is the

CPR program offered to health professionals and the public. Learners are not certified until they are able to demonstrate proficiency in performing the procedures of CPR. In addition, to remain certified, the learner must be evaluated on a yearly basis. Admittedly, CPR is a very special case. Rarely does the topic of a continuing nursing education program have such documentation of effectiveness and need and such support from the medical establishment. Although it is unrealistic to expect all continuing nursing education programs to be as rigorously evaluated, CPR can serve as a model program as far as the evaluation of learners is concerned.

For clients, the motivating force is usually to improve a condition or at least prevent a condition from deteriorating. This motivation is not always high. In some situations, the best that can happen is to slow the disease process or maintain the client in a state that the individual finds undesirable. Thus, lack of motivation can be a serious problem in client education. Even if a client understands the reasons for treatment and can demonstrate the ability to participate in the treatment, it does not mean that the client will conscientiously perform it. It should never be taken for granted that clients will comply in following their treatment plans. Follow-up evaluation is extremely important. We are all clients at one time or another. Thus, the client population is as varied as the population at large. Some clients cannot read, others have physical disabilities that may prevent them from being able to see, hear, or do many motor tasks. These limitations must be considered in both the educational program and evaluation measures used.

SUMMARY

The nature of the learner or learner group does influence and affect evaluation procedures. Evaluations should be matched with learner characteristics and educational programs for evaluation results to guide intelligent decision making. Primary decisions to be made based on evaluation data for graduate and undergraduate nursing students relate to program advancement and graduation. Grading is a by-product of the evaluation process. Whether or not to award continuing education units is the primary concern of the continuing nursing education provider. Decisions relating to clients usually center around whether the client has achieved critical self-care, health maintenance, and health promotion objectives and making recommendations for further teaching and care.

Intrinsic learner motivation is a critical variable in evaluation. Nurse-teachers need to recognize this fact and try to help learners understand the purpose for evaluations and their benefits. Follow-up evaluation is a necessary component of any evaluation program.

TEACHER EVALUATION

Teacher evaluation should not be just an assessment of a teacher's "classroom" performance. Nurse-teacher evaluation is much broader and should include, as appropriate, the quality of planning, teaching materials prepared and used, teaching-learning climate, student or client rapport, student advising provided, and clinical teaching. A complete evaluation of a nurse-teacher as a faculty member also considers scholarly contributions, research, and academic and community service.

The most common reason for nurse-teacher evaluation in academic settings is review for promotion and tenure. This evaluation usually incorporates some criterion-referenced standards, such as a certain number of publications and research, although these are not always formally stated.

Besides these summative reasons, teacher evaluation is also conducted for teacher improvement. Here the teacher is asking for feedback about how teaching behaviors can be improved to meet the needs of the students and how teaching and learner evaluation materials can be designed and used effectively. The primary source for information on teaching effectiveness is learner judgments. Students provide useful information about certain important aspects of teaching, like the enthusiasm of the teacher, self-assessment of their understanding of the material taught, clarity of the teacher's expression, and so forth. There are some areas in which students are not a good source of information, however. Students are not good judges of the importance of the content provided in an educational program or class; they have only a limited amount of experience. Only rarely do they have enough experience to make valid judgments regarding the importance of a content area. Often students report back to teachers that it was only after they had been actually in practice that they realized how important the content was.

Another area that students should not be asked to evaluate is the teacher's understanding of the content area. A very knowledgeable teacher may appear to students to have a poor grasp of content for a number of reasons. For instance, the teacher might have difficulty expressing thoughts at the level of the students or have difficulty organizing content in a manner that students find helpful. While these are obviously weaknesses, they may not be related to content knowledge. Peer or subject matter experts are better sources for this type of evaluative data.

Professional educators can also provide useful information about most of the noncontent aspects of teaching, such as lecture delivery style, design of teaching materials, selection of teaching strategies, and psychometric soundness of test items. Peers or subject matter experts can provide valuable feedback about the appropriateness of objectives, textbooks, test items, handouts, and other aspects of teaching. Thus, careful consideration should be given to what sources are appropriate for obtaining the different types of data desired.

When to collect teacher evaluation data depends, again, on what purpose the data will serve. If the data are to be formative, it is usually best to collect data well before the end of the course. While end-of-course data can be formative for future course offerings, it is not useful for improving that particular course offering. Summative data are usually best collected at the end of the course after all course activities have been completed.

Much has been written on procedures for classroom evaluation, including the advice that an independent third party should administer, collect, and tally the evaluation forms. See the appendix for examples of forms that can be used to facilitate evaluation of teaching effectiveness. Such forms can be used as an adjunct to video-recorded teaching episodes for self-evaluation of teaching effectiveness.

SUMMARY

Evaluation of teaching effectiveness is both formative and summative. Formative data should be collected before the end of a teaching experience. The purpose of formative evaluation is to judge strengths and weaknesses to improve teaching to meet learner needs. It focuses on evaluating planning, teaching-learning climate, lesson design, management, teaching materials and strategies, content, and evaluation methodologies.

Summative evaluation focuses on collecting relevant data to improve all aspects of teaching in the future and to obtain data to make decisions regarding promotion and tenure. Students, peers, and "outside" experts can assist with various aspects of evaluating teaching effectiveness. Self-evaluation is also an important data-gathering measure.

MATERIALS EVALUATION

There is a wide array of different materials, devices, and strategies that nurses can use to assist learners to achieve learning objectives. These include textbooks, handouts, slides, video and audio programs, models, displays, programed instruction, and computer-assisted instruction. Teaching materials can play a very important role in the quality of instruction provided to learners, and as such, influence learning either positively or negatively.

Poor teaching materials reflect negatively on the teacher and can be detrimental to the learning process. Thus, it is important that teaching materials be carefully evaluated in advance of use. In many cases, flaws can be identified by a relatively quick inspection. In other cases, they may not be apparent until the materials are actually used. If proper precautions are observed, however, it is unlikely that flawed materials will actually be used.

The basic decision to be made in any evaluation of materials is to determine the suitability of the materials for a particular application. The application is the critical element. Materials suitable for one application may not be suitable for another. This decision must include consideration of the audience (learner characteristics), the format, cost, availability, content, technical quality, educational level, the setting for use, and the extent to which the materials are based on sound learning principles. Other considerations may also be necessary, depending on the particular application.

All materials should be previewed and evaluated prior to use. Often colleagues are involved in the review process and the nurse-teacher will ask colleagues for help in identifying appropriate materials. Reviews of print and nonprint materials are available through AVLINE and in many professional journals. AVLINE, a computer-based listing and description of available audiovisual materials, is supported by the National Library of Medicine.

Materials evaluation typically involves a teacher or group of teachers who review the appropriateness of materials for a particular use. Often, an evaluation form is completed as part of the evaluation (see the Appendix for examples). If suitable materials cannot be found, the nurse-teacher can prepare or adapt materials, sometimes with the help of specialists. In this case, a sample of the potential learner group should review the material prior to full implementation with the target population. Self-contained materials, such as self-instructional texts, computer-assisted instruction, learning activity packages, modular instruction, and so on, should also undergo a formal review by colleagues, as well as the learner sample. The purpose of this formative evaluation is to debug the materials and aid in the revision process.

Review of materials is largely a matter of determining the appropriateness or suitability for the intended use. This includes consideration of whether the materials provide the conditions necessary for achievement of learning outcomes. A material may be rejected because it does not reinforce, provide feedback, practice, or repetition, because it is poorly organized, or it has too much or too little information, its language or content is too difficult or too easy, it does not allow the learner control over the rate of presentation that one wants, or the price is too high. In the case of audiovisual materials, technical quality should be considered. Actors may not be appropriate for the roles they play, voices may have the wrong accents, or auditory or visual quality may be substandard. In addition, teacher preferences and biases influence decision making. The "not-invented-here syndrome" causes some teachers to reject materials simply because they were developed at another institution. Materials evaluation should be as objective as possible to reduce unnecessary expenditure and duplication of effort.

An additional problem is that the reliability and validity of published materials is seldom reported by publishers and distributors. The reputation of the reviewers as experts is the appeal generally used to establish credibility. Conscientious evaluation of materials, including use of evaluation forms, may strengthen the credibility of the review.

SUMMARY

Identifying, selecting, and evaluating materials—those that embody and transmit conditions that promote achievement of learning outcomes—are primary actions of the nurse-teacher. These direct and contrived strategies used by the nurse-teacher influence teaching and learning effectiveness. Therefore, evaluating the strengths and weaknesses of materials in relationship to learner characteristics and preferences, critical tasks, objectives, content, setting, and physical and environmental conditions related to format and setting is an important teaching action. As with any type of evaluation, the purposes of materials evaluation are both formative and summative. The goal is to determine the suitability of materials for a particular teaching-learning experience. A fairly large body of research and practical experience is available to guide decision making. In addition, colleagues, learners, and materials specialists can assist in review and evaluation process. Reviews of selected commercial materials are available through online computer systems, such as AV-LINE, professional journals, distributors' and publishers' flyers and catalogs of software. Obtaining information on the reliability and validity of materials is a major problem, however, even though this data is extremely important for intelligent decison making.

Nurse-teachers can obtain most materials for preview. Materials evaluation forms are available to help make appraisal more objective. Data from multiple evaluators can be compiled and analyzed to guide decisions, and evaluation files can be kept for future reference.

It is important that all materials selected and prepared for use, including nurse-teacher-prepared materials, undergo evaluation by colleagues, as well as target population samples prior to and following implementation.

PROGRAM EVALUATION

Program evaluation is more than student evaluation of teaching. It is an assessment of the quality and effectiveness of an instructional session, course, conference, workshop, curriculum, or school. The decisions based on a program evaluation are aimed at the improvement of the program (formative evaluation) or go/no-go decisions (summative evaluation). Examples of several types of summative decisons include: accredit a program or not, offer a course again or not, and approve a program for continuing education credit or not.

Information for program evaluation can come from practically any source that is associated with the program, including learners, alumni, instructors, administrators, and other audiences affected, such as parents, community, and other professionals in the field.

There are many methods of program evaluation. Historically, the most common one focuses on whether prespecified learner objectives have been attained. This is the pretest-posttest model. A more recent approach to evaluation, goal-free, denies the evaluator the list of objectives and forces the evaluator to conduct an investigation to find out the actual effects produced by the program. Although the various evaluation models differ, most contemporary models stress that the evaluation information collected be useful and address important issues. Qualitative evaluation models are especially worth investigating.

Some examples may help illustrate how program evaluations are conducted. Formal accreditation evaluations typically consist of an internal self-study, which is followed by a site visit by a team of experts. Evaluations of conferences and continuing-education programs often consist only of a participant survey. More rigorous evaluations assess the degree of learners' gain in knowledge, skills, and attitudes as a result of the program.

Dixon describes four levels that indicate effectiveness of continuing-nursing-education programs.[5] The first level consists of participant and program staff satisfaction. The next level addresses changes in knowledge, skills, or attitudes of participants. The third level measures change in actual participant behavior in practice. The final level indicates improvement in the health status of clients treated. These four levels have correlates for most programs and can be useful in planning the type of evidence of program success that is necessary.

If program survival is at stake in an evaluation, it is recommended that an evaluator from outside the program be sought to conduct the evaluation and that the most convincing indicators of program success be examined. In less dramatic cases, a rough idea of program success can be obtained by examining first level indicators, including participant evaluation of the experience and discussions with program personnel.

It is beyond the scope of this chapter to discuss the many facets of program evaluation. Suffice it to say that programs are usually complicated and require a great deal of effort to thoroughly evaluate. For readers who are interested in program evaluation, some excellent texts are available.[6,7]

SUMMARY

Evaluation is a primary function of all nurse-teachers. The nurse evaluates learners, teaching effectiveness, materials, and programs. Program evaluation is necessary to determine the overall quality and effectiveness of an educational experience, whether it be an individualized learning episode, a class presentation, an entire course, a conference, a curriculum, or an entire educational program. A program evaluation generates data on which to base decisions as to whether a program should be continued and whether it enables learners to achieve program goals and social obligations. A program evaluation pinpoints strengths and weaknesses and is a dynamic force for change.

RESEARCH IMPLICATIONS

The area of evaluation and measurement offers many interesting topics for research. Researchers are attempting to determine the effectiveness of the different types of evaluation instruments, methodologies, and processes. For instance, Albanese, Kent, and Whitney compared the difficulty, reliability, and validity of four types of evaluative items and found that multiple true-false items were more reliable than complex multiple-choice items.[8] Ongoing research is needed in this area as well as many others. One area that is particularly in need of further study is determining how to effectively measure problem-solving processes. While various approaches have been explored, none of them has proven satisfactory. Research on measuring the effectiveness of communication skills is also needed. These skills are very important in nursing practice, yet our methods of assessing communication skills are not well developed.

Wider availability of microcomputers has opened up new avenues of research on instruction, but research on the use of the computer as an evaluation tool has only scratched the surface. The use of microcomputers to adapt tests to individual learner needs is likely to be an area of continuing research activity.

Another area in need of investigation is the assessment of client compliance. The effectiveness of health education programs is often best assessed through client compliance; however, present methods of assessing compliance have many weaknesses. There is also need for developing an effective method of setting cutting scores on criterion-referenced tests. The limitations of existing methods have been a major factor limiting the use of criterion-referenced tests.

These few examples should provide a sense of the broad range of measurement and evaluation issues researchers are addressing. While much progress has been made in recent years, there is still a great deal left to accomplish. The nurse who is able to keep abreast of the advances in evaluation methodologies and research will be the more effective teacher.

POSTTEST

MULTIPLE-CHOICE

1. Which of the following errors is more likely to affect an essay test than a multiple-choice test?
   a. The situation is artificial
   b. Questions contain inadvertent clues to the correct answer
   c. Content sampled is insufficiently representative
2. What type of data is primarily used to establish the base-line level of a learner's knowledge?
   a. Formative evaluation
   b. Needs assessment
   c. Summative evaluation
3. Assigning grades to a learner is most likely what type of evaluation data?
   a. Needs assessment
   b. Formative evaluation
   c. Summative evaluation
4. What relationship does a test score have to the actual level of knowledge possessed by a student?
   a. The score is an estimate of the student's knowledge
   b. The score is equivalent to the student's knowledge
   c. The score is unrelated to the student's knowledge

TRUE OR FALSE

5. For purposes of giving feedback to the learner, assessment data should be more accurate than when the results are used to assign grades. *True* *False*
6. Program evaluation is limited to student evaluation of teaching. *True* *False*

SHORT ANSWER

7. Cite one assumption about prerequisite skills possessed by learners when a multiple-choice test is administered.
8. Bill took a written test on the mechanics of administering an injection and made a perfect score. Immediately afterward, he was observed by his instructor as he performed an injection on a fellow student. Bill received a failing grade from the instructor based on the observation. Cite three reasons for the discrepancy between the written test results and the performance rating.
9. What is meant by cumulative assessment?
10. What is meant by interference?
11. Compare and contrast normative- and criterion-referenced interpretation of assessment results.
12. What are two advantages of using multiple-choice test items?
13. What are two disadvantages of multiple-choice items?
14. What is the definitive feature of open-response questions?
15. Describe a situation in which a test composed of supply-type items would be more appropriate than one composed of multiple-choice items.
16. What is the primary advantage of the fill-in-the-blank item over the essay and short-answer essay?
17. What precautions should be taken to minimize subjectivity in grading supply-type tests?
18. What distinguishes a perception from an attitude?
19. Describe what a Likert-type, attitudinal item looks like.
20. In selecting a format for an attitude item, what should be the single most important consideration?
21. Describe two undesirable influences on attitudinal measures.
22. Under what circumstances is it better to use a simulation to teach a skill than to provide practice in the clinical setting with actual clients?
23. Why is it better to introduce a skill in a simulated situation rather than in actual client care when students are just beginning to learn the skill?
24. List and define two types of instruments used to evaluate clinical skills.
25. Describe two important administrative issues that should be regularly performed when using rating scales to evaluate clinical skills.
26. What is an anecdotal record?

27. What are two weaknesses of anecdotal reports?
28. What are several ways to maximize the usefulness of the information recorded in anecdotal reports?
29. Students are *not* a good source of information for what sort of teaching effectiveness data?
30. What precautions can be taken to avoid using flawed teaching materials?

POSTTEST ANSWER KEY

1. c
2. b
3. c
4. a
5. True
6. False
7. You could have stated one of the following:
   a. Learners can read.
   b. Learners have the psychomotor skills necessary to do the mechanics of making a response.
8. You could have listed any of the following:
   a. Passing a written test does not indicate that one has the necessary skills to actually perform a psychomotor task.
   b. Test items may have contained many clues to the correct answers.
   c. The instructor observing performance may have had unrealistically high standards of proficiency.
   d. The test may have been trivial with many self-evident items.
9. The assessment incorporates previously tested content.
10. New information becomes confused with old, causing a decline in performance.
11. A normative-referenced interpretation compares learner performance with that of peers, whereas a criterion-referenced interpretation compares the learner's performance with a standard of performance.
12. a. A large amount of content can be tested in a relatively short amount of time.
    b. Tests can be machine scored.
13. You may have listed any of the following:
    a. Completing multiple-choice items bears little resemblance to the demands of actual nursing practice.
    b. Good multiple-choice items are difficult to write.
    c. Good multiple-choice items are time-consuming to write.
    d. There is a definite possibility students will select the correct answer by guessing.

14. The student must supply the answer without the aid of any list of answers.
15. You may have described one of the following:
    a. A creative writing test.
    b. If the purpose of the test is to determine how well a student can express him or herself in writing.
    c. If the goal of the test is to see how well a student can synthesize a large amount of information into a coherent summary.
    d. If it is extremely important to minimize the incidence of giving credit for correct answers arrived at by guessing.
16. A broader range of content can usually be sampled.
17. a. Students' names should be covered.
    b. A list of acceptable responses with the amount of credit to be given for each should be specified in advance.
18. Perceptions reflect how learners view some experience, whereas attitudes reflect some belief or value that is held.
19. A statement followed by response options ranging from strongly agree to strongly disagree.
20. How the attitude can be most clearly expressed.
21. a. The halo effect, which is the tendency of learners to rate uniquely different characteristics according to their own overall perceptions.
    b. Social desirability, which is the tendency of individuals to avoid making a response that they feel will reflect undesirably on themselves.
22. a. When the need to use the skill is infrequently encountered during the course of normal patient care.
    b. When the skill involves a procedure that is unpleasant or dangerous for the patient.
    c. When students are just beginning to learn a skill.
23. The simulation is cleaner and does not introduce complications arising from the idiosyncrasies of individual patients.
24. You may have described two of the following:
    a. The checklist, which is a detailed list of steps necessary to be performed as part of a skill.
    b. The logbook, which is used to check off clinical experiences in which students have participated.
    c. The rating scale, which is a listing of characteristics, each of which is evaluated as to its quality based on a range of options.
25. a. All raters should be instructed in the use of the rating form.
    b. The rating form and how it is used should be reviewed on a regular basis.
26. An anecdotal record is a narrative report of a student's behavior that a nurse-teacher has observed.
27. You may have listed two of the following:
    a. They are time-consuming to complete.
    b. Anecdotal reports reflect the personal biases and reporting style of the nurse-teacher.
    c. Results from anecdotal reports are difficult to summarize.

28. a. Concentrate on observable behavior and avoid references to inferred personality characteristics.
    b. Record as many details as possible during the observation period, e.g., date, time, location, others present.
    c. Comment on the good aspects of a student's performance as well as the bad.
29. a. Importance of content presented.
    b. The instructor's command of the material.
    c. Relevance of content to the profession.
30. a. Review of materials by the nurse-teacher before use.
    b. Review of materials by teaching colleagues.
    c. Pilot test materials with learners like those who will be the intended audience.

SUGGESTED APPLICATION ACTIVITIES

1. Prepare at least one evaluation instrument composed of several types of items for a particular purpose and learner population. Try it out on a sample of the target population.
2. Review the chapter again and outline the evaluation instruments/items according to type for each of the three domains of learning. Check your outline with the one that follows this list of activities.
3. Discuss the decisions that can be based on evaluation results.
4. Conduct a needs assessment to determine the current status of a learner or learner group. Use the data to design learning events that meet the needs revealed in the assessment.
5. Design a plan for evaluating a course, class, or program of interest.
6. Describe a system for monitoring whether students have had a minimum set of clinical experiences.
7. Prepare an anecdotal record as you observe a student in clinical practice. Then share your notes with the student in a debriefing session.
8. Conduct an AVLINE search for materials on a topic of interest.
9. Review and evaluate at least two commercial materials on a particular topic to determine if they are appropriate for use with a particular learner or learner group.
10. Design a plan for evaluating materials you have developed for client education.
11. Explore the topics of program and teacher evaluation further.
12. Debate the issue of grading versus nongrading.
13. Conduct a literature search to find what research has been done on evaluation in the field of nursing.
14. Design a research study on some aspect of evaluation.

OUTLINE FOR APPLICATION ACTIVITY 2

I. Knowledge
    A. Written
        1. Multiple-choice
        2. Open-response/supply-type
            a. Fill-in-the-blank
            b. Short-answer essay
            c. Essay
        3. Simulation
    B. Oral examination
II. Attitudes and perceptions
    A. Written
        1. Likert-type
        2. Semantic differential
    B. Oral interview
III. Skills
    A. Simulation
    B. Checklist
    C. Rating scale
    D. Anecdotal report

REFERENCES

1. Mehrens WA, Lehmann IJ: Measurement and Evaluation in Education and Psychology, ed 3. New York, Holt, Rinehart & Winston, 1984.
2. McGuire CH, Solomon LM, Bashook PG: Construction and Use of Written Simulations. New York, Psychological Corporation, 1976.
3. Yang JC: A Reliability Study of Oral Examinations Administered to Third Year Medical Students During Their Obstetrics and Gynecology Clerkship. Unpublished doctoral dissertation, The University of Iowa, 1982.
4. Nunnally J: Psychometric Theory, ed 2. New York, McGraw-Hill Book Co., 1978.
5. Dixon J: Evaluation Criteria in Studies of Continuing Education in the Health Professions: A Critical Review and Suggested Strategy. Evaluation and the Health Professions 1 (4):47–65, 1978.
6. Guba EG, Lincoln YS: Effective Evaluation. San Francisco, Jossey-Bass, Inc., Publishers, 1981.
7. Patton MQ: Qualitative Evaluation Methods. Beverly Hills, CA, Sage Publications Inc., 1980.
8. Albanese MA, Kent TH, Whitney DA: A Comparison of the Difficulty, Reliability and Validity of Complex Multiple-Choice, Multiple-Choice, Multiple Response and Multiple True-False Items. Unpublished research report, University of Iowa, July 1977.

BIBLIOGRAPHY

Aleamoni LM: Student Ratings of Instruction. In J Millman (ed): Handbook of Teacher Evaluation. Beverly Hills, CA, Sage Publications Inc., 1981.

Anderson SB, Ball S, et al.: Encyclopedia of Educational Evaluation. San Francisco, Jossey-Bass Inc., Publishers, 1975.

Borg WR, Call MD: Educational Research, ed 4. New York, Longman Inc., 1983.

Bradburn NM, Sudman S: Improving Interview Method and Questionnaire Design. San Francisco, Jossey-Bass Inc., Publishers, 1981.

Campbell, JP, Dunnette MD, Arvey RD, Hellervik LW: The Development and Evaluation of Behaviorally Based Rating Scales. Journal of Applied Psychology 57:15–22, 1973.

Cronbach, LJ: Essentials of Psychological Testing, ed 3. New York, Harper & Row, Publishers Inc., 1970.

Doyle KS Jr: Student Evaluation of Instruction. Lexington, MA, D.C. Heath & Co., 1975.

Ellis H: Fundamentals of Human Learning and Cognition. Dubuque, IA, Wm. C. Brown Co., Publishers, 1972.

Foster J, Abramson S, Lass S, Girard R, Garris R: Analysis of an Oral Examination used in Specialty Board Certification. Journal of Medical Education 44 (10):951–954, 1969.

Friedman CP, Stritter FT, Talbert LM: A Systematic Comparison of Teaching Hospital and Remote-Site Clinical Education. Journal of Medical Education 53:565–573, 1978.

Gronlund NE, Constructing Achievement Tests. Englewood Cliffs, NJ, Prentice-Hall, Inc., 1968.

Guba, EG, Lincoln YS: Effective Evaluation. San Francisco, Jossey-Bass Inc., Publishers, 1981.

House ER: Evaluating With Validity. Beverly Hills, CA, Sage Publications Inc., 1980.

Issac S, Michael WB: Handbook in Research and Evaluation, ed 2. San Diego, EdITS, 1981.

Kelley PR, Mathews JH, Schumacher CF: Analysis of the Oral Examination of the American Board of Anesthesiology. Journal of Medical Education 46 (11):982–988, 1971.

Likert RA: A Technique for the Measurement of Attitudes. Arch Psychol 40:448, 1932.

McGreal TL: Successful Teacher Evaluation. Alexandria, VA, Association for Supervision and Curriculum Development, 1983.

McGuire CH: The Oral Examination: A Measure of Professional Competence. Journal of Medical Education 41:267–274, 1966.

McGuire CH, Solomon LM, Bashook PG: Construction and Use of Written Simulations. New York, Psychological Corporation, 1976.

McKeachie WJ: Teaching Tips, ed 7. Lexington, MA, D.C. Heath & Co., 1978.

Mehrens WA, Ebel RL: Some Comments on Criterion-Referenced and Norm-Referenced Achievement Tests. Measurement in Education 10 (1): 1979.

Mehrens WA, Lehmann IJ: Measurement and Evaluation in Education and Psychology, ed 3. New York, Holt, Rinehart & Winston, 1984.

Nedelsky L: Absolute Grading Standards for Objective Tests. Educational and Psychological Measurement 14 (1):13–19, 1954.

Nunnally J: Psychometric Theory, ed 2. New York, McGraw-Hill Book Co., 1978.

Stake RE (ed): Evaluating the Arts in Education: A Responsive Approach. Columbus, OH, Charles E. Merrill Publishing Co., 1975.

Stritter FT, Flair MD: Effective Clinical Teaching. Atlanta, GA, US Department of Health, Education, and Welfare, National Library of Medicine, National Medicine Audiovisual Center, 1980.

Thorndike RL, Hagen EP: Measurement and Evaluation in Psychology and Education, ed 4. New York, John Wiley & Sons, Inc., 1977.

Appendix

STRATEGY ANALYSIS AND APPRAISAL INVENTORY

STRATEGY TITLE/SERIES: ____________________

AUTHOR/EDITOR: ____________________ PUBLISHER/COPYRIGHT: ____________________

CURRICULUM AREA: ____________________

CONCEPT: ____________________ SKILL: ____________________ COST: ____________________

PURPOSE/OBJECTIVES:

INTENDED USE
___ Client teaching/health promotion
___ Nursing education
___ Other: ____________________

AUDIENCE LEVEL
___ Preschool
___ Primary
___ Intermediate
___ Secondary
___ Undergraduate
___ Graduate

AUDIENCE SIZE
___ Large group (over 50)
___ Medium-to-small group
___ Individual

FORMAT
___ 16mm film
___ 8mm film
___ Video
___ Filmstrip
___ Slides (2×2)
___ Sound-filmstrip
___ Game
___ Model/mock-up
___ Book, text
___ Kit
___ Overhead transparency
___ Audiocassette
___ Audio reel
___ Phonorecord
___ Chart/poster/picture
___ Braille
___ Programed instruction
___ Computer-assisted instruction
___ Object/specimen
___ Workbook, worktext
___ Activity
___ Other: ____________________

FORMAT CHARACTERISTICS
___ color
___ black and white
___ still
___ silent
___ sound

Sequencing
___ fixed
___ flexible

Length
___ 5–15 min.
___ 15–30 min.
___ over 30 min.
___ frames
___ pages
___ items

SENSORY RECEPTION (INPUT)
___ Auditory
___ Visual
___ Auditory and visual
___ Tactile
___ Visual/tactile
___ Auditory/tactile
___ Other: ____________________

RESPONSE MODE (OUTPUT)

OVERT
___ speak
___ write
___ manipulate
___ mark
___ Other: ____________________

COVERT
___ listen only
___ view only
___ listen and view
___ Other: ____________________

INSTRUCTIONAL DESIGN
___ Self-instructional
___ Instructor-directed
___ Combination
___ Instructor's manual or guide
___ Validation information included

PREREQUISITE LEARNING NEEDED:

ADDITIONAL EQUIPMENT/SUPPLIES NEEDED:

ADDITIONAL PERSONNEL NEEDED:

ADDITIONAL FACILITIES NEEDED:

SYNOPSIS:

S	U	CONTENT QUALITY
		Accuracy
		Currency
		Consistency
		Scope/range
		Sequencing
		Agreement of objectives with purpose and content
		Social fairness (sex role, ethnic)
		Bias
		Longevity

		INSTRUCTIONAL DESIGN QUALITY
		Objectives clearly stated
		Objectives measurable
		Directions clearly stated
		Introduction provided (set)
		Provision for practice
		Provision for student response
		Prompts and primes
		Appropriateness of medium
		Appropriateness of visuals
		Evaluation instrument provided
		Activities provided
		Summary provided (closure)
		Student reaction
		Reinforcement provided
		Feedback provided
		Repetition
		Organization
		Rate of presentation

		TECHNICAL QUALITY
		Audio
		Visual
		Durability

		OTHER
		Cost
		Adaptability
		Editability
		Maintenance

INFORMATION LOAD
___ Too high
___ High
___ Average
___ Too low

OVERALL RATING

Low 1 2 3 4 5 High

☐ ACCEPT

☐ REJECT

STRATEGY ATTRIBUTES CHECKLIST

STRATEGY ____

SOURCE: ______________________________ COST: ______________

ATTRIBUTES: (Check all that apply.)

_____ Conveys color stimuli.
_____ Conveys movement.
_____ Magnifies actions and objects.
_____ Alters normal time-place relationships.
_____ Message is in a fixed sequence and can't be easily rearranged beyond forward and reverse.
_____ Message is flexible, permitting relatively easy change in order of information.
_____ Conveys visual input.
_____ Conveys auditory and visual input.
_____ Conveys tactile input.
_____ Conveys visual/tactile input.
_____ Conveys auditory/tactile input.
_____ Provides for learner response, feedback, and reinforcement.
_____ Facilitates overt response (doing).
_____ Facilitates covert response (listen, view).
_____ Facilitates active overt practice.
_____ Provides repetition.
_____ Primes or prompts response.
_____ Information load appropriate for learner(s).
_____ Provides deductive organization of information.
_____ Provides inductive organization of information.
_____ Establishes set.
_____ Facilitates cognitive closure.
_____ Primarily a self-instructional or independent strategy.
_____ Primarily a direct instructor-directed strategy.
_____ Can be used for group study.
_____ Permits revelation of message bit by bit and allows retention of prior bits as further bits are revealed.
_____ Pacing or rate of message can be controlled by the learner.
_____ Pacing or rate of message is controlled by the equipment.
_____ Can be repeated or reused in part or whole.
_____ Facilitates immediacy and objectivity.
_____ Conveys reality (size, shape, etc.).
_____ Requires technical know-how to use.
_____ Expands time (slow motion).
_____ Compresses, contracts, or condenses time (time-lapse photography).
_____ Projection or display equipment is needed. List type: ______________
_____ Equipment relatively simple to operate.
_____ Equipment readily available.
_____ Special facilities are needed. Explain: ______________
_____ Darkening of room required.

SELECTED SOURCES OF TEACHING MATERIALS

Associations, Societies, Foundations

Addiction Research Foundation, 33 Russell St., Toronto, Canada, M5S2S1
American Academy of Orthopaedic Surgeons, P.O. Box 7195, Chicago, IL 60680
American Academy of Pediatrics, 1801 Hinman Ave., Evanston, IL 60204
American Association for Maternal and Child Health, Inc., Box 965, Los Altos, CA 94022
American Cancer Society, 219 E. 42nd St., New York, NY 10017
American Diabetes Association, 1 W. 48th St., New York, NY 10020
American Heart Association, 44 E. 23rd St., New York, NY 10010
American Red Cross, 5816 Seminary Road, Falls Church, VA 22041
American Society of Hospital Pharmacists, 4630 Montgomery Ave., Washington, DC 20014
American Thoracic Society, American Lung Association, 1740 Broadway, New York, NY 10019
Arthritis Foundation, 475 Riverside Dr., New York, NY 10027
Children's Hospital National Medical Center, Washington, DC 20009
Drug Abuse Council, 1828 L. St., NW, Washington, DC 20036
Emphysema Anonymous, Inc., 1364 Palmetto Ave., Box 66, Fort Myers, FL 33902
Epilepsy Foundation of America, 1828 L. St., NW, Suite 406, Washington, DC 20036
March of Dimes Materials and Supply Division, 1275 Mamaroneck Avenue, White Plains, NY 10605
National Association for Mental Health, Inc., 1800 N. Kent St., Arlington, VA 22209
National Braille Association, Inc., 85 Godwin Ave., Midland Park, NJ 07432
National Foundation for Ileitis and Colitis, Inc., 295 Madison Ave., New York, NY 10017
National Hemophilia Foundation, 25 W. 39th St., New York, NY 10018
National Multiple Sclerosis Society, 257 Park Ave. S., New York, NY 10010
National Safety Council, 4255 N. Michigan Ave., Chicago, IL 60611
US Government Printing Office, Public Documents Distribution Center, Dept. 14, Pueblo, CO 81009

Producers and Distributors

Abbott Laboratories, Abbott Park, IL 60064
ABC Wide World of Learning, 1330 Avenue of the Americas, New York, NY 10019
Aldine Publishing Co., 529 S. Wabash Ave., Chicago, IL 60605
Alfred Higgins Productions, Inc., 9100 Sunset Blvd., Los Angeles, CA 90069
American Journal of Nursing, Educational Services Division, 555 W. 57th St., New York, NY 10019
Appleton-Century-Crofts, 25 Van Zant St., East Norwalk, CT 06855
Association Films, Inc., 866 Third Ave., New York, NY 10022
Audio Visual Narrative Arts, Inc., Box 9, Pleasantville, NY 10570
AVC Nursing Series, P.O. Box H, Novato, CA 94947
Ayerst Laboratories, 685 Third Avenue, New York, NY 10017
Bio-Communications Corp., P.O. Box 5547, Garden Grove, CA 92645
Career Aids, Inc., 8950 Lurline Ave., Department P5, Chatsworth, CA 91311
Carolina Biological Supply, 2700 York Rd., Burlington, NC 27215
Cassettes Unlimited, Roanoke, TX 76262

Centron Films, 1621 W. 9th, Box 687, Lawrence, KS 66044
Churchill Films, 662 N. Robertson Blvd., Los Angeles, CA 90069-9990
CIBA Pharmaceutical Co., P.O. Box 195, Summit, NJ 07901
Concept Media, Box 19542, Irvine, CA 92713-9542
Crisis Communications Corporation, Ltd. Box 904, Garden Grove, CA 92642
CRM/McGraw-Hill Films, 110 15th St., Del Mar, CA 92014
Eli Lilly and Co., P.O. Box 100B, Indianapolis, IN 46206
Eye Gate Media, Inc., 146-01 Archer Ave., Jamaica, NY 11435
Guidance Associates, 757 Third Ave., New York, NY 10017
Harcourt Brace Jovanovich Films, Polk and Geary, San Francisco, CA 94109
Harper & Row, 2350 Virginia Ave., Hagerstown, MD 21740
The Hartley Film Foundation, Inc., Cat Rock Rd., Cos Cob, CT 06807
Heshi Computing, 17 Cedar Lawn, Galveston, TX 77550
Health Sciences Consortium, 103 Laurel Ave., Carrboro, NC 27510
Human Development Institute, 450 E. Ohio St., Chicago, IL 60611
Human Relations Media, 175 Tompkins Ave., Pleasantville, NY 10570
Human Sciences Press, Inc., 72 Fifth Ave., New York, NY 10011
IBIS Media, P.O. Box 308, Pleasantville, NY 10570
Intercollegiate Center for Nursing Education, Learning Resources Unit, West 2917 Fort George Wright Dr., Spokane, WA 99204-5291
J.B. Lippincott Co., East Washington Square, Philadelphia, PA 19105
Johnson & Johnson Baby Products, Grand View Rd., Skillman, NJ 08558
Medcom, Inc. P.O. Box 116, Garden Grove, CA 92642 (formerly Trainex Corp.)
Medfact, Inc., P.O. Box 418, Massillon, OH 44648
Medi-Sim, Inc., P.O. Box 13267, Edwardsville, KS 66113
Medi Visuals, 4 Midland Ave., Hicksville, NY 11801
Medical Electronic Educational Services, Inc., 1802 W. Grant Rd., Suite 119, Tucson, AZ 85705
The Micro Center, Dept. MF717, Box 6, Pleasantville, NY 10570
C.V. Mosby Company, Mosby Software Division, 11830 Westline Industrial Dr., P.O. Box 28430, St Louis, MO 63146
MTI Teleprograms, Inc., 3710 Commercial Ave., Northbrook, IL 60062
NASCO, 901 Janesville Ave., Fort Atkinson, WI 53538
National Audio Visual Center, Information Services ME, Washington, DC 20409
Parent's Magazine Films, Inc., 52 Vanderbilt Ave., New York, NY 10017
Pleasantville Media, Suite E-61, Box 415, Pleasantville, NY 10570
Southerby Productions Inc., 5000 E. Anaheim St., Long Beach, CA 90804
Spenco Medical Corp., Box 8113, Waco, TX 76714-8113
Sunburst Communications, Rm. G7474, 39 Washington Ave., Pleasantville, NY 10570
W.B. Saunders Co., West Washington Square, Philadelphia, PA 19105

EVALUATING TEACHING EFFECTIVENESS

Rate each item on the following scale: 1 = unsatisfactory; 2 = below average; 3 = average; 4 = above average; 5 = very good; 6 = excellent; 7 = exceptional.

A. Establishing mind-set	1	2	3	4	5	6	7
B. Clarity of objectives	1	2	3	4	5	6	7
C. Organization of content	1	2	3	4	5	6	7
D. Pace of presentation	1	2	3	4	5	6	7
E. Suitability of content	1	2	3	4	5	6	7
F. Appropriateness of strategies	1	2	3	4	5	6	7
G. Use of examples to clarify content	1	2	3	4	5	6	7
H. Student involvement in learning	1	2	3	4	5	6	7
I. Stimulation of thinking and future study	1	2	3	4	5	6	7
J. Attitude toward students	1	2	3	4	5	6	7
K. Evidence of prior planning	1	2	3	4	5	6	7
L. Establishing closure	1	2	3	4	5	6	7
M. Time on task	1	2	3	4	5	6	7
N. Overall rating	1	2	3	4	5	6	7

EVALUATING CLINICAL TEACHING EFFECTIVENESS

Rate the following items on a scale of 1 to 5 according to the behaviors described.

5	4	3	2	1
Orients students and presents clinical objectives to be accomplished.		Partially orients students or incompletely states objectives to be accomplished.		Does not orient students or state objectives to be accomplished.
5	4	3	2	1
Thoroughly plans clinical assignments and communicates plans to students.		Plans clinical assignments, but doesn't communicate them well to students.		Does not thoroughly plan clinical assignments or communicate assignments to students.
5	4	3	2	1
Provides student supervision at all times.		Haphazardly supervises students.		Does not supervise students as required.
5	4	3	2	1
Fosters smooth relationships with clinical staff.		Occasional rifts with clinical staff evidenced, but tries to foster working relationships.		Does not cooperate with clinical staff.
5	4	3	2	1
Safeguards clients' rights at all times.		Occasionally is negligent in safeguarding the rights of clients.		Does not safeguard the rights of clients.

5	4	3	2	1
Participates with students in direct client care, exhibiting effective communication and teaching behaviors.		Inappropriately participates with students in client care or exhibits ineffective communication and teaching behaviors some of the time.		Does not participate with students in client care and does not exhibit effective communication and teaching behaviors.
5	4	3	2	1
Evaluates student performance using appropriate evaluation methods; provides constructive feedback to students on performance.		Occasionally evaluates student performance inappropriately or gives inappropriate feedback to students.		Does not evaluate student performance or uses inappropriate evaluation methods; does not provide constructive feedback to students.

Index